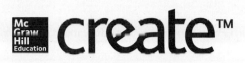

Taking Sides: Clashing Views
in Health and Society, 12/e

Eileen L. Daniel

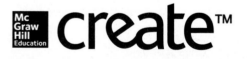

http://create.mheducation.com

ISBN-10: 1259394042   ISBN-13: 9781259394041

Contents

Detailed Table of Contents

Unit: The Health Care Industry

Issue: Is the Affordable Care Act Successful?
Yes: **Gordon Whitman**, from "Six Things Every Sane Person Should Know About the Healthcare Debate", *huffingtonpost.com* (2012).
No: **Peter Suderman**, from "Obamacare's Phony Success Story", *Reason* (2014).

Political correspondent Gordon Whitman believes the Affordable Care Act is the best hope Americans have for making our health care system better. *Reason* magazine senior editor Peter Suderman counters that the law increased health spending, missed enrollment targets, and continues to experience problems with the website.

Issue: Should the Healthcare System Continuously Strive to Extend Life?
Yes: **Miguel Faria**, from "Bioethics and Why I Hope to Live Beyond Age 75 Attaining Wisdom!-A Rebuttal to Dr. Ezekiel Emanuel's 75 Age Limit", *haciendapublishing.com* (2014).
No: **Ezekiel J. Emanuel**, from "Why I Hope to Die at 75: An Argument That Society and Families—and You—Will Be Better Off if Nature Takes Its Course Swiftly and Promptly", *The Atlantic* (2014).

Physician Miguel Faria contends that lives can be productive and fulfilling and worthwhile past age 75 and that there is a difference between aging and infirmity and illness. Physician, bioethicist, and vice provost of the University of Pennsylvania Ezekiel Emanuel disagrees and claims that society and families would be better off if we died at 75 rather than be incapacitated and unable to live a full life.

Issue: Does the Affordable Health Care Act Violate Religious Freedom by Requiring Employers' Health Insurance Plans to Cover Birth Control?
Yes: **Wesley J. Smith**, from "What About Religious Freedom: The Other Consequences of Obamacare", *The Weekly Standard* (2012).
No: **Elizabeth Sepper and Alisha Johnson**, from "Rhetoric Versus Reality: The Contraception Benefit and Religious Freedom", *religionandpolitics.org* (2013).

Senior fellow in the Discovery Institute's Center on Human Exceptionalism Wesley J. Smith believes birth control cases are just the beginning of far more intrusive violations of religious liberty to come, e.g., requiring businesses to provide free abortions to their employees. Law professor Elizabeth Sepper and research assistant and law student Alisha Johnson counter that the Affordable Care Act strikes a delicate balance by providing broad protection for religiously affiliated employers, while at the same time it protects the freedom of all Americans to live out their own religious and moral convictions.

Unit: Health and Society

Issue: Is the Cost of Treating Cancer Unsustainable?
Yes: **Lee N. Newcomer**, from "Myths and Realities in Cancer Care: Another Point of View", *Health Affairs* (2014).
No: **Dana P. Goldman and Tomas Philipson**, from "Five Myths About Cancer Care In America", *Health Affairs* (2014).

UnitedHealthcare's vice president for oncology, physician Lee Newcomer believes that the cost to treat cancer will be unsustainable in the near future and will undermine the progress made in cancer treatment. Professor of public policy Dana Goldman and professor of health economics Tomas Philipson maintain that it's a myth that treatment costs are unsustainable and that restricting patients' treatments is socially wasteful and will likely discourage research innovations.

Issue: Should Marijuana Be Legalized for Medicinal Purposes?
Yes: **Kevin Drum**, from "The Patriot's Guide to Legalization", *Mother Jones* (2009).
No: **Abigail Sullivan Moore**, from "This Is Your Brain on Drugs", *The New York Times* (2014).

Political columnist and blogger Kevin Drum contends that medical marijuana is now legal in more than a dozen states without any serious problems or increased usage. Journalist Abigail Sullivan Moore counters that young people who smoke marijuana frequently are more likely to have mental health problems and learning difficulties.

Issue: Is the Use of "Smart" Pills for Cognitive Enhancement Dangerous?
Yes: **Alan Schwarz**, from "Drowned in a Stream of Prescriptions", *The New York Times* (2013).
No: **Joshua Gowin**, from "How 'Smart Drugs' Enhance Us", *Psychology Today* (2009).

Pulitzer Prize-nominated reporter Alan Schwarz maintains that "smart pills" such as Adderall can significantly improve the lives of children and others with ADHD but that too many young adults who do not have the condition fake the symptoms and get prescriptions for the highly addictive and dangerous drugs. Psychologist Joshua Gowin argues that these drugs aren't much different from a cup of coffee and should be treated accordingly.

Issue: Should Embryonic Stem Cell Research Be Permitted?
Yes: **Jeffrey Hart**, from "NR on Stem Cells: The Magazine Is Wrong", *National Review* (2004).
No: **Ramesh Ponnuru**, from "NR on Stem Cells: The Magazine Is Right", *National Review* (2004).

Professor Jeffrey Hart contends there are many benefits to stem cell research and that a ban on funded cloning research is unjustified. Writer Ramesh Ponnuru argues that a single-celled human embryo is a living organism, which directs its own development and should not be used for experimentation.

Unit: Mind-Body Relationships

Issue: Should Addiction to Drugs Be Labeled a Brain Disease?
Yes: **Alan I. Leshner**, from "Addiction Is a Brain Disease", *Issues in Science and Technology* (2001).
No: **Alva Noë**, from "Addiction Is Not a Disease of the Brain", *National Public Radio* (2011).

Alan I. Leshner, director of the National Institute on Drug Abuse at the National Institute of Health, believes that addiction to drugs and alcohol is not a behavioral condition but a treatable disease. Professor Alva Noë counters that addiction is a phenomenon that can only be understood in terms of the life choices, needs, and understanding of the whole person.

Issue: Do Religion and Prayer Benefit Health?
Yes: **Thomas J. Cottle**, from "Our Thoughts and Our Prayers", *The Antioch Review* (2006).
No: **Michael Shermer**, from "Prayer and Healing: The Verdict Is In and the Results Are Null", *Skeptic* (2006).

Psychologist and educator Thomas J. Cottle believes that prayer can fill patients with a spirit of security when confronted with illness. Author Michael Shermer contends that intercessory prayer offered by strangers on the health and recovery of patients undergoing coronary bypass surgery is ineffective. He also addresses flaws in studies showing a relationship between prayer and health.

Unit: Sexuality and Gender Issues

Issue: Is It Necessary for Pregnant Women to Completely Abstain from All Alcoholic Beverages?
Yes: **National Organization on Fetal Alcohol Syndrome**, from "Is It Completely Safe and Risk-Free to Drink a Little Alcohol While Pregnant, Such as a Glass of Wine?", *nofas.org* (2013).
No: **Emily Oster**, from "I Wrote That It's OK to Drink While Pregnant. Everyone Freaked Out. Here's Why I'm Right", *slate.com* (2013).

The National Organization on Fetal Alcohol Syndrome provides evidence that even moderate quantities of alcohol can damage a developing fetus and cites new research indicating that even small amounts of alcoholic beverages consumed during pregnancy may be harmful. Economics professor Emily Oster argues that there are almost no studies on the effects of moderate drinking during pregnancy and that small amounts of alcohol are unlikely to have much effect.

Issue: Should Pro-Life Health Providers Be Allowed to Deny Prescriptions on the Basis of Conscience?
Yes: **John A. Menges**, from "Public Hearing on HB4346 Before the House State Government Administration Committee", Illinois House State Government Administration Committee (2006).
No: **R. Alta Charo**, from "The Celestial Fire of Conscience--Refusing to Deliver Medical Care", *The New England Journal of Medicine* (2005).

Pharmacist John Menges believes that it is his right to refuse to dispense any medication that is designed to end a human life. Attorney R. Alta Charo argues that health care professionals who protect themselves from the moral consequences of their actions may do so at their patients' risk.

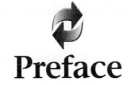

Preface

This textbook offers debates on controversial issues on health and society. Each issue consists of opposing viewpoints presented in a YES–NO format. Most of the questions that are included here relate to health topics of modern concern, such as universal health insurance, abortion, and drug use and abuse. The authors of these articles take strong stands on specific issues and provide support for their positions. While we may not agree with a particular point of view, each author clearly defines his or her stand on the issues.

This book is divided into units containing related issues. Each issue is preceded by an Introduction, which sets the stage for the debate, gives historical background on the subject, provides learning outcomes, and provides a context for the controversy. Each issue concludes with further exploration of the issue, which offers a summary of the debate and some concluding observations and suggests further readings on the subject. The summary also raises further points, since most of the issues have more than two sides.

Contributors to this volume are identified, which gives information on the physicians, professors, journalists, theologians, and scientists whose views are debated here.

Taking Sides: Clashing Views in Health and Society is a tool to encourage critical thought on important health issues. Readers should not feel confined to the views expressed in the articles. Some readers may see important points on both sides of an issue and may construct for themselves a new and creative approach, which may incorporate the best of both sides or provide an entirely new vantage point for understanding.

Changes to this edition: This edition of *Taking Sides: Clashing Views in Health and Society* includes some important changes from previous editions: For some issues, I have kept the topic, but have replaced one or both of the articles in order to make it more current or more clearly focus the controversy. I also added new topics and selections that reflect current controversies in health and society.

Editor of This Volume

Eileen L. Daniel, a registered dietitian and licensed nutritionist, is a professor in the Department of Health Science and associate vice provost for academic affairs at the State University of New York College at Brockport. She received a BS in nutrition and dietetics from the Rochester Institute of Technology, an MS in community health education from SUNY College at Brockport, and a PhD in health education from the University of Oregon. A member of the American Dietetics Association, the New York State Dietetics Society, and other professional and community organizations, she has published over 40 articles in professional journals on issues of health, nutrition, and health education. She is also the editor of *Annual Editions: Health*.

Acknowledgments

Special thanks to my family. Also, thanks to my colleagues at the State University of New York College at Brockport for all their helpful contributions. I was also assisted in preparing this edition by the valuable suggestions from the adopters of this book. Many of your recommendations were incorporated into this edition. Finally, I appreciate the assistance of the staff at McGraw-Hill for all their help.

Academic Advisory Board Members

Members of the Academic Advisory Board are instrumental in the final selection of articles for each edition of TAKING SIDES. Their review of articles for content, level, and appropriateness provides critical direction to the editor and staff. We think that you will find their careful consideration well reflected in this volume.

Douglas Abbott
University of Nebraska, Lincoln

Harold Abramowitz
Charles Drew University

Isaac Addai
Lansing Community College

David Anderson
George Mason University

Steven Applewhite
University of Houston

Judith Ary
North Dakota State University

Faye Avard
Mississippi Valley State University

Alice Baldwin-Jones
The City College of New York

Barry Brock
Barry University

Elaine Bryan
Georgia Perimeter College

Cynthia Cassell
University of North Carolina, Charlotte

Jeanne Clerc
Western Illinois University

Marilyn Coleman
University of Missouri

Scarlett Conway
University of South Carolina Upstate

J. Sunshine Cowan
University of Central Oklahoma

Susan Crowley
North Idaho College

Peter Cruise
Mary Baldwin College

Michelle D'Abundo
University of North Carolina, Wilmington

Evia L. Davis
Langston University

Geoffrey Davison
Lyndon State College

Joanne Demyun
Eastern University

Karen Dennis
Illinois State University

Kathi Deresinski
Triton College

Diane Dettmore
Fairleigh Dickinson University

Jonathan Deutsch
Kingsborough Community College

Johanna Donnenfield
Scottsdale Community College

Karen Dorman
St. Johns University

Wilton Duncan
ASA College

William Dunscombe
Union County College

Neela Eisner
Cuyahoga Community College

Ifeanyi Emenike
Benedict College

Marie Emerson
Washington County Community College

Brad Engeldinger
Sierra College

David Evans
Pennsylvania College of Technology

Susan Farrell
Kingsborough Community College

Jenni Fauchier
Metropolitan Community College

Christine Feeley
Adelphi University

Catherine Felton
Central Piedmont Community College

Paul Finnicum
Arkansas State University

Eunice Flemister
Hostos Community College, Cuny

Deborah Flynn
Southern Conn State University

Mary Flynn
Brown University

Amy Frith
Ithaca College

Bernard Frye
University of Texas, Arlington

Stephen Gambescia
Drexel University

Kathie Garbe
University of North Carolina, Asheville

Jeff Goodman
Union College

Aleida Gordon
California State Polytechnic University, Pomona

Deborah Gritzmacher
Clayton State University

Dana Hale
Itawamba Community College

Jeffrey Hampl
Arizona State University

Leslie Hellstrom
Tidewater Community College

George Hertl
Northwest Mississippi Community College

Martha Highfield
California State University, Northridge

Marc D. Hiller
University of New Hampshire

Cathy Hix-Cunningham
Tennessee Technological University

Loreen Huffman
Missouri Southern State University

Kevin Hylton
University of Maryland, Baltimore County

Allen Jackson
Chadron State College

Leslie Jacobson
Brooklyn College

Pera Jambazian
California State University, Los Angeles

Barry Johnson
Davidson County Community College

Marcy Jung
Fort Lewis College

Melissa Karolides
San Diego City College

Leroy Keeney
York College of Pennsylvania

John Kowalczyk
University of Minnesota, Duluth

Sylvette La Touche-Howard
University of Maryland, College Park

Robert Lavery
Montclair State University

Hans Leis
Louisiana College

Craig Levin
National American University

Linda Levin-Messineo
Carlow University

Karen Lew
University of Miami

Michelle Lewis
Fairleigh Dickinson University

Xiangdong Li
New York City College of Technology

Cindy Manjounes
Lindenwood University

Hal Marchand
Western Illinois University

Willis McAleese
Idaho State University

Michael McDonough
Berkeley College

James McNamara
Alverno College

Julie Merten
University of North Florida

James Metcalf
George Mason University

Eric Miller
Kent State University

Lloyd Mitchell III
Elizabeth City State University

Kara Montgomery
University of South Carolina

Martha Olson
Iowa Lakes Community College

Anna Page
Johnson County Community College

Judy Peel
North Carolina State University

Tina M. Penhollow
Florida Atlantic University

Jane Petrillo
Kennesaw State University

Regina Pierce
Davenport University

Roger Pinches
William Paterson University

Roberta L. Pohlman
Wright State University

M. Paige Powell
University of Alabama, Birmingham

Elizabeth Quintana
West Virginia University

Leon Ragonesi
California State University, Dominguez Hills

Ralph Rice
Wake Forest University School of Medicine

Leigh Rich
Armstrong Atlantic State University

Andrea Salis
Queensborough Community College

Kathryn Schneider
Pacific Union College

Elizabeth Schneider
Keiser University, Ft. Lauderdale

Allan Simmons
Jackson State University

Donna Sims
Fort Valley State University

Carrie Lee Smith
Millersville University

Cynthia Smith
Central Piedmont Community College

Kathleen Smyth
College of Marin

Stephen Sowulewski
J. Sargeant Reynolds Community College

Caile Spear
Boise State University

Diane Spokus
Penn State University, University Park

Betsy Stern
Milwaukee Area Technical College

Craig Stillwell
Southern Oregon University

Susan Stockton
University of Central Missouri

Meg Stolt
John Jay College

Lori Stolz
Oakland City University

Winona Taylor
Bowie State University

Michael Teague
University of Iowa

Julie Thurlow
University of Wisconsin, Madison

Theresa Tiso
Stony Brook University

Terry Weideman
Oakland Community College

Peggie Williamson
Central Texas College

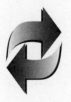

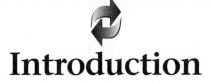

Introduction

What Is Health?

Traditionally, being healthy meant the absence of illness. If an individual did not have a disease, then he or she was considered healthy. The overall health of a nation or specific population was determined by data measuring illness, disease, and death rates. Today, this rather negative view of assessing individual health, and health in general, is changing. A healthy person is one who is not only free from disease but also fully well.

Being well, or wellness, involves the interrelationship of many dimensions of health: physical, emotional, social, mental, and spiritual. This multifaceted view of health reflects a holistic approach, which includes individuals taking responsibility for their own well-being.

Our health and longevity are affected by the many choices we make every day: Medical reports tell us that if we abstain from smoking, drugs, excessive alcohol, fat, and cholesterol consumption and get regular exercise, our rate of disease and disability will significantly decrease. These reports, while not totally conclusive, have encouraged many people to make positive lifestyle changes. Millions of people have quit smoking, alcohol consumption is down, and more and more individuals are exercising regularly and eating low-fat diets. While these changes are encouraging, many people who have been unable or unwilling to make these changes are left feeling worried and/or guilty over continuing their negative health behaviors.

But disagreement exists among the experts about the exact nature of positive health behaviors, which causes confusion. For example, some scientists claim that overweight Americans should make efforts to lose weight, even if it takes many tries. Many Americans have unsuccessfully tried to lose weight by eating a low-fat diet, though the experts debate which is best: a low-fat, high-carbohydrate diet or a low-carbohydrate diet which includes ample protein and fat. Other debatable issues include whether or not people should utilize conventional medicine or seek out alternative therapies.

Health status is also affected by society and government. Societal pressures have helped pass smoking restrictions in public places, mandatory safety belt legislation, and laws permitting condom distribution in public schools. The government plays a role in the health of individuals as well, although it has failed to provide minimal health care for many low-income Americans.

Unfortunately, there are no absolute answers to many questions regarding health and wellness issues. Moral questions, controversial concerns, and individual perceptions of health matters all can create opposing views. As you evaluate the issues in this book, you should keep an open mind toward both sides. You may not change your mind regarding the morality of abortion or the limitation of health care for the elderly or mentally handicapped, but you will still be able to learn from the opposing viewpoint.

The Health Care Industry

In the United States, approximately 40 million Americans have no health insurance, there has been a resurgence in infectious diseases such as TB, and antibiotic-resistant strains of bacterial infections which threaten thousands of Americans all put pressure on the current system, along with AIDS, diabetes, and other chronic diseases. Those enrolled in government programs such as Medicaid often find few, if any, physicians who will accept them as patients since reimbursements are so low and the paperwork is so cumbersome. On the other hand, Americans continue to live longer and longer, and for most of us, the health care available is among the best in the world. While many Americans agree that there are some situations in which limited health care dollars should be rationed, it's unclear by whom or how these decisions should be made. Other issues in this section address the issue of the health care system's role in extending life.

Health and Society

This section introduces current issues related to health from a societal perspective. The controversial issues of whether or not schools should be required to track the body mass index of students and report those data to parents, the debate over the cost of the "war" on cancer, should marijuana be legalized for medicinal purposes, and should embryonic stem cell research be allowed are addressed. Stem cell technology offers the *potential* to cure or treat diseases such as Parkinson's and multiple sclerosis and others. While there are pros and cons to the use of stem cells, ethical and moral questions also arise.

Mind–Body Issues

Important issues related to the relationship between mind and body are discussed in this section. Millions of Americans use and abuse drugs that alter their minds and affect their bodies. These drugs range from illegal substances, such as crack cocaine and opiates, to the widely used legal drugs, alcohol and tobacco. Increasingly, prescription drugs obtained either legally or not are becoming substances of abuse. Use of these substances can lead to physical and psychological addiction and the related problems of family dysfunction, reduced worker productivity, and crime. Are addictions within the control of individuals who abuse drugs? Or are they an actual disease of the brain which needs treatment? The role of spirituality in the prevention and treatment of disease is discussed in this section. Many studies have found that religion and prayer play a role in recovery from sickness. Should health providers encourage spirituality for their patients? Does prayer really help to prevent disease and hasten recovery from illnesses?

Sexuality and Gender Issues

There is much advice given to pregnant women to help ensure they have healthy babies. Research indicates that women who avoid drugs, alcohol, and tobacco reduce the risk of complications. If a pregnant woman does not consume any alcohol, her child will not be born with fetal alcohol syndrome. For some women, however, avoiding alcohol during pregnancy is particularly difficult and they question whether or not it's safe to have a moderate amount of alcohol. For years, physicians and other health providers have cautioned that even one drink consumed at the wrong time could negatively affect the outcome of the pregnancy. This obviously created much concern for women, especially those who drank before they knew they were pregnant.

Other issues debate the conscience clause relative to health providers and whether or not the cervical cancer vaccine for girls should be mandatory. Should pro-life doctors and pharmacists have the right to refuse to prescribe and/or dispense birth control or morning after pills if their beliefs and conscience do not support the use of these drugs. Also in this section are arguments over the validity of routine male circumcision and whether or not there's a downside to delaying pregnancy.

Public Health Issues

Debate continues over fundamental matters surrounding many health concerns. Topics addressed in this section include issues related to immunizations and a possible link to autism, and the ongoing debate over the health impacts of "fracking." While this process of natural gas extraction offers considerable economic benefits, there appears to be a downside related to water pollution and potential human health concerns.

The threat of bio-terrorism has resurrected the risk of smallpox, thought to be eradicated in the late 1970s. Should all parents be forced to have their children immunized against smallpox, which carries certain risks? At the turn of the century, millions of American children developed childhood diseases such as tetanus, polio, measles, and pertussis (whooping cough). Many of these children died or became permanently disabled because of these illnesses. Today, vaccines exist to prevent all of these conditions; however, not all children receive their recommended immunizations. Some do not get vaccinated until the schools require them, and others are allowed exemptions. More and more, parents are requesting exemptions for some or all vaccinations based on fears over their safety and/or their effectiveness. The pertussis vaccination seems to generate the biggest fears. Reports of serious injury to children following the whooping cough vaccination (usually given in a combination of diphtheria, pertussis, and tetanus, or DPT) have convinced many parents to forgo immunization. As a result, the rates of measles and pertussis have been climbing after decades of decline. Is it safer to be vaccinated than to risk getting the disease? Is there a relationship between vaccination and the development of autism? Is the research linking the two valid? Also included in this section is the health issues linked to breastfeeding. Is it the best way to feed babies? What about women who are unable to nurse their babies? Two authors disagree on this concern.

On September 2012, New York City's Board of Health voted to ban the sale of sugary drinks in containers larger than 16 ounces in restaurants and other venues, in a move meant to combat obesity and encourage residents to live healthier lifestyles. That topic is debated in this section. Are restrictions on sugar and sugary beverages justified? Finally, the topic of a theoretical relationship between cell phone usage and cancer is addressed. As the number of cell phones continues to rise, questions about their safety are raised.

Consumer Health Issues

This section introduces questions about particular issues related to consumer choices about health issues or products. As Americans grow increasingly overweight, the most effective means of weight control continues to be debated. Along with that debate is the controversy over whether or not it's possible to lose weight and actually keep it off. The risk associated with the use of alcoholic energy drinks is an increasingly important topic, and many college students consume this beverage.

Will the many debates presented in this book ever be resolved? Some issues may resolve themselves because of the availability of resources. An overhaul of the health care system to provide care for all while keeping costs down seems inevitable, as most Americans agree that the system should be changed. While there's agreement it should be changed, the Affordable Care Act remains controversial even though many Americans now have health insurance. Other controversies may require the test of time for resolution. The debates over the health effects of global warming and the long-term benefits of medical marijuana may also take years to be fully resolved.

Other controversies may never resolve themselves. There may never be a consensus over the right of health providers to be allowed to deny care based on their beliefs, the abortion issue, rationing health care, or the cancer–cell phone connection. This book will introduce you to many ongoing controversies on a variety of sensitive and complex health-related topics. In order to have a good grasp of one's own viewpoint, it is necessary to be familiar with and understand the points made by the opposition.

Eileen L. Daniel
SUNY College at Brockport

Unit 1

UNIT

The Health Care Industry

*T*he United States currently faces many challenging health and health care concerns, including lack of universal health insurance for all its citizens. Unlike other major industrialized nations, the United States doesn't have a single payer plan to fund national health coverage, and millions of Americans are without health insurance. The Affordable Care Act is an attempt to provide more Americans with health care coverage though the Act remains controversial relative to its mandate to provide women with birth control. While some see it as a step in the right direction, others don't believe it offers the kind of universal coverage available in most other developed nations.

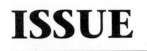

Selected, Edited, and with Issue Framing Material by:
Eileen L. Daniel, *SUNY College at Brockport*

ISSUE

Is the Affordable Care Act Successful?

YES: Gordon Whitman, from "Six Things Every Sane Person Should Know About the Healthcare Debate," *huffingtonpost.com* (2012)

NO: Peter Suderman, from "Obamacare's Phony Success Story," *Reason* (2014)

Learning Outcomes
After reading this issue, you will be able to:
• Discuss the provisions of the Affordable Care Act.
• Assess the impact of the Act on health care access.

ISSUE SUMMARY

YES: Political correspondent Gordon Whitman believes the Affordable Care Act is the best hope Americans have for making our health care system better.

NO: *Reason* magazine senior editor Peter Suderman counters that the law increased health spending, missed enrollment targets, and continues to experience problems with the website.

The Patient Protection and Affordable Care Act (PPACA), also known as "Obama Care" or the Affordable Care Act, is a federal statute signed into law by President Obama in the spring of 2010. The Act aims to both increase the rate of Americans with health insurance and lower the overall costs of health care. The PPACA includes several components including mandates, subsidies, and tax credits to help and encourage employers and individuals to increase the coverage rate. Additional reforms seek to improve health care outcomes and streamline the delivery of health care. The Congressional Budget Office predicts that the PPACA will reduce both future deficits and spending for Medicare.

Polls indicate support of health care reform in general, but became more negative in regards to specific plans during legislative debates. The Act that was ultimately signed into law in 2010 remains controversial with opinions falling along party lines. Opinions are clearly divided by age and party affiliation, with a solid majority of seniors and Republicans opposing the bill while a solid majority of Democrats and those younger than 40 are in favor. In a 2010 poll conducted by CNN, 62% of respondents said they thought the PPACA would "increase the amount of money they personally spend on health care," 56 percent said the bill "gives the government too much involvement in health care," and only 19 percent said they thought they and their families would be better off with the legislation.

The Act mandates that insurance companies cover all applicants at the same rates regardless of preexisting conditions or gender. In addition, a provision mandates that all insurance policies cover birth control without a co-pay as part of preventive care. The Act requires that all insurance policies cover *all* forms of basic preventive care without a co-pay, including well-woman, well-baby, and well-child visits, as well as other basic prevention care for men and women. This coverage is intended to save costs and promote public health. Basic preventive reproductive and sexual health care services, including contraception, are therefore also covered without a co-pay. As part of the mandate, all insurance plans must provide coverage without a co-pay for all methods of contraception approved by the Food and Drug Administration (FDA). Employees *earn* their salaries and their benefits, and many pay for all or a portion of their health care premiums out of their salaries. As such, none of this coverage is "free," but is rather covered by the policies they are earning or for which they are paying.

For many Americans, the Affordable Care Act is synonymous with a dysfunctional website. But the president's health care law has insured far more people outside the private insurance exchanges—upward of 10 million, beginning with 1 million children with preexisting conditions who were covered with the law's 2010 passage, and 3 million young adults who have secured coverage on their parents' health plans. The law never got a public option, but a huge portion of its new enrollees are now on Medicaid, the publicly funded health plan. In the 26 states participating in its expansion, Medicaid now offers comprehensive coverage for anyone earning less than 138 percent of poverty income—$16,105 for individuals or $27,310 for a family of three. More than 4.5 million low-income Americans have already gained coverage, and with no enrollment deadline that figure will only grow. Meanwhile, outreach efforts have also brought nearly 2 million very poor Americans to sign up for Medicaid benefits for which they would already have been eligible.

The law's impact is even greater than these enrollment numbers might indicate. Before the law, insurers previously rejected nearly one in five applicants; today an estimated 120 million Americans with a preexisting health condition cannot be denied coverage. The Affordable Care Act also guarantees zero-co-pay preventive care for policies bought on its exchanges. For some young women with modest incomes who take the Pill, the value of these benefits (up to $1,200) is greater than the yearly premiums on a very basic plan (roughly $1,100). Addiction treatment, mental-health care, and maternity coverage are all now guaranteed. Even seniors are coming out ahead, having already pocketed an average $1,265 in savings on prescription drugs bought under Medicare.

While the numbers indicate success, the Act has never been well received by the public. Many people feel there are many downsides to the law including the belief that the law actually forces plans to cover more and more (children must be covered to age 27) that everyone was forced to pay into. In addition, many feel there are too many loopholes which have had negative impacts including employers who have cut back hours or reduced staff to avoid covering their health insurance costs.

Initially, the bill was hyped as a means to both cover the uninsured and help reduce costs for everyone. Many, however, believe that the reality is that the goal of insuring all the uninsured isn't going to be met. The Congressional Budget Office projected that by 2023—more than a decade after implementation—that 31 million people will still be uninsured. Finally, for many Americans, the very fact that the law is run by the government is a reason it is failing. They believe that the government is incapable of ever running anything cost-efficiently or effectively.

YES ↵

Gordon Whitman

Six Things Every Sane Person Should Know About the Healthcare Debate

With all of the silly signs outside the Supreme Court and philosophizing inside, it can be easy to miss how catastrophic it would be for the country if the justices strike down the Affordable Care Act. While still a work-in-progress, the new health law is almost certainly the last best hope we have for attacking the fatal flaws in the American healthcare system. Take away the law, and we are stuck for a generation or more with the reality of a healthcare system that each year will cost more, deliver less and exclude more people.

Here are six things that every sane person should know about the healthcare debate.

1. **The legislation is not as big and complicated as we've been made to think.** Think of the law as a triangle that does three basic things: First, it tightens the screws on insurance companies so that none of us is at risk of being cutoff or denied coverage when we or our loved ones get sick and need it most. Second, it brings almost everyone into the system by providing individuals with subsidies to buy coverage and expanding the Medicaid program to cover all people at or just above the poverty level. And third, it promotes a set of promising local and state innovations designed to improve the delivery of care in order to reduce the cost and improve quality.

   Rather than see the Affordable Care Act as a big federal takeover of healthcare, as it has been politically attacked, it is more accurate to understand the law as a framework for states, local communities, healthcare providers, businesses and ordinary citizens to tackle the urgent task of fixing the American healthcare system. We should not be fighting about the framework, which represents a set of compromises between conservatives and progressives, but about how to implement the law.

2. **The Affordable Care Act is already helping tens of millions of people get better health.** In 2011 more than 86 million Americans received free preventive care such as mammograms and colonoscopies. More than three and a half million Medicare beneficiaries have saved more than $2.1 billion on prescription drugs. Small businesses are better able to provide coverage to their employees, and parents of children with preexisting conditions no longer have to worry their children will be denied coverage. More young adults (2.5 million) are able to stay healthy by remaining on their parents' health insurance plans. In the coming years millions more Americans will gain the physical and financial security of having health coverage.

3. **There is no real alternative.** With all of the talk about repeal, there is no viable alternative on either the right or the left that would plausibly result in a healthcare system that provides coverage to all Americans and slows the growth in healthcare spending. If the Roberts Court strikes the mandate, it will probably also eliminate popular rules that prohibit insurance companies from denying people coverage for preexisting conditions. This would take the heart out of the law. The Roberts Court could still leave in place the expansion of Medicaid, which extends health coverage to as many as 16 million low-income uninsured people. That would still be an important step forward for the country that shouldn't be sneezed at.

   Regardless of whether the Roberts Court takes a scalpel or a sledge hammer to the law, it will be extraordinarily difficult to find any common ground in Congress to pass new healthcare legislation. And federal politicians will go back to avoiding the issue like the plague, as they did after the Clinton effort failed. After all of the political capital invested by President Obama, who would try again anytime soon?

4. **People will die.** I found it sickening to read of Justices Scalia and Alito's concern about the financial health of insurance companies and the amount of reading their clerks might have to do in contrast to their seemingly heartless

disregard for human life and the pressures on families who cannot afford health insurance. Each year about 40,000 people die prematurely because they lack health coverage. Many hundreds of thousands of people delay needed care and live with unnecessary pain and stress. The justices (who sit in the warm embrace of government-provided healthcare) are happy to philosophize over broccoli. They need to be reminded that their decisions on this case will have life or death consequences of people in the United States.

5. **Costs will go through the roof.** The Affordable Care Act does not do enough to limit the long-term growth in health spending in the United States. But it does put the country on the right path by changing how healthcare is paid for to reward medical providers for getting and keeping people healthy rather than for more tests and procedures. It also enables states to create healthcare exchanges that will bring transparency to the healthcare market and be a boon for people who purchase coverage on their own. More will need to be done, but almost all of the policies that control healthcare costs build on what is already in the new health law.

6. **If it looks like judicial activism and smells like judicial activism, it is.** Seventy-five years ago the U.S. Supreme Court relented on its stubborn opposition to regulations designed to protect children and families from the vicissitudes of an increasingly complex national economy. Since then, the Court has allowed Congress and the President to regulate the national economy without judicial meddling. If the Roberts Court decides to strike down the healthcare mandate or the entire healthcare law, it will not be because it faces a novel question, but because Justice Roberts and his conservative colleagues have made a decision to use their powers to remake the country along their personal preferences. And they know that.

The Roberts Court's Citizens United jurisprudence on money in politics has already fundamentally eroded American democracy. In June we'll know if the Court has done the same thing to our social safety net.

Let's pray for Justice Kennedy—the court's swing vote—to find the wisdom and compassion to understand the real world, human consequences of his legal analysis. If he fails, our nation will not only miss out on an opportunity to save tens of thousands of Americans from shorter and more painful lives, it will move one step further in losing the Supreme Court as an instrument of justice, fairness and social progress.

GORDON WHITMAN is a political correspondent.

Peter Suderman 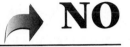 **NO**

Obamacare's Phony Success Story

After year one, the health care overhaul is riddled with problems.

IT COULD HAVE been worse.

In the first weeks after Obamacare's health insurance exchanges launched on October 1, 2013, almost nothing worked. The main federal exchange, which served as an insurance hub for 36 states, was down more often than it was up, and when it was online, it didn't work. Many exchanges run by state governments were in disarray as well. Millions of people with individual health insurance policies received letters indicating that their existing coverage would be canceled. The law's mandated small business exchange had been delayed, as had its Spanish language website. Thousands of applications were stranded inside the glitchy exchange systems. It seemed entirely plausible that between the cancellations and the website failures, Obamacare's expansion of insurance coverage—the main selling point of a $2 trillion overhaul of the health care system—might end up making no meaningful dent in the uninsured rate at all.

The rollout was bad enough that the Obama administration was gritting its teeth in full crisis-P.R. mode, assuring Americans that, despite a few bumps in the road, all was okay. "This system is not failing," embattled White House Press Secretary Jay Carney told CNN in October. "Hundreds of thousands of Americans are submitting their applications successfully to get into the system and enroll in Obamacare, and they are doing it through a variety of means, through state exchanges and through the call-in centers and that's going to continue."

Behind the scenes, however, the White House was terrified. Reporting would later come out that top officials were actively considering scrapping the health exchange system they had spent three years building, and starting over from scratch. More than a few Republicans in Congress confidently predicted that the law would soon collapse under its own weight. Obamacare looked doomed.

But in December, following a series of frantic all-hands-on-deck repair efforts by the administration's tech team, the federal exchange began to function normally. An end of year sign-up surge showed not only that the system could handle increased traffic volume, but that there might be real demand for the insurance being sold. Exchanges run by densely populated states such as California and New York were reporting brisk traffic and hundreds of thousands of sign-ups. In January, the administration fired the technology contractor that had built the federal exchange. Progress was being made.

At the end of March, Obamacare's first open enrollment period—the timeframe during which anyone is allowed to sign for coverage each year—came to a close, providing an opportunity to benchmark the controversial new system's performance. That final week brought a surge in people applying for coverage, taking the total number of sign-ups to just over 8 million—better than the 7 million enrollments that the Congressional Budget Office (CBO) had predicted when the law passed, and far better than the revised estimate of 6 million the CBO predicted after the website crashed. Relying on a daily tracking poll, Gallup reported that the nation's uninsurance rate had dropped to its lowest point since 2008.

The administration's spin quickly went from cautiously optimistic to cocky. "I think it is fair to say we surpassed everybody's expectations," Carney said in April.

Critics who wanted to overturn the law had been definitively proven wrong. "The point is the repeal debate is and should be over," President Obama said in a press conference a few days later. "The Affordable Care Act is working." White House senior adviser Dan Pfeiffer tweeted that the health care law was an "amazing comeback story."

The administration's belated claims of success rested heavily on two pillars: the 8 million sign-up figure and the exceedingly low expectations established by the exchanges' disastrous launch. The White House was selling an unlikely underdog story in which the plucky little health care law, backed only by the entire executive branch of the federal government, came from behind to score an unexpected victory.

But judged by other metrics, such as rising health spending, state-by-state sign-ups, demographic balance, and public opinion, the law looks less like a success story and more like an enormous national experiment still struggling out of the gate. Yes, it could have been worse. But it also could have been a lot better. And beyond the headline successes, more than a few potential problems remain.

Sign-Ups vs. Enrollments

The administration's single most prominent piece of evidence that Obamacare is a success is that it surpassed expectations by signing up 8 million people for coverage. That statistic, however, leaves out an important detail: how many of those 8 million have actually enrolled.

For now, what the administration knows for sure is that 8 million people "selected a plan": they successfully logged on to a website, looked at the insurance choices that were available to them, and clicked a box indicating which plan they'd like to buy. What's less clear is how many of those people followed up by paying their first month's premium, a requirement for coverage.

When pressed, federal officials have responded that only insurers have complete information about payment rates. For their part, insurers say they don't know with absolute precision, either. But it's possible to arrive at a rough estimate.

At the end of April, Karen Ignagni, the CEO of the health insurance trade group America's Health Insurance Plans, told a Politico briefing that about 85 percent of sign-ups had paid. In testimony before Congress in May 2014, several insurance company executives put their payment rates at between 80 and 90 percent. Officials in California, which has more sign-ups than any other state and is widely regarded as producing the most successful implementation of Obamacare, have also estimated an 85 percent payment rate.

Prior to the launch of the exchanges, the administration had targeted 7 million enrollments by the end of open enrollment. In June 2013, Health and Human Services (HHS) Secretary Kathleen Sebelius told reporters, "We're hopeful that 7 million is a realistic target." A September 2013 memo from the Centers for Medicare and Medicaid Services projected 7.066 million enrollments by the end of March. Right before the exchanges opened for business, Sebelius told NBC that "success looks like at least 7 million people having signed up by the end of March 2014."

If 85 percent of the 8 million sign-ups end up paying, then the true exchange-enrollment total is more like 6.8 million. Even a 10 percent reduction would still knock 800,000 off the administration's sign-up total—far better than prospects looked in the law's darkest days, but still substantially less than the headline figure the administration advertised.

Getting the Right Demographic Mix

It's not enough to have millions of people signed up for insurance though. It matters what kind of people sign up.

Because the Affordable Care Act restricts how insurers can price based on age and health history, the law needs a substantial portion of younger, healthier people to sign up for coverage in order to balance out the higher costs of insuring older and sicker people.

Even the Obama administration has suggested that getting the right demographic mix is more important than getting lots of people into the exchanges. "Whatever the total figure is of people who enroll by March 31st, the aggregate number," Carney said in January, "the total number is not as important as the overall makeup that you see in that population."

That's why you saw so many ads over the winter targeting young people: If the Obamacare exchanges were filled disproportionately with people who were old and sick, then premiums would rise, and fewer people would purchase insurance, which could cause premiums to rise again, potentially resulting in a meltdown of the insurance pool.

In background briefings with various reporters in the summer of 2013, the White House said that the goal, based on estimates by the CBO, was to have 39 percent of all enrollees to be between the ages of 18 and 35. So what was the final total? Just 28 percent of sign-ups were in that age range.

The exchange enrollees are not just older; they're probably sicker, too. An April study by pharmacy benefits manager Express Scripts found that use of expensive specialty drugs by early exchange enrollees is 47 percent higher than is typical for those enrolled in employer health insurance, usually a sign of a less healthy population.

State-by-State Enrollment Targets

Even under a federal law like Obamacare that features a main federal exchange, insurance markets are still regulated and separated by state lines. So the experience of the Affordable Care Act will differ dramatically by region, with some states seeing robust enrollment figures and healthy risk pools, and others struggling to make do despite low enrollment.

By the middle of April, 22 states had met or exceeded their initial enrollment targets, according to a May analysis by the health policy consulting group Avalere Health (which assumed an 85 percent payment rate among signups). A few of those states far exceeded their aims, including California and Florida, which enrolled 186 percent and 199 percent of their goals, respectively.

That left slightly more than half the states below their stated targets. Some of the stragglers, such as Indiana, Arizona, Illinois, and Kansas, came in reasonably close, hitting at least 85 percent of their goals. But a handful of states missed the mark by wide margins. Wisconsin enrolled just 57 percent of its goal, and West Virginia just 61 percent. New York and Hawaii both enrolled fewer than half their target numbers.

Some of the states with low enrollment can expect to face serious problems maintaining viable, affordable insurance markets under Obamacare. West Virginia in particular has been pegged as likely to see big premium hikes, for its combination of low enrollment, sicker than expected population, and weak insurer competition. "West Virginia sticks out as really worrisome," Avalere Health Vice President Caroline Pearson told National Journal in May. "Their exchange is not having great luck."

Complicating matters further is that several of the state-run exchanges continue to struggle with major technical malfunctions throughout open enrollment, and a few are essentially inoperable.

Website Still Incomplete

At the center of Obamacare's botched launch last October was a broken federal exchange system, housed at Healthcare.gov, which covers insurance sign-ups in 36 states. For all practical purposes, the system did not work for two months. After an all-in effort to fix the mess, the administration deemed the site largely repaired. "We believe we have met the goal of having a system that will work smoothly for the vast majority of users," HHS stated in an early December report.

But the technical troubles were far from over. The administration's repair effort had focused on repairing the front end of the system—the part that could be seen and used by insurance shoppers—at the expense of everything else. The result was that the crucial components of the back end, the guts of the system designed to communicate critical data and manage the law's complex web of payments and subsidies, remained not broken but almost entirely unbuilt.

In November, Henry Chao, the top HHS tech official working on the exchanges, testified before Congress that 30–40 percent of the federal exchange, including payment processing capabilities, had still not been completed. At the time, he said that the administration expected to finish the job by January.

But when January arrived, the work was still not done. The administration fired its tech contractor, CGI Federal, and hired a new one, Accenture, relying on a no-bid contract that the administration indicated was necessary to speed up the typically slow federal contracting process.

"Failure to deliver" payment functionality "by mid-March 2014," the administration warned in a document justifying the contract, "will result in financial harm to the Government. If this functionality is not complete by March 2014, the Government could make erroneous payments to providers and insurers." Without a finished system, "the entire healthcare reform program is jeopardized." Missing the mid-March deadline would "significantly increase" a variety of risks for the program, and could "potentially [put] the entire health insurance industry at risk."

Yet March, too, came and went, and the back end remained incomplete. As late as May, the White House refused to provide any expected deadline for total functionality. An administration spec sheet said that insurers should prepare to rely on manually created workaround estimates at least through September.

Meanwhile, the related tech-headaches continued to mount. In May, *The Washington Post* reported that more than one million insurance sign-ups under the law had resulted in incorrect subsidy payments. Obamacare subsidies are based on income, but in many cases, the incomes submitted on the insurance applications did not match the incomes on file with the Internal Revenue Service. Normally, such a problem would be resolved through a follow-up check, in which individuals with discrepancies could submit paperwork. But the system to process that paperwork had not been completed, either. So the verification process had to be completed by hand. Federal officials told the *Post* that they did not expect discrepancy-check functionality until summer, after other verification issues were sorted out.

Bailing Out Insurers?

Among the crucial payment systems left unbuilt as of mid-May was the mechanism for managing a program buried within the law known as risk corridors. This initially obscure provision became far more prominent when

Republican critics started labeling it a built-in bailout for the insurance industry.

At its most basic, the risk corridors program is a process for sharing risk between the federal government and the health insurers participating in Obamacare. Each year, insurers set targets for health claims spending within their plans. If spending comes in at 97 percent or less of their expected costs, then they pay the savings into the federal government. If claims costs come in at 103 percent or more above target, then the federal government pays the insurer, covering a portion of the unanticipated costs.

In theory, some insurers pay in, others are paid out, and it all balances out, with no net cost to the feds. That's how the program was expected to work when the law was written, and federal health officials affirmed this year that they intend to run it revenue neutral. But what happens if most or all of the insurers spend more than expected, and the federal government ends up on the hook?

Such a scenario is not outside the realm of possibility. Multiple insurers have issued warning signals that the exchange business may not be financially stable yet. A January Securities and Exchange Commission (SEC) filing from Humana told investors that the exchange population was "more adverse"—sicker and more expensive—than expected. Cigna CEO David Cordani said in February that the company does not expect Obamacare to be "a money maker." Aetna CEO Mark Bertolini said flatly in February that the company expects "to lose money in the first year."

The ratings agency Moody's cut its health insurer outlook to negative in January as a result of "uncertainty over the demographics of those enrolling in individual products through the exchanges." And in perhaps the most telling sign of all, insurers have mounted an aggressive lobbying campaign defending the necessity of the risk corridors.

If insurers have a bad year, the administration says it has them covered. An HHS regulation issued in May indicated that the government would find "other sources of funding" if needed in order to pay risk corridor claims. That promise, however, is "subject to the availability of appropriations." That last caveat could be a problem. According to a January 2013 Congressional Research Service memo, there are no appropriations available for the risk corridors, which means the administration may have made a promise it does not have the legal authority to keep.

Pushing the Boundaries of Executive Authority

When it comes to Obamacare, legal authority has never proven much of a constraint for the White House. Since the law's passage in March 2010, the Obama administration

has repeatedly relied on executive authority to alter the law's requirements and implementation procedures.

According to an ongoing count by the Galen Institute, a free market policy group focused on health care, the administration has used executive authority to change the law on 22 separate occasions. Those changes include extending Obamacare's "hardship waivers," which exempt certain individuals from the law's insurance requirement, to people whose health plans were cancelled; extending the enrollment deadline into April via the creation of a "special enrollment period"; allowing some people who purchase individual coverage outside the exchanges to access subsidies; and delaying the creation of the law's small-business exchange.

Some of the changes have had the effect of undermining the law's policy scheme. In March, for example, the administration allowed insurers two additional years to offer certain individual health plans that do not comply with Obamacare's requirements, and therefore were previously slated to be cancelled. The move was a political response to the outcry over a wave of health plan cancellations that directly contradicted the president's repeated promise that, under the law, people could keep health plans they liked.

But the result of letting otherwise disqualifying policies live on is that the new exchanges will be more heavily weighted toward people who didn't previously have insurance and are therefore more likely to be sick—meaning that insurers will be faced with smaller, less healthy, and less viable risk pools in the near term, and thus more likely to depend on risk corridor payouts from the administration.

Other changes were almost certainly illegal. In July 2013, the administration delayed for one year the law's requirement that employers with 50 or more employees provide qualifying health coverage or pay a penalty. In February of this year, that requirement was delayed an additional year for employers with between 50 and 100 employees, and the penalty was reduced for larger firms, conveniently moving the full, presumably painful implementation into 2015, beyond November's mid-term elections.

As Case Western University Law Professor Jonathan Adler wrote in The Washington Post at the time, "whatever the stated reason for the new delay, it is illegal." The text of the health care law states clearly that the employer requirement "shall apply" after December 31, 2013.

Even some supporters of the law agreed that the change was beyond die president's lawful power. Writing in *The New England Journal of Medicine,* University of Michigan Law School Professor Nicholas Bagley wrote that "the delays appear to exceed the traditional scope of the President's enforcement discretion," and "set a troubling precedent" of selective enforcement, one that could potentially be invoked by future administrations opposed to the law.

In the meantime, regardless of legality, it's unclear whether the administration will ever enforce the provision. "I don't think the employer mandate will go into effect," former White House Press Secretary Robert Gibbs predicted in April. "I think it will be one of the first things to go."

Health Spending Increases

Among the least discussed of the many Obamacare promises that have already been broken is the law's supposed dampening effect on national health spending. Obamacare, President Obama promised in March 2010, would "bring down the cost of health care for families, for businesses, and for the federal government." If anything, though, large hikes in overall health spending look to have returned after a very brief hiatus.

Between 2009 and 2012, the annual growth rate of health care spending did indeed decrease to less than 4 percent—its lowest rate in years, prompting Obamacare supporters to claim credit. "The bottom line is this," President Obama said at the end of March, "under this law, the share of Americans with insurance is up and the growth of health care costs is down."

But even then, there were signs that the spending slowdown would not last. It may already be ending. The federal Bureau of Economic Analysis reported that health spending in the fourth quarter of 2013 grew at 5.6 percent, up from 2.3 percent in the fourth quarter of the previous year. That faster-paced growth appears to be driven largely by increased use of health services, and it has continued into this year. National health spending in March 2014 grew 7.1 percent faster than in March 2013, the fastest annual rate since 2005, according to researchers at the Altarum Institute. In March, health spending as a share of the economy reached 17.9 percent—an all-time high.

The Debate Isn't Over

Of all the problems that have bedeviled Obamacare supporters, perhaps the most frustrating one is how to get Americans to like the law. Since before the Affordable Care Act was passed, it has struggled in the court of public

opinion, rendering the law politically unstable even if its policy scheme proves workable. And all the while prominent Democrats have been predicting that a majority of the public will finally support the law any day now.

But for the last four years, polls have consistently shown that more of the public disapproves of the health law than approves of it, and large segments of the population support repealing it entirely. Democrats had bet that the law would become more popular once its biggest benefits kicked in, but if anything, opposition has only grown. On average, polls show that just over 52 percent of the public opposed Obamacare as of May, according to RealClearPolitics. That's up slightly from an average of about 48 percent between the summer of 2012 and summer 2013. At the same time, 48 percent of the public wants Obamacare wiped from the books entirely, according to a May Politico poll, and another 35 percent say they want the law fixed and modified. Just 16 percent think it should be left alone.

"Based on what you know now," the poll asked, after noting the president's defense of the law and Republicans' ongoing criticism, "do you believe that the debate on Obamacare should be over, or not?" Some 60 percent of respondents said they believed discussion about the law's merits should continue.

President Obama may believe, as he insists, that the debate over Obamacare is now over, but as his power wanes, the public continues to disagree.

It seemed entirely plausible that between the cancellations and the website failures, Obamacare's expansion of insurance coverage" the main selling point—might end up making no meaningful dent in the uninsured rate at all.

If insurers have a bad year, the administration says it has them covered. An HHS regulation issued in May indicated that the government would find "other sources of funding" if needed in order to pay risk corridor claims.

Legal authority has never proven much of a constraint for the White House. Since the law's passage, the Obama administration has repeatedly relied on executive authority to alter its requirements and implementation procedures.

Obamacare was supposed to "bring down the cost of health care for families, for businesses and for the federal government." But in March, health spending as a share of the economy reached 17.9 percent—an all-time high.

PETER SUDERMAN is senior editor of *Reason* magazine.

EXPLORING THE ISSUE

Is the Affordable Care Act Successful?

Critical Thinking and Reflection

1. Why are so many Americans opposed to the Affordable Care Act when millions have no health insurance?
2. How will the Affordable Care Act be able to significantly increase the number of uninsured Americans? Explain.
3. Describe why many Americans believe the government should not be involved in providing health insurance.

Is There Common Ground?

The government estimated that the Affordable Care Act legislation will lower the number of the uninsured by 32 million, leaving 23 million uninsured residents by 2019 after the bill's mandates have all taken effect. Among the people in this uninsured group will be approximately 8 million illegal immigrants, individuals eligible but not enrolled in Medicare, and the mostly young and single men and women not otherwise covered who choose to pay the annual penalty instead of purchasing insurance.

Early experience under the Act was that, as a result of the tax credit for small businesses, some businesses offered health insurance to their employees for the first time. On September 13, 2011, the Census Bureau released a report showing that the number of uninsured 19- to 25-year-olds (now eligible to stay on their parents' policies) had declined by 393,000, or 1.6%. A later report from the Government Accountability Office in 2012 found that of the 4 million small businesses that were offered the tax credit only 170,300 businesses claimed it. Due to the effect of the U.S. Supreme Court ruling, states can opt in or out of the expansion of Medicaid.

Also, a component ensuring children could remain included on their parents' plans until age 26 remains a popular, fairly noncontroversial part of the bill. The contraceptive coverage, however, remains contentious. The Affordable Care Act includes a contraceptive coverage mandate that, with the exception of churches and houses of worship, applies to all employers and educational institutions. These regulations made under the Act rely on the recommendations of the Institute of Medicine which concluded that access to contraception is medically necessary "to ensure women's health and well-being."

Additional Resources

Dickinson, T. (2014). Obamacare: It's working! *Rolling Stone, 1207,* 32–35.

Muller, L. A., Isely, P., & Levin, A. (2015). Employer reactions to the Affordable Care Act. *Benefits Quarterly, 31*(1), 51–63.

Obama, B. (2014). The Affordable Care Act: The rollout has been rough. *Vital Speeches of the Day, 80*(1), 25–26.

Slade, S. (2013). The Not-So-Affordable Care Act. *U.S. News Digital Weekly, 5*(27), 17.

Wilensky, G. (2015). Why does the Affordable Care Act remain so unpopular? *Journal of the American Medical Association, 313*(10), 1002–1003.

Internet References . . .

Health Care

www.healthcare.gov

Health Care Law and You

www.healthcare.gov/law/

Medicaid

http://medicaid.gov/affordablecareact/affordable
-care-act.html

Selected, Edited, and with Issue Framing Material by:
Eileen L. Daniel, *SUNY College at Brockport*

ISSUE

Should the Health Care System Continuously Strive to Extend Life?

YES: Miguel Faria, from "Bioethics and Why I Hope to Live Beyond Age 75 Attaining Wisdom!—A Rebuttal to Dr. Ezekiel Emanuel's 75 Age Limit," *haciendapublishing.com* (2014)

NO: Ezekiel J. Emanuel, from "Why I Hope to Die at 75: An Argument That Society and Families—and You—Will Be Better Off if Nature Takes Its Course Swiftly and Promptly," *The Atlantic* (2014)

Learning Outcomes

After reading this issue, you will be able to:

- Discuss the quality versus quantity of life issues.
- Identify the reasons Americans are living longer.
- Assess the economic impact of extended lifespans.

ISSUE SUMMARY

YES: Physician Miguel Faria contends that lives can be productive and fulfilling and worthwhile past age 75 and that there is a difference between aging and infirmity and illness.

NO: Physician, bioethicist, and vice provost of the University of Pennsylvania Ezekiel J. Emanuel disagrees and claims that society and families would be better off if we died at 75 rather than be incapacitated and unable to live a full life.

In 1980, 11 percent of the U.S. population was over age 65, but they accounted for about 29 percent ($219 billion) of the total American health care expenditures. By the beginning of the new millennium, the percentage of the population over 65 had risen to 12 percent, which consumed 31 percent of total health care expenditures, of $450 billion. It has been projected that by the year 2040, people over 65 will represent 21 percent of the population and they will consume 45 percent of all health care expenditures.

Medical expenses at the end of life appear to be extremely high in relation to other health care costs. Studies have shown that nearly one-third of annual Medicare costs are for the 5 percent of beneficiaries who die that year. Expenses for dying patients increase significantly as death nears, and payments for health care during the last weeks of life make up 40 percent of the medical costs for the entire last year of life. Some studies have shown that up to 50 percent of the medical costs incurred during a person's entire life are spent during their last year!

Many surveys have indicated that most Americans do not want to be kept alive if their illness is incurable and irreversible, for both economic and humanitarian reasons. Many experts believe that if physicians stopped using high technology at the end of life to prevent death, then we would save billions of dollars, which could be used to insure the uninsured and provide basic health care to millions. In England the emphasis of health care is on improving the quality of life through primary care medicine, well-subsidized home care, and institutional programs for the elderly and those with incurable illnesses, rather than through life-extending acute care medicine. The British seem to value basic medical care for all rather than expensive technology for the few who might benefit from it. As a result, the British spend a much smaller proportion of their gross national product (6.2 percent) on health services than do Americans (10.8 percent) for a nearly identical health status and life expectancy.

While the economics of extending life is certainly a major issue, the quality of life after a certain age is also a major consideration. Americans are living longer lives leading to a real increase in life expectancy. This is mainly the result of the many scientific and technological discoveries as well as education about our health. Though we are living longer, for many older Americans, their older years are often spent suffering from one or more chronic diseases causing pain and disability. But how does an individual decide which takes precedence, the actual number of years lived or quality of life of those years? How does a person determine what is more important, the quality or quantity of life? While it is a person's own prerogative to decide which they value more, there may be many personal factors that play a role in an individual's decision. No one can make this determination for another person, not even the scientists that have made miraculous breakthroughs in regards to health care. It is a personal decision that is a unique choice for each person to make for themselves.

According to the latest U.S. Census predictions, our country's population of individuals over the age of 65 will increase 1% to 3% per year. If these predictions are accurate, by the year 2030, one in five persons in the United States will be over the age of 65 and this age group will represent 25 percent of the U.S. population. In addition, the United States has a higher number of individuals over 100 than any other nation and approximately 70,000 centenarians exist in our population today. The number of people that are living to be 100 years old is increasing at such a rapid rate that by the year 2050 there will be an estimated 850,000 individuals in the United States over the age of 100.

As a result of these demographic changes, there will be many shifts in health care that will be necessary to care for this growing population. Transportation, home health care, and housing are among the factors that will need to be addressed in order to accommodate those over age 65. Also affected will be Social Security income, Medicare, and Medicaid. These increases in our population can have serious implications on our country as a whole.

For many reasons there is an increase in the average life expectancy of the American population. Life expectancy has risen due to the many advances in public health, science, technology, nutrition, and medicine, and researchers are finding new ways to treat chronic conditions.

Each individual should ask the question of whether they would rather live a longer life that may require the utilization of various forms of medical intervention which may be able to slow or lessen the effects of various diseases. Or would they rather live quality years that are free from all of these various products and inventions of science that may prolong the years that are actually lived, but with the sacrifice of feeling ultimately healthy? This can be a difficult decision for an individual to make, and it may take a person some time to weigh the pros and cons of their unique situation to determine the ultimate choice that is right for them.

Overall, it appears that the best way that a person can ensure that they are living their life with the quality that they desire is to educate himself or herself about the importance of maintaining an overall healthy well-being. This includes taking care of oneself, both physically and mentally. A person should stay up to date with health care professionals when it comes to annual exams and procedures that need to be performed. It is important for each person to listen to their body, and hear what it is telling them. Only a person knows their own body and can tell how they are feeling. It is imperative to know what needs to be done and what changes need to be made to ensure an ultimate healthy well-being. This is where the education that has been provided can take the reins and lead an individual to their optimal health.

YES ↵

Miguel Faria

Bioethics and Why I Hope to Live Beyond Age 75 Attaining Wisdom!—A Rebuttal to Dr. Ezekiel Emanuel's 75 Age Limit

For several decades, American bioethicists have been providing persuasive arguments for rationing medical care via the theory of the necessary "rational allocation of finite health care resources."(2) More recently, assisted by various sectors of organized medicine, they have developed multiple approaches to justify what they see as the necessary curtailment of services and specialized treatments deemed not medically necessary. The problem persists, though, and the need for rationing health services in increasingly socialized medical systems, including ObamaCare, requires more ingenious approaches, particularly in the U.S., where patients are accustomed to receiving the best medical care that third-party payers are willing to pay for, regardless of whether the payer is the insurance company or the government.(6)

Furthermore, government planners, supported by the ever-accommodating bioethicists, posit that with increasing longevity and augmentation of the population of American elderly, more drastic actions will be required to prevent the bankruptcy of the public financing of medical care. They believe therefore that outright government-imposed euthanasia, not only for the terminally ill but also for the inconvenient infirm and the superfluous elderly, will become necessary.(1,4,8,10)

It is in this context that the individual-based, patient-oriented ethics of Hippocrates, including his fundamental dictum, "First Do No Harm," are seen as an obstacle by the bioethics movement. Obtrusive and in their way, time-honored medical ethics are being eroded and supplanted by the more convenient, collectivist, population-based ethics propounded by today bioethicists. As early as the 1980s, some bioethicists, including Daniel Callahan, then Director of the Hastings Center; Peter Singer, bioethics professor at Stanford University; and John Hardwick of East Tennessee State University, openly insisted that elderly patients who had lived a full life had a "duty to die" for the good of society and the proper utilization of societal health resources.(2) Dr. Callahan pointedly asserted, "Denial of nutrition, may, in the long run, become the only effective way to make certain that a large number of biologically tenacious patients actually die."(11) Likewise, Dr. Hardwick dropped all pretenses regarding their real intentions at about the time of the Clinton health care debate and the tentative formulation of HillaryCare, affirming a "duty to die" was necessary for those citizens whose lives had become not worth living because of chronic disease or advanced age.(7,10) Such openness was not well-received by the American people, and Hardwick's proposals were ignored, or like HillaryCare ostensibly discarded, thrown by the wayside. But appearances can be deceiving. Many proposals of the bioethics movement have quietly and gradually been implemented. Here is an insightful report by Pope Benedict XVI in his address to the Pontifical Academy for Life:

"Some ethicists warn that modern bioethics is in fact a new normative system of ethics that, based on principles of utilitarianism, can never be compatible with Natural Law principles. In the last few decades, bioethics has largely supplanted traditional, Natural Law-based medical ethics in hospitals and ethics boards in most western countries. Under traditional medical ethics, the guiding principle is 'do no harm.' But contemporary bioethics abandons this . . . in an effort to find the utilitarian goal of the 'greatest good for the greatest number.' Under these principles, preserving the life of the human patient is not considered paramount."(12) He is largely correct in his assessment. Moreover, the bioethics movement has recently received more impetus with President Barack Obama's creation of the Presidential Commission for the Study of Bioethical Issues.(9)

But their proposals have not all been fully implemented. To do so, today's bioethicists, although equally determined, are more subtle, and the foremost exponent of the new trend in bioethics is Dr. Ezekiel J. Emanuel.(3) Although 57 years of age and in good health,

Dr. Emanuel says he hopes and wants to live to age 75 and die. He has lived a fulfilled and a good life and it is time to exit. After age 75, Emanuel claims life is a downhill spiral and not worth living. His family disagrees with him and says he is "crazy,"(3) yet the fact remains Dr. Emanuel is a respected bioethicist, the Director of the Clinical Bioethics Department at the U.S. National Institutes of Health, the recipient of numerous awards, but the danger here is he encapsulates the views many bioethicists hold today. He insists that the productivity of creative people reach a peak at age 40 and plateau by age 60. In other words, after age 60, even productive people, create and produce little of value to society.(3) I beg to differ. In a recent conversation with my friend Dr. Russell Blaylock, who has also written on this subject,(1) he opined, "The reason very smart, creative people no longer produce earth-shattering discoveries later in life is because after their great accomplishments, they become department heads, drowning in administrative duties that prevent creative activities." I agree with Dr. Blaylock. Moreover, as we age and mellow and reach retirement, we also achieve satisfaction from a productive life well spent, and begin the contemplation and enjoyment of life that is only possible with the leisure that comes with retirement.

Dr. Emanuel, in stressing the relatively young age in which productive people reach the apex of their creativity, e.g., novelists, poets, and physicists, argues as if becoming poet laureates and Noble Prize winners were the universal aspirations of the average citizen. Most people do not aspire to reach those dizzying heights! The more realistic goals in life, instead, are more mundane, namely, fulfillment and contentment, qualities that are attained by being good citizens, and the satisfaction of leading good and productive lives; men and women performing their occupations and respective jobs, whether menial, artistic or intellectual, and doing them well—in short, being the best we can be in this transitory phase of our existence!

In his article Dr. Emanuel writes that if we live longer than age 75, "we are no longer remembered as vibrant and engaged but as feeble, ineffectual, even pathetic."(3) And as far as suicide or euthanasia, Dr. Emmanuel claims he is against those options, although it escapes him logical reasoning will lead many people to pursue exactly those options when afflicted with depression, physical illness, or merely reaching that lethal age of 75—or even worse. By which I refer to the State compulsorily implementing exactly those policies, purportedly as pragmatic and "sound" health care policies, when in fact they may be implemented for political expediency or budgetary considerations. This is particularly ominous when the State is involved in administering and funding medical care, as in socialized medicine or ObamaCare.(6,7)

In the same vein toward the end of his paper, Dr. Emanuel claims he is not advocating compulsory end of life at age 75 "in order to save resources, ration health care, or address public-policy issues," but that is exactly what he is inferring. In fact, in the next breath, he admits his proposals do have at least two policy implications and that these implications do refer to reducing life expectancy.(3)

Dr. Emanuel complains that Americans are obsessed with performing physical and mental exercises, undertaking diets, taking vitamins and supplements, "all in a valiant effort to cheat death and prolong life as long as possible."(3) In fact, leading healthy lifestyles and sticking to healthy diets are exactly what Americans should be doing, not only to prolong their lives, but even more importantly to improve the quality of their lives, while saving their own health care costs.

"Doing mental puzzles," which people have done to exercise brain function and which Dr. Emanuel derides, (3) may not exactly translate to the highest intellectual exercise. But not so other intellectual pursuits. I refer to reading and studying the classics of history and literature for their own sake; listening to good music in moments of contemplation for mere enjoyment; spending more leisure time with our families—in short enjoying all of those happy activities of leisure and exercising those fundamental virtues, which eluded us in our earlier, more active and hectic years of youth and adulthood. It is in our advancing years that we have the leisure to spend the time in just those intellectual activities that engage the mind and sooth the soul.

Others find happiness and satisfaction in doing what they have always done in life. This is particularly true of those who have answered a professional calling, who obtain intellectual rewards in continuing to practice their professions to the very end or until they are impaired by age or disability. That was the case with my father, a physician. It is the case, I suspect, with Dr. James I. Ausman, editor-in-chief of *Surgical Neurology International*, who at age 76 remains a scholar and an incorrigible multitasker and who seems to gather ever more speed in life as he gets older!

The key to meaningful longevity, then, is to remain active, exercising our intellectual faculties for their own sake, as well as for the preservation of brain plasticity. Dr. Emanuel admits the neural connections that are most utilized are reinforced and preserved, while those connections and synapses not used degenerate and atrophy. However, he is incorrect when he states that we cannot learn as we get older because no new neural connections and re-wirings are possible. Brain plasticity allows us to continue to learn well beyond age 75 for those who remain active, although it is true that in extremely advanced age, learning, creative thoughts, and memory retention become progressively more difficult as degeneration of neural connections and neuronal death take place.

Thus, I am curious as well as perplexed. Has Dr. Emanuel ever had the interest or time to read Thucydides and Herodotus? I wonder if he ever read Plutarch, Livy, Virgil, or any of the poems of Sappho or Elizabeth Barrett Browning? I wonder if he ever read Plato, Aristotle, or understands the meaning of the Aristotelian good life, and the time and activities that are necessary for the attainment of real happiness and wisdom? The ultimate good life is not necessarily found in our hard-working, intensive, utilitarian, and productive years, but in our years of leisure and contemplation that in today's stressful and fast-moving society can be attained only in our advancing years. One can also spend those years continuing to fulfill the duties of citizenship, improving his/her communities, insisting on better government—e.g., preserving and increasing liberty—for one's children and grandchildren, hoping they live in a better world. In this sense, Dr. Emanuel's attitude reflects selfishness and lack of concern for the welfare of others around him or who may come after he's gone! Contrary to Dr. Emanuel's opinion about "faltering and declining" years past age 75, it is idleness, selfishness, and wasteful lives associated with diseases of the soul primarily that are the culprits for moral and intellectual decrepitude, rather than physical decline and reaching a certain capricious chronological age.

I'm not arguing here against individuals exercising their right to medical autonomy, especially those suffering from chronic disease and terminal illness. End-of-life decisions should be left to individual patients, their families, and their physicians. What I'm saying is that lives can be productive and fulfilling, worthy of living past age 75. I'm also cautioning bioethicists from propounding the utilitarian concept of "a duty to die" because a certain lethal age has been reached or chronic illness has become manifest. We cannot separate, nor does Dr. Emanuel distinguish, the process of aging from infirmity and illness. Certainly one leads to the other, and the duty to die at age 75 becomes the duty to die at any age, once a life is deemed not worth living. Death then is prescribed by the government planners and the doctors and bioethicists employed by the State, whether one reaches a certain age or is afflicted by illness.(1,4,8–11)

With the advances in medical care, life expectancy has been prolonged and the quality of life has been made immensely better. Yet, Dr. Emanuel argues: "Since 1960, however, increases in longevity have been achieved mainly by extending the lives of people over 60. Rather than saving more young people, we are stretching out old age." Furthermore, he asserts this is wrong because we are saving the life of older people with a myriad of medical problems and residual disabilities.(3) While I admit this is partly true, many of these people can be returned to normal or near normal life with proper medical and nursing care. Moreover, medical and Judeo-Christian ethics, not to mention the lessons of history, have taught us that we should treat with compassion the sick and the most vulnerable segments of our society. Societies that do not do this descend into cruelty and barbarism. Once again, we must recollect the lessons of fairly recent history. Dr. Leo Alexander, the leading psychiatrist and Chief U.S. Medical Consultant at the Nuremberg War Crimes Trials, in his classic 1949 *New England Journal of Medicine* article described how German physicians became willing accomplices with the Nazis in Ktenology, "the science of killing." This was done, we learn, for the good of German society and the improvement of "the health of the German nation." And in this light, Dr. Alexander asked the critical question: "If only those whose treatment is worthwhile in terms of prognosis are to be treated, what about the other ones? The doubtful patients are the ones whose recovery appears unlikely, but frequently if treated energetically, they surprise the best prognosticators." Once the rational allocation of scarce and finite resources enters the decision-making process in the doctor's role as physician, the next logical step is: "Is it worthwhile to do this or that for this type of patient," or for those who have reached a certain age?(5)

As much as Dr. Emanuel insists he is against euthanasia, his arguments lead inexorably to utilitarian ethics, the idea of lives deemed not worth living, and ultimately to euthanasia. Under the utilitarian ethics of the rational allocation of resources, productive lives whose only merit was considered benefit to society, Hitler issued his first order for active euthanasia in Germany on September 1, 1939. And yet it must be pointed out the road to euthanasia was paved before the Nazis came to power. German physicians in the social democracy of the Weimar Republic, as early as 1931, had openly held discussions about the sterilization of undesirables and euthanasia of the chronically mentally ill. So when the National Socialists (Nazis) came to power, "humanitarian" groups had already been set up, ostensibly for the promotion of health. These misguided groups with arguably "good intentions" had taken the first steps and were very useful serving as cover for the subsequent Nazi mass-killing program. And so it was that years before the onset of World War II and the Final Solution had been implemented, 275,000 non-Jewish citizens were put to death in Germany's "mercy-killing" program. From small beginnings and seemingly "well-intended" proposals, the values of the medical profession as well as an entire society were (and may be again) subverted by deliberately evil or misguided, well-intentioned men working in tandem with the State. Dr. Alexander was correct: "Corrosion begins in microscopic proportions."(5)

In conclusion, the resurgent bioethics movement—stressing "futility of care," conservation of resources, and "the duty to die," while rejecting Hippocrates' dictum of "First Do No Harm" and refusing to stand for what is in the best interest of the individual and the dignity of human life—is transmogrifying the time-honored, individual-based, patient-oriented medical ethics of Hippocrates into a collectivist, population-based ethic derived from the current thinking of the bioethics movement in the United Kingdom and most of Europe, as well as the United States. This resurgent ethic, presently propounded with subtle and dissimulating persuasion, is particularly well exemplified by Dr. Ezekiel Emanuel, today its foremost proponent. This bioethics "duty to die" movement is buttressed by a utilitarian, population-based ethic concerned primarily with the conservation of resources in the administration of socialized medicine by the State, rather than with the individual patient—and represents the first step down the slippery slope of determining who lives and who dies, rationing by death, and euthanasia. Doctors, patients, and the public at large must be made aware of the direction present society is headed.

References

1. Blaylock RL. National Health Insurance (Part II): Any Social Utility in the Elderly? *HaciendaPublishing.com*, September 26, 2009.

2. Callahan D. *Setting Limits: Medical Goals in an Aging Society*. New York: Simon and Schuster, 1988.

3. Emanuel EJ. Why I Hope to Die at 75: An argument that society and families—and you—will be better off if nature takes its course swiftly and promptly. *The Atlantic*, September 17, 2014.

4. Faria MA. Bioethics—The Life and Death Issue. *HaciendaPublishing.com*, October 24, 2012.

5. Faria MA. Euthanasia, Medical Science, and the Road to Genocide. *Medical Sentinel* 1998;3(3):79–83

6. Faria MA. Getting US in line for ObamaCare and medical rationing. *GOPUSA.com*, March 18, 2010.

7. Faria MA. ObamaCare: Another step toward corporate socialized medicine in the U.S. *Surg Neurol Int* 2012;3:71.

8. Faria MA. Slouching Towards a Duty to Die. *Medical Sentinel* 1999;4(6):208–210.

9. Faria MA. The road being paved to neuroethics: A path leading to bioethics or to neuroscience medical ethics? *Surg Neurol Int* 2014;5:146.

10. Smith WJ. *Culture of Death: The Assault on Medical Ethics in America*. San Francisco, CA, Encounter Books, 2000.

11. Wickham ED. *Repackaging Death as Life—The Third Path to Imposed Death*. Presented at the Annual Life Conference Raleigh, North Carolina, October 23, 2010. Citing Bioethicist Daniel Callahan, 1983, "On Feeding the Dying," *Hastings Center Report* 13(5):22.

12. Wickham ED. *Repackaging Death as Life—The Third Path to Imposed Death*. Presented at the Annual Life Conference Raleigh, North Carolina, October 23, 2010. Citing Pope Benedict XVI's 2010 address to the Pontifical Academy for Life.

MIGUEL FARIA is an associate editor-in-chief and a world affairs editor of *Surgical Neurology International*. He is a retired neurosurgeon and neuroscientist, editor and author, medical historian and ethicist, and public health critic.

Ezekiel J. Emanuel   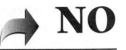 **NO**

Why I Hope to Die at 75: An Argument That Society and Families—and You—Will Be Better Off if Nature Takes Its Course Swiftly and Promptly

SEVENTY-FIVE.

That's how long I want to live: 75 years.

This preference drives my daughters crazy. It drives my brothers crazy. My loving friends think I am crazy. They think that I can't mean what I say; that I haven't thought clearly about this, because there is so much in the world to see and do. To convince me of my errors, they enumerate the myriad people I know who are over 75 and doing quite well. They are certain that as I get closer to 75, I will push the desired age back to 80, then 85, maybe even 90.

I am sure of my position. Doubtless, death is a loss. It deprives us of experiences and milestones, of time spent with our spouse and children. In short, it deprives us of all the things we value.

But here is a simple truth that many of us seem to resist: living too long is also a loss. It renders many of us, if not disabled, then faltering and declining, a state that may not be worse than death but is nonetheless deprived. It robs us of our creativity and ability to contribute to work, society, the world. It transforms how people experience us, relate to us, and, most important, remember us. We are no longer remembered as vibrant and engaged but as feeble, ineffectual, even pathetic.

By the time I reach 75, I will have lived a complete life. I will have loved and been loved. My children will be grown and in the midst of their own rich lives. I will have seen my grandchildren born and beginning their lives. I will have pursued my life's projects and made whatever contributions, important or not, I am going to make. And hopefully, I will not have too many mental and physical limitations. Dying at 75 will not be a tragedy. Indeed, I plan to have my memorial service before I die. And I don't want any crying or wailing, but a warm gathering filled with fun reminiscences, stories of my awkwardness, and celebrations of a good life. After I die, my survivors can have their own memorial service if they want—that is not my business.

Let me be clear about my wish. I'm neither asking for more time than is likely nor foreshortening my life. Today I am, as far as my physician and I know, very healthy, with no chronic illness. I just climbed Kilimanjaro with two of my nephews. So I am not talking about bargaining with God to live to 75 because I have a terminal illness. Nor am I talking about waking up one morning 18 years from now and ending my life through euthanasia or suicide. Since the 1990s, I have actively opposed legalizing euthanasia and physician-assisted suicide. People who want to die in one of these ways tend to suffer not from unremitting pain but from depression, hopelessness, and fear of losing their dignity and control. The people they leave behind inevitably feel they have somehow failed. The answer to these symptoms is not ending a life but getting help. I have long argued that we should focus on giving all terminally ill people a good, compassionate death—not euthanasia or assisted suicide for a tiny minority.

I am talking about how long I *want* to live and the kind and amount of health care I will consent to after 75. Americans seem to be obsessed with exercising, doing mental puzzles, consuming various juice and protein concoctions, sticking to strict diets, and popping vitamins and supplements, all in a valiant effort to cheat death and prolong life as long as possible. This has become so pervasive that it now defines a cultural type: what I call the American immortal.

I reject this aspiration. I think this manic desperation to endlessly extend life is misguided and potentially destructive. For many reasons, 75 is a pretty good age to aim to stop.

What are those reasons? Let's begin with demography. We are growing old, and our older years are not of high quality. Since the mid-19th century, Americans have been living longer. In 1900, the life expectancy of an average American at birth was approximately 47 years. By 1930, it was 59.7; by 1960, 69.7; by 1990, 75.4. Today, a newborn can expect to live about 79 years. (On average, women live longer than men. In the United States, the gap is about five years. According to the National Vital Statistics Report, life expectancy for American males born in 2011 is 76.3, and for females it is 81.1.)

In the early part of the 20th century, life expectancy increased as vaccines, antibiotics, and better medical care saved more children from premature death and effectively treated infections. Once cured, people who had been sick largely returned to their normal, healthy lives without residual disabilities. Since 1960, however, increases in longevity have been achieved mainly by extending the lives of people over 60. Rather than saving more young people, we are stretching out old age.

The American immortal desperately wants to believe in the "compression of morbidity." Developed in 1980 by James F. Fries, now a professor emeritus of medicine at Stanford, this theory postulates that as we extend our life spans into the 80s and 90s, we will be living healthier lives—more time before we have disabilities, and fewer disabilities overall. The claim is that with longer life, an ever smaller proportion of our lives will be spent in a state of decline.

Compression of morbidity is a quintessentially American idea. It tells us exactly what we want to believe: that we will live longer lives and then abruptly die with hardly any aches, pains, or physical deterioration—the morbidity traditionally associated with growing old. It promises a kind of fountain of youth until the ever-receding time of death. It is this dream—or fantasy—that drives the American immortal and has fueled interest and investment in regenerative medicine and replacement organs.

But as life has gotten longer, has it gotten healthier? Is 70 the new 50?

NOT QUITE. It is true that compared with their counterparts 50 years ago, seniors today are less disabled and more mobile. But over recent decades, increases in longevity seem to have been accompanied by increases in disability—not decreases. For instance, using data from the National Health Interview Survey, Eileen Crimmins, a researcher at the University of Southern California, and a colleague assessed physical functioning in adults, analyzing whether people could walk a quarter of a mile; climb 10 stairs; stand or sit for two hours; and stand up, bend, or kneel without using special equipment. The results show that as people age, there is a progressive erosion of physical functioning. More important, Crimmins found that between 1998 and 2006, the loss of functional mobility in the elderly increased. In 1998, about 28 percent of American men 80 and older had a functional limitation; by 2006, that figure was nearly 42 percent. And for women the result was even worse: more than half of women 80 and older had a functional limitation. Crimmins's conclusion: There was an "increase in the life expectancy with disease and a decrease in the years without disease. The same is true for functioning loss, an increase in expected years unable to function."

This was confirmed by a recent worldwide assessment of "healthy life expectancy" conducted by the Harvard School of Public Health and the Institute for Health Metrics and Evaluation at the University of Washington. The researchers included not just physical but also mental disabilities such as depression and dementia. They found not a compression of morbidity but in fact an expansion—an "increase in the absolute number of years lost to disability as life expectancy rises."

How can this be? My father illustrates the situation well. About a decade ago, just shy of his 77th birthday, he began having pain in his abdomen. Like every good doctor, he kept denying that it was anything important. But after three weeks with no improvement, he was persuaded to see his physician. He had in fact had a heart attack, which led to a cardiac catheterization and ultimately a bypass. Since then, he has not been the same. Once the prototype of a hyperactive Emanuel, suddenly his walking, his talking, his humor got slower. Today he can swim, read the newspaper, needle his kids on the phone, and still live with my mother in their own house. But everything seems sluggish. Although he didn't die from the heart attack, no one would say he is living a vibrant life. When he discussed it with me, my father said, "I have slowed down tremendously. That is a fact. I no longer make rounds at the hospital or teach." Despite this, he also said he was happy.

As Crimmins puts it, over the past 50 years, health care hasn't slowed the aging process so much as it has slowed the dying process. And, as my father demonstrates, the contemporary dying process has been elongated. Death usually results from the complications of chronic illness—heart disease, cancer, emphysema, stroke, Alzheimer's, diabetes.

Take the example of stroke. The good news is that we have made major strides in reducing mortality from strokes. Between 2000 and 2010, the number of deaths from stroke declined by more than 20 percent. The bad news is that many of the roughly 6.8 million Americans who have survived a stroke suffer from paralysis or an inability to speak. And many of the estimated 13 million more Americans who have survived a "silent" stroke suffer from more-subtle brain dysfunction such as aberrations in thought processes, mood regulation, and cognitive functioning. Worse, it is projected that over the next 15 years there will be a 50 percent increase in the number of Americans suffering from stroke-induced disabilities. Unfortunately, the same phenomenon is repeated with many other diseases.

So American immortals may live longer than their parents, but they are likely to be more incapacitated. Does that sound very desirable? Not to me.

The situation becomes of even greater concern when we confront the most dreadful of all possibilities: living with dementia and other acquired mental disabilities. Right now approximately 5 million Americans over 65 have Alzheimer's; one in three Americans 85 and older has Alzheimer's. And the prospect of that changing in the next few decades is not good. Numerous recent trials of drugs that were supposed to stall Alzheimer's—much less reverse or prevent it—have failed so miserably that researchers are rethinking the whole disease paradigm that informed much of the research over the past few decades. Instead of predicting a cure in the foreseeable future, many are warning of a tsunami of dementia—a nearly 300 percent increase in the number of older Americans with dementia by 2050.

Half of people 80 and older with functional limitations. A third of people 85 and older with Alzheimer's. That still leaves many, many elderly people who have escaped physical and mental disability. If we are among the lucky ones, then why stop at 75? Why not live as long as possible?

Even if we aren't demented, our mental functioning deteriorates as we grow older. Age-associated declines in mental-processing speed, working and long-term memory, and problem-solving are well established. Conversely, distractibility increases. We cannot focus and stay with a project as well as we could when we were young. As we move slower with age, we also think slower.

It is not just mental slowing. We literally lose our creativity. About a decade ago, I began working with a prominent health economist who was about to turn 80. Our collaboration was incredibly productive. We published numerous papers that influenced the evolving debates around health-care reform. My colleague is brilliant and continues to be a major contributor, and he celebrated his 90th birthday this year. But he is an outlier—a very rare individual.

American immortals operate on the assumption that they will be precisely such outliers. But the fact is that by 75, creativity, originality, and productivity are pretty much gone for the vast, vast majority of us. Einstein famously said, "A person who has not made his great contribution to science before the age of 30 will never do so." He was extreme in his assessment. And wrong. Dean Keith Simonton, at the University of California at Davis, a luminary among researchers on age and creativity, synthesized numerous studies to demonstrate a typical age-creativity curve: creativity rises rapidly as a career commences, peaks about 20 years into the career, at about age 40 or 45, and then enters a slow, age-related decline. There are some, but not huge, variations among disciplines. Currently, the average age at which Nobel Prize-winning physicists make their discovery—not get the prize—is 48. Theoretical chemists and physicists make their major contribution slightly earlier than empirical researchers do. Similarly, poets tend to peak earlier than novelists do. Simonton's own study of classical composers shows that the typical composer writes his first major work at age 26, peaks at about age 40 with both his best work and maximum output, and then declines, writing his last significant musical composition at 52. (All the composers studied were male.)

This age-creativity relationship is a statistical association, the product of averages; individuals vary from this trajectory. Indeed, everyone in a creative profession thinks they will be, like my collaborator, in the long tail of the curve. There are late bloomers. As my friends who enumerate them do, we hold on to them for hope. It is true, people can continue to be productive past 75—to write and publish, to draw, carve, and sculpt, to compose. But there is no getting around the data. By definition, few of us can be exceptions. Moreover, we need to ask how much of what "Old Thinkers," as Harvey C. Lehman called them in his 1953 *Age and Achievement*, produce is novel rather than reiterative and repetitive of previous ideas. The age-creativity curve—especially the decline—endures across cultures and throughout history, suggesting some deep underlying biological determinism probably related to brain plasticity.

We can only speculate about the biology. The connections between neurons are subject to an intense process of natural selection. The neural connections that are most heavily used are reinforced and retained, while those that are rarely, if ever, used atrophy and disappear over time. Although brain plasticity persists throughout life, we do not get totally rewired. As we age, we forge a very extensive network of connections established through a lifetime of experiences, thoughts, feelings, actions, and memories. We are subject to who we have been. It is difficult, if not impossible, to generate new, creative thoughts, because we don't develop a new set of neural connections that can supersede the existing network. It is much more difficult for older people to learn new languages. All of those mental puzzles are an effort to slow the erosion of the neural connections we have. Once you squeeze the creativity out of the neural networks established over your initial career, they are not likely to develop strong new brain connections to generate innovative ideas—except maybe in those Old Thinkers like my outlier colleague, who happen to be in the minority endowed with superior plasticity.

MAYBE MENTAL FUNCTIONS—processing, memory, problem-solving—slow at 75. Maybe creating something novel is very rare after that age. But isn't this a peculiar obsession? Isn't there more to life than being totally physically fit and continuing to add to one's creative legacy?

One university professor told me that as he has aged (he is 70) he has published less frequently, but he now contributes in other ways. He mentors students, helping them translate their passions into research projects and advising them on the balance of career and family. And people in other fields can do the same: mentor the next generation.

Mentorship is hugely important. It lets us transmit our collective memory and draw on the wisdom of elders. It is too often undervalued, dismissed as a way to occupy seniors who refuse to retire and who keep repeating the same stories. But it also illuminates a key issue with aging: the constricting of our ambitions and expectations.

We accommodate our physical and mental limitations. Our expectations shrink. Aware of our diminishing capacities, we choose ever more restricted activities and projects, to ensure we can fulfill them. Indeed, this constriction happens almost imperceptibly. Over time, and without our conscious choice, we transform our lives. We don't notice that we are aspiring to and doing less and less. And so we remain content, but the canvas is now tiny. The American immortal, once a vital figure in his or her profession and community, is happy to cultivate avocational interests, to take up bird watching, bicycle riding, pottery, and the like. And then, as walking becomes harder and the pain of arthritis limits the fingers' mobility, life comes to center around sitting in the den reading or listening to books on tape and doing crossword puzzles. And then . . .

Maybe this is too dismissive. There is more to life than youthful passions focused on career and creating. There is posterity: children and grandchildren and great-grandchildren.

But here, too, living as long as possible has drawbacks we often won't admit to ourselves. I will leave aside the very real and oppressive financial and caregiving burdens that many, if not most, adults in the so-called sandwich generation are now experiencing, caught between the care of children and parents. Our living too long places real emotional weights on our progeny.

Unless there has been terrible abuse, no child wants his or her parents to die. It is a huge loss at any age. It creates a tremendous, unfillable hole. But parents also cast a big shadow for most children. Whether estranged, disengaged, or deeply loving, they set expectations, render judgments, impose their opinions, interfere, and are generally a looming presence for even adult children. This can be wonderful. It can be annoying. It can be destructive. But it is inescapable as long as the parent is alive. Examples abound in life and literature: Lear, the quintessential Jewish mother, the Tiger Mom. And while children can never fully escape this weight even after a parent dies, there is much less pressure to conform to parental expectations and demands after they are gone.

Living parents also occupy the role of head of the family. They make it hard for grown children to become the patriarch or matriarch. When parents routinely live to 95, children must caretake into their own retirement. That doesn't leave them much time on their own—and it is all old age. When parents live to 75, children have had the joys of a rich relationship with their parents, but also have enough time for their own lives, out of their parents' shadows.

But there is something even more important than parental shadowing: memories. How do we want to be remembered by our children and grandchildren? We wish our children to remember us in our prime. Active, vigorous, engaged, animated, astute, enthusiastic, funny, warm, loving. Not stooped and sluggish, forgetful and repetitive, constantly asking "What did she say?" We want to be remembered as independent, not experienced as burdens.

At age 75 we reach that unique, albeit somewhat arbitrarily chosen, moment when we have lived a rich and complete life, and have hopefully imparted the right memories to our children. Living the American immortal's dream dramatically increases the chances that we will not get our wish—that memories of vitality will be crowded out by the agonies of decline. Yes, with effort our children will be able to recall that great family vacation, that funny scene at Thanksgiving, that embarrassing faux pas at a wedding. But the most-recent years—the years with progressing disabilities and the need to make caregiving arrangements—will inevitably become the predominant and salient memories. The old joys have to be actively conjured up.

Of course, our children won't admit it. They love us and fear the loss that will be created by our death. And a loss it will be. A huge loss. They don't want to confront our mortality, and they certainly don't want to wish for our death. But even if we manage not to become burdens to them, our shadowing them until their old age is also a loss. And leaving them—and our grandchildren—with memories framed not by our vivacity but by our frailty is the ultimate tragedy.

SEVENTY-FIVE. That is all I want to live. But if I am not going to engage in euthanasia or suicide, and I won't, is this all just idle chatter? Don't I lack the courage of my convictions?

No. My view does have important practical implications. One is personal and two involve policy.

Once I have lived to 75, my approach to my health care will completely change. I won't actively end my life. But I won't try to prolong it, either. Today, when the doctor recommends a test or treatment, especially one that will extend our lives, it becomes incumbent upon us to give a good reason why we don't want it. The momentum of medicine and family means we will almost invariably get it.

My attitude flips this default on its head. I take guidance from what Sir William Osler wrote in his classic turn-of-the-century medical textbook, *The Principles and Practice of Medicine:* "Pneumonia may well be called the friend of the aged. Taken off by it in an acute, short, not often painful illness, the old man escapes those 'cold gradations of decay' so distressing to himself and to his friends."

My Osler-inspired philosophy is this: At 75 and beyond, I will need a good reason to even visit the doctor and take any medical test or treatment, no matter how routine and painless. And that good reason is not "It will prolong your life." I will stop getting any regular preventive tests, screenings, or interventions. I will accept only palliative—not curative—treatments if I am suffering pain or other disability.

This means colonoscopies and other cancer-screening tests are out—and before 75. If I were diagnosed with cancer now, at 57, I would probably be treated, unless the prognosis was very poor. But 65 will be my last colonoscopy. No screening for prostate cancer at any age. (When a urologist gave me a PSA test even after I said I wasn't interested and called me with the results, I hung up before he could tell me. He ordered the test for himself, I told him, not for me.) After 75, if I develop cancer,

I will refuse treatment. Similarly, no cardiac stress test. No pacemaker and certainly no implantable defibrillator. No heart-valve replacement or bypass surgery. If I develop emphysema or some similar disease that involves frequent exacerbations that would, normally, land me in the hospital, I will accept treatment to ameliorate the discomfort caused by the feeling of suffocation, but will refuse to be hauled off.

What about simple stuff? Flu shots are out. Certainly if there were to be a flu pandemic, a younger person who has yet to live a complete life ought to get the vaccine or any antiviral drugs. A big challenge is antibiotics for pneumonia or skin and urinary infections. Antibiotics are cheap and largely effective in curing infections. It is really hard for us to say no. Indeed, even people who are sure they don't want life-extending treatments find it hard to refuse antibiotics. But, as Osler reminds us, unlike the decays associated with chronic conditions, death from these infections is quick and relatively painless. So, no to antibiotics.

Obviously, a do-not-resuscitate order and a complete advance directive indicating no ventilators, dialysis, surgery, antibiotics, or any other medication—nothing except palliative care even if I am conscious but not mentally competent—have been written and recorded. In short, no life-sustaining interventions. I will die when whatever comes first takes me.

As for the two policy implications, one relates to using life expectancy as a measure of the quality of health care. Japan has the third-highest life expectancy, at 84.4 years (behind Monaco and Macau), while the United States is a disappointing No. 42, at 79.5 years. But we should not care about catching up with—or measure ourselves against—Japan. Once a country has a life expectancy past 75 for both men and women, this measure should be ignored. (The one exception is increasing the life expectancy of some subgroups, such as black males, who have a life expectancy of just 72.1 years. That is dreadful, and should be a major focus of attention.) Instead, we should look much more carefully at children's health measures, where the U.S. lags, and shamefully: in preterm deliveries before 37 weeks (currently one in eight U.S. births), which are correlated with poor outcomes in vision, with cerebral palsy, and with various problems related to brain development; in infant mortality (the U.S. is at 6.17 infant deaths per 1,000 live births, while Japan is at 2.13 and Norway is at 2.48); and in adolescent mortality (where the U.S. has an appalling record—at the bottom among high-income countries).

A second policy implication relates to biomedical research. We need more research on Alzheimer's, the growing disabilities of old age, and chronic conditions—not on prolonging the dying process.

Many people, especially those sympathetic to the American immortal, will recoil and reject my view. They will think of every exception, as if these prove that the central theory is wrong. Like my friends, they will think me crazy, posturing—or worse. They might condemn me as being against the elderly.

Again, let me be clear: I am not saying that those who want to live as long as possible are unethical or wrong. I am certainly not scorning or dismissing people who want to live on despite their physical and mental limitations. I'm not even trying to convince anyone I'm right. Indeed, I often advise people in this age group on how to get the best medical care available in the United States for their ailments. That is their choice, and I want to support them.

And I am not advocating 75 as the official statistic of a complete, good life in order to save resources, ration health care, or address public-policy issues arising from the increases in life expectancy. What I am trying to do is delineate my views for a good life and make my friends and others think about how they want to live as they grow older. I want them to think of an alternative to succumbing to that slow constriction of activities and aspirations imperceptibly imposed by aging. Are we to embrace the "American immortal" or my "75 and no more" view?

I think the rejection of my view is literally natural. After all, evolution has inculcated in us a drive to live as long as possible. We are programmed to struggle to survive. Consequently, most people feel there is something vaguely wrong with saying 75 and no more. We are eternally optimistic Americans who chafe at limits, especially limits imposed on our own lives. We are sure we are exceptional.

I also think my view conjures up spiritual and existential reasons for people to scorn and reject it. Many of us have suppressed, actively or passively, thinking about God, heaven and hell, and whether we return to the worms. We are agnostics or atheists, or just don't think about whether there is a God and why she should care at all about mere mortals. We also avoid constantly thinking about the purpose of our lives and the mark we will leave. Is making money, chasing the dream, all worth it? Indeed, most of us have found a way to live our lives comfortably without acknowledging, much less answering, these big questions on a regular basis. We have gotten into a productive routine that helps us ignore them. And I don't purport to have the answers.

But 75 defines a clear point in time: for me, 2032. It removes the fuzziness of trying to live as long as possible. Its specificity forces us to think about the end of our lives and engage with the deepest existential questions and ponder what we want to leave our children and grandchildren, our community, our fellow Americans, the world. The deadline also forces each of us to ask whether our consumption is worth our contribution. As most of us learned in college during late-night bull sessions, these questions foster deep anxiety and discomfort. The specificity of 75 means we can no longer just continue to ignore them and maintain our easy, socially acceptable agnosticism. For me, 18 more years with which to wade through these questions is preferable to years of trying to hang on to every additional day and forget the psychic pain they bring up, while enduring the physical pain of an elongated dying process.

Seventy-five years is all I want to live. I want to celebrate my life while I am still in my prime. My daughters and dear friends will continue to try to convince me that I am wrong and can live a valuable life much longer. And I retain the right to change my mind and offer a vigorous and reasoned defense of living as long as possible. That, after all, would mean still being creative after 75.

EZEKIEL J. EMANUEL is a physician, bioethicist, and vice provost of the University of Pennsylvania.

EXPLORING THE ISSUE

Should the Health Care System Continuously Strive to Extend Life?

Critical Thinking and Reflection

1. Does Ezekiel has a valid point about hoping to die by age 75?
2. What are the common causes of pain and disability during the senior years?
3. Should health resources be used to extend life after age 75 at the expense of health care for younger individuals?

Is There Common Ground?

In October 1986 Dr. Thomas Starzl of Pittsburgh, Pennsylvania, transplanted a liver into a 76-year-old woman at a cost of over $200,000. Soon after that, Congress ordered organ transplantation to be covered under Medicare, which ensured that more older persons would receive this benefit. At the same time these events were taking place, a government campaign to contain medical costs was under way, with health care for the elderly targeted.

Not everyone agrees with this means of extend life at all costs. In a recent study, the majority of older people surveyed accept the withholding of life-prolonging medical care from the hopelessly ill but that few would deny treatment on the basis of age alone.

Currently, about 40 million Americans have no medical insurance and are at risk of being denied basic health care services. At the same time, the federal government pays most of the health care costs of the elderly. While it may not meet the needs of all older people, the amount of medical aid that goes to the elderly is greater than any other demographic group, and the elderly have the highest disposable income.

Most Americans have access to the best and most expensive medical care in the world. As these costs rise, some difficult decisions may have to be made regarding the allocation of these resources. As the population ages and more health care dollars are spent on care during the last years of life, medical services for the elderly or the dying may become a natural target for reduction in order to balance the health care budget.

Additional Resources

Carstensen, L. L. (2015). The new age of much older age. *Time*, *185*(6/7), 68–70.

Digangi, P. (2014). Health span vs. life span for baby boomers. *Rdh*, 74–98.

Easterbrook, G. (2014). What happens when we all live to 100? *Atlantic*, *314*(3), 60–72.

Faria, M. A. (2014). The road being paved to neuroethics: A path leading to bioethics or to neuroscience medical ethics? *Surgical Neurology International, 5,* 146.

Human sustainability: A manifesto for living the good, long life. (2014). *Vital Speeches of the Day, 80*(7), 240–242.

Internet References . . .

American Academy of Family Physicians-Geriatrics

www.aafp/org/geriatric/html

Coalition to Extend Life

www.coalitiontoextendlife.org/

American Association of Retired Persons

www.aarp.org

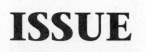

Selected, Edited, and with Issue Framing Material by:
Eileen L. Daniel, *SUNY College at Brockport*

ISSUE

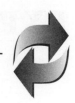

Does the Affordable Care Act Violate Religious Freedom by Requiring Employers' Health Insurance Plans to Cover Birth Control?

YES: **Wesley J. Smith**, from "What About Religious Freedom: The Other Consequences of Obamacare," *The Weekly Standard* (2012)

NO: **Elizabeth Sepper and Alisha Johnson**, from "Rhetoric Versus Reality: The Contraception Benefit and Religious Freedom," *religionandpolitics.org* (2013)

Learning Outcomes

After reading this issue, you will be able to:

- Discuss the provisions of the Affordable Care Act.
- Assess the impact of the Act on religious liberty.
- Discuss the importance of access to affordable birth control.

ISSUE SUMMARY

YES: Senior fellow in the Discovery Institute's Center on Human Exceptionalism Wesley J. Smith believes birth control cases are just the beginning for far more intrusive violations of religious liberty to come, for example, requiring businesses to provide free abortions to their employees.

NO: Law professor Elizabeth Sepper and research assistant and law student Alisha Johnson counter that the Affordable Care Act strikes a delicate balance by providing broad protection for religiously affiliated employers, while at the same time it protects the freedom of all Americans to live out their own religious and moral convictions.

T he Patient Protection and Affordable Care Act (PPACA), also known as "Obama Care" or the Affordable Care Act, is a federal statute signed into law by President Obama in the spring of 2010. The Act aims to both increase the rate of Americans with health insurance and lower the overall costs of health care. The PPACA includes several components including mandates, subsidies, and tax credits to help and encourage employers and individuals to increase the coverage rate. Additional reforms seek to improve health care outcomes and streamline the delivery of health care. The Congressional Budget Office predicts that the PPACA will reduce both future deficits and spending for Medicare.

Polls indicate support of health care reform in general, but became more negative in regards to specific plans during legislative debates. While the Act that was ultimately signed into law in 2010, it remains controversial, with opinions falling along party lines. Opinions are clearly divided by age and party affiliation, with a solid majority of seniors and Republicans opposing the bill while a solid majority of Democrats and those younger than 40 in favor. In a 2010 poll conducted by CNN, 62 percent of respondents said they thought the

PPACA would "increase the amount of money they personally spend on health care," 56 percent said the bill "gives the government too much involvement in health care," and only 19 percent said they thought they and their families would be better off with the legislation.

The Act mandates that insurance companies cover all applicants at the same rates regardless of preexisting conditions or gender. In addition, a controversial provision mandates that all insurance policies cover birth control without a co-pay as part of preventive care. The Act requires that all insurance policies cover *all* forms of basic preventive care without a co-pay, including well-woman, well-baby, and well-child visits, as well as other basic prevention care for men and women. This coverage is intended to save costs and promote public health. Basic preventive reproductive and sexual health care services, including contraception, are therefore also covered without a co-pay; as part of the mandate, all insurance plans must provide coverage without a co-pay for all methods of contraception approved by the Food and Drug Administration (FDA). Employees *earn* their salaries and their benefits, and many pay for all or a portion of their health care premiums out of their salaries. As such, none of this coverage is "free," but is rather covered by the policies they are earning or for which they are paying.

In January 2013, the Obama administration issued a rule that most employers, including religiously affiliated institutions such as Catholic universities and hospitals, must provide health care coverage that includes contraceptive services for all women employees and their dependents, at no cost to the employee. A narrow exemption exists for some religious employers, limited in most cases to houses of worship. The requirement only affects health care plans created after March 23, 2010. Plans in effect before that date do not have to meet the new rules.

While women's health advocates applauded the new rule, intense pressure from prominent religious organizations, including the U.S. Conference of Catholic Bishops, immediately followed. In response the Obama administration issued a compromise. Objecting nonprofit religious employers will not be required to pay for contraceptive services, instead shifting the cost to the employer's health insurance company. Those opposed to the compromise find the mandate a stark contradiction to the First Amendment to the U.S. Constitution: "Congress shall make no law respecting an establishment of religion." In addition, many Catholic organizations say that shifting the cost of birth control to the insurer does not resolve the moral objection, because they are self-insured, meaning the insurance provider and the organization are one and the same. Opponents also feel the government should have permission to come in and force an organization to violate its religious beliefs. While there is religious opposition, there are some strong proponents of the mandate who maintain that no one is denying anybody's religious rights. Religious activists hold that while protecting religious liberties is an important responsibility of government, blocking a plan designed to serve all people based on the values of one faith system becomes a violation of her rights. Those who favor the bill also contend that the bill is about women's right to comprehensive and preventive health care with equal access regardless of cost and it's just good health care.

In the spring of 2013, 18 for-profit companies have filed lawsuits to avoid complying with the birth control benefit in the Affordable Care Act (ACA) based on several claims. One is that providing insurance policies that cover birth control violates the religious freedom of the companies' owners. The owners of these companies share the belief that a woman is pregnant as soon as there is a fertilized egg (the medical definition of pregnancy is successful implantation of an embryo in the uterine wall) and that a fertilized egg has the same rights as a born person. They also claim that the ACA forces them to cover "abortifacients," with most pointing to emergency contraception methods such as Plan B to make their case. Emergency contraception, however, prevents ovulation, and therefore fertilization, and does not work after an egg has been fertilized. These lawsuits, now in various phases of litigation, are posing a critical challenge to the Affordable Care Act. Wesley J. Smith believes birth control cases are just the beginning for far more intrusive violation of religious liberty to come and is concerned over a slippery slope where businesses might be required to provide free abortions to their employees. Attorney and editor Aram A. Schvey argues that access to affordable contraception is a cornerstone of women's independence and equality and that the Affordable Care Act does not violate religious freedom.

YES ↵

Wesley J. Smith

What About Religious Freedom: The Other Consequences of Obamacare

Obamacare won't just ruin health care. It is also a cultural bulldozer. Before the law is even fully in effect, Health and Human Services bureaucrats have begun wielding their sweeping new powers to assault freedom of religion in the name of their preferred social order.

The promulgation of the free birth control rule indicates the regulatory road ahead. The government now requires every covered employer to provide health insurance that offers birth control and sterilization surgeries free of charge—even if such drugs and procedures violate the religious beliefs of the employer. Only houses of worship and monastic communities are exempt. Religious institutions have until August 1, 2013, to comply.

The lawsuits are flying. In August, the Catholic owners of Hercules Industries, a Colorado air conditioning and heating manufacturer, won a preliminary injunction against enforcement of the free birth control rule against their company (*Newland v. Sebelius*). The case hinges on the meaning of the Religious Freedom Restoration Act (RFRA), enacted in 1993 to remedy a Supreme Court decision allowing federal drug laws of "general applicability" to supersede Native American religious ceremonies in which peyote is used. Since many laws not aimed at stifling a specific faith can be construed to do so, the threat to religious liberty was clear. A Democratic Congress passed, and President Clinton signed, RFRA.

RFRA states that the government "shall not substantially burden a person's exercise of religion" unless it can demonstrate that the law "is in furtherance of a compelling governmental interest." The *Newland* trial judge found that forcing Hercules to pay for birth control—the company is self-insured—did indeed constitute a substantial burden on the owners' free exercise of their Catholic faith. Since no compelling government interest was found, the judge protected the company from the rule pending trial. The Department of Justice has appealed.

Alas, in a nearly identical case, *O'Brien v. U.S. Department of Health and Human Services*, U.S. District Judge Carol E. Jackson reached the opposite legal conclusion. Frank O'Brien is the Catholic owner of O'Brien Industrial Holdings, LLC, a mining company in St. Louis. Demonstrating the sincerity and depth of O'Brien's faith, a statue of the Sacred Heart of Jesus greets visitors in the company's lobby, and the mission statement on its website affirms the intent "to make our labor pleasing to the Lord."

Despite acknowledging "the sincerity of plaintiff's beliefs" and "the centrality of plaintiff's condemnation of contraception to their exercise of the Catholic religion," Jackson dismissed O'Brien's case on the basis that forcing his company to buy insurance covering contraception was not a "substantial burden" on his religious freedom.

Here is the philosophical core of the ruling:

> The challenged regulations do not demand that plaintiffs alter their behavior in a manner that will directly and inevitably prevent plaintiffs from acting in accordance with their religious beliefs. Frank O'Brien is not prevented from keeping the Sabbath, from providing a religious upbringing for his children, or from participating in a religious ritual such as communion. Instead plaintiffs remain free to exercise their religion, by not using contraceptives and by discouraging employees from using contraceptives.

Excuse me, but that's a lot like a judge telling a Jewish butcher that his freedom of religion is not violated by a regulation requiring him to carry nonkosher wares in his shop. After all, the government wouldn't be requiring *the butcher* to eat nonkosher meat.

More to the point, Jackson embraced the Department of Justice's reasoning. If this view prevails, it will shrivel the "free exercise of religion" guaranteed by the First Amendment into mere "freedom of worship," limiting RFRA's protections to personal morality, domestic activities, and religious rites behind closed doors. Worse, the court ruled that O'Brien is the aggressor in the matter, *that it is he who is seeking to violate the rights of his employees.*

"RFRA is a shield, not a sword," Judge Jackson wrote, "it is not a means to force one's religious practices upon others."

How does O'Brien's desire not to involve himself in any way with contraception force Catholicism upon his employees? He hasn't threatened anyone's job for not following Catholic moral teaching. He hasn't tried to prevent any employee from using birth control. He hasn't compelled employees to go to confession or get baptized. He merely chooses not to be complicit in what he considers sinful activities.

But that analysis presupposes that O'Brien's religious freedom extends to his actions as an employer. It doesn't, sayeth the Obama administration: "By definition, a secular employer does not engage in any 'exercise of religion,'" the Department of Justice argued in the *Newland* case. In other words, according to the Obama administration, the realm of commerce is a religion-free zone.

Some might dismiss these employers' concerns because birth control is hardly controversial outside of orthodox religious circles. But these birth control cases are stalking horses for far more intrusive violations of religious liberty to come, e.g., requiring businesses to provide free abortions to their employees. Consider the Democratic party's 2012 platform:

> The Democratic party strongly and unequivocally supports *Roe v. Wade* and a woman's right to make decisions regarding her pregnancy, including a safe and legal abortion, *regardless of ability to pay*. [Emphasis added.]

If Democrats regain the control of Congress and the presidency they enjoyed in 2009 and 2010, look for the Affordable Care Act to be amended consistent with their platform. After that, it won't take long for HHS to promulgate a free abortion rule along lines similar to the free birth control mandate.

And what could be done about it? According to Judge Jackson's thinking, ensuring free access to abortion would not prevent employers from "keeping the Sabbath." They would not be prohibited from "providing a religious upbringing" for their children or "participating in a religious ritual such as communion." Rather, they would be barred from "forcing their religious practices" on employees by leaving employees to pay for their own terminations. In time, why shouldn't in-vitro fertilization, assisted suicide, and sex change operations be added to the list?

If higher courts accept this radically antireligious view, the only corrective will be to amend RFRA to spell out that its protections extend to the actions of employers. In fact, why not take that step now and short circuit what could be years of litigation defending religious liberty in the public square?

WESLEY J. SMITH is a senior fellow in the Discovery Institute's Center on Human Exceptionalism and consults for the Patients Rights Council and the Center for Bioethics and Culture.

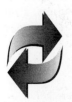

Elizabeth Sepper and Alisha Johnson

➡ **NO**

Rhetoric Versus Reality: The Contraception Benefit and Religious Freedom

The Catholic bishops argue that the Affordable Care Act's requirement that health plans include contraception violates religious freedom for both religious and secular corporations. Their counsel, Anthony Picarello, has indicated they will not rest until even a Taco Bell franchise owned by a Catholic is exempted from the law. For-profit businesses have joined religiously affiliated non-profits in filing suit to avoid providing their employees coverage for contraception. Most prominently, Hobby Lobby, a for-profit crafts store chain with 13,000 employees, has defied the insurance requirements in the name of free exercise of religion.

To hear these claims, one might think that religious freedom is under attack. But the rhetoric does not match reality. The contraception benefit rule strikes a delicate balance. It provides broad protections for religiously affiliated employers. At the same time, it protects the freedom of all Americans to live out their own religious and moral convictions.

Under the Affordable Care Act, health insurance plans must cover preventive services for women without cost-sharing. This includes all FDA-approved contraceptives from birth control pills to sterilization. This contraception benefit rule addresses pressing problems of gender inequality in healthcare and barriers to obtaining contraception. It recognizes that more than half of women between 18 and 34 cannot afford birth control. Due in large part to the price of contraception, almost half of all pregnancies in the U.S. are unintended. These pregnancies lead to poorer health outcomes for mother and child, and higher costs. Our workforce also suffers, as women abandon their professional and educational goals to have children before they are ready.

In acknowledgement of the varied religious teachings on contraception, the rule, especially with its latest proposed exemptions, provides generous accommodation for religious employers. Those that primarily employ and serve co-adherents, like churches, are entirely exempted from the rule and are not required to provide contraception coverage. Religiously affiliated non-profits, like hospitals, universities, and social service providers, also enjoy broad exemptions. They may exclude contraception from their plans and will not have to contract, arrange, pay, or refer for coverage. But their employees will still have access to contraception through a separate policy provided by the insurance company. Although one might think that the employer ultimately pays for this policy, contraception coverage saves at least as much as it costs and, therefore, is cost-free.

Secular, for-profit corporations, by contrast, must comply with the contraception benefit rule. A wide range of businesses, including food processors and craft stores, have objected to this requirement. They argue that the law forces them to either conduct business in a way that violates their religious beliefs or pay hefty penalties to the government.

But can for-profit companies exercise religion? Companies do not have beliefs or attend services. For-profits are not designed to bring believers together or carry out the mission of a church. They exist to maximize profit; their concern is the bottom line. Our legal system recognizes this difference, and regularly subjects for-profit businesses to regulation while exempting some religious non-profits.

Some say that the shareholders, or owners, of corporations nonetheless have religious beliefs that are burdened by the rule. But our laws do not require exemptions for every claim of religious belief. Instead, under the Religious Freedom Restoration Act, laws are only suspect if they produce substantial burdens on free exercise of religion. Where the law furthers a compelling government interest, as the contraception benefit does, even substantial burdens can be justified.

Here, any burden on the owners' free exercise is insubstantial. It is the corporation, not its owners, that must offer a plan with contraceptive coverage or pay higher taxes. As the Supreme Court has noted, the very purpose of incorporating a business is to create a distinct legal entity with legal rights and obligations separate from the individuals who own it.

Owners of for-profit corporations do not have to purchase or take contraception. They may speak against it and live their lives in accordance with their religious beliefs. Their involvement in the perceived wrongdoing of purchasing or using contraception is highly attenuated.

The employer's alleged burden becomes even weaker when we consider that health insurance, like wages, is compensation that employees earn. When a corporation purchases a health plan that its employees and their families use to buy contraception, it is no more paying for contraception than it does when employees use their wages to buy it. A basic principle of health economics is that there is a tradeoff between wages and insurance. As a recent study in Massachusetts showed, employees pay almost the full cost of their insurance benefits through lower wages.

A serious burden, however, would fall on employees if their employers were excused from compliance with the contraception benefit rule due to their religious objections. Secular, for-profit corporations could then successfully use religion as a shield against any number of laws that promote workers' health and safety. Some businesses might resist coverage of prenatal care for unmarried pregnant women or STD screening, based on the belief that non-marital sex is immoral. Others might challenge vaccinations or depression screening on religious grounds.

As the Supreme Court has observed, bowing to an employer's objection to an insurance scheme for employees ultimately "operates to impose the employer's religious faith on the employees." The contraception benefit rule instead safeguards the religious freedom of each individual. Women, men, and their families will be free to decide whether to use contraception based on their own conscientious beliefs.

ELIZABETH SEPPER is an associate professor of law at Washington University, St. Louis, MO.
ALISHA JOHNSON is a law student at Washington University.

EXPLORING THE ISSUE

Does the Affordable Care Act Violate Religious Freedom by Requiring Employers' Health Insurance Plans to Cover Birth Control?

Critical Thinking and Reflection

1. Why might affordable birth control be considered the cornerstone of women's independence and equality?
2. Does the Affordable Care Act violate religious freedom?
3. Describe how providing birth control through the Affordable Care Act might be perceived as a violation of religious liberty.

Is There Common Ground?

The government estimated that the Affordable Care Act legislation will lower the number of the uninsured by 32 million, leaving 23 million uninsured residents by 2019 after the bill's mandates have all taken effect. Among the people in this uninsured group will be approximately 8 million illegal immigrants, individuals eligible but not enrolled in Medicare, and mostly the young and single men and women not otherwise covered who choose to pay the annual penalty instead of purchasing insurance.

Early experience under the Act was that, as a result of the tax credit for small businesses, some businesses offered health insurance to their employees for the first time. On September 13, 2011, the Census Bureau released a report showing that the number of uninsured 19- to 25-year-olds (now eligible to stay on their parents' policies) had declined by 393,000, or 1.6 percent. A later report from the Government Accountability Office in 2012 found that of the 4 million small businesses that were offered the tax credit only 170,300 businesses claimed it. Due to the effect of the U.S. Supreme Court ruling, states can opt in or out of the expansion of Medicaid.

Also, a component ensuring children could remain included on their parents' plans until age 26 remains a popular, fairly noncontroversial part of the bill. The contraceptive coverage, however, remains contentious. The Affordable Care Act includes a contraceptive coverage mandate that, with the exception of churches and houses of worship, applies to all employers and educational institutions. These regulations made under the Act rely on the recommendations of the Institute of Medicine, which concluded that access to contraception is medically necessary "to ensure women's health and well-being."

The initial regulations proved controversial among Christian hospitals, Christian charities, Catholic universities, and other enterprises owned or controlled by religious organizations that oppose contraception on doctrinal grounds. To accommodate those concerns while still guaranteeing access to contraception, the regulations were adjusted to "allow religious organizations to opt out of the requirement to include birth control coverage in their employee insurance plans. In those instances, the insurers themselves will offer contraception coverage to enrollees directly, at no additional cost." Unfortunately, this didn't entirely satisfy religious organizations who still believe their beliefs are being compromised.

Additional Resources

Burlone, S., Edelman, A. B., Caughey, A. B., Trussell, J., Dantas, S., & Rodriguez, M. I. (2013). Extending contraceptive coverage under the Affordable Care Act saves public funds. *Contraception, 87*(2), 143–148.

Church & State. (2015). Priests for Life vows defiance after losing birth control case. *Church & State, 68*(1), 19.

Churchill, S. (2015). Whose religion matters in corporate RFRA claims after *Burwell v. Hobby Lobby stores, Inc.*, 134 S. CT. 2751 (2014)? *Harvard Journal of Law & Public Policy, 38*(1), 437–450.

Morse, E. A. (2013). Lifting the fog: Navigating penalties in the Affordable Care Act. *Creighton Law Review, 46*(2), 207–257.

Richey, W. (2014). Affordable Care Act and birth control: Can corporations assert religious rights? *Christian Science Monitor*, March 23.

Internet References . . .

Health Care

www.healthcare.gov

Health Care Law and You

www.healthcare.gov/law/

Planned Parenthood

www.plannedparenthood.org

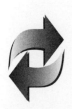

Unit 2

UNIT

Health and Society

*H*uman health is complex, influenced not only by the biology and chemistry of the body but also by societal structures, culture, and politics and economics. Interestingly, public policy and medical ethics have not always kept pace with rapidly growing technology and scientific advances, especially if we consider the impact of recent biomedical research. Some developments, for example, those associated with reproductive technologies such as in vitro fertilization and cloning, seem to present us with ethical problems and the need for public policy that are unprecedented. More often, however, the advance of biomedical research has simply added complexity to old problems and created a sense of urgency with regard to their solution. Euthanasia and health care rationing are not new problems, but our ability to save the lives of individuals who would have died in the past has certainly added new dimensions which include the economic impact of treatment.

Selected, Edited, and with Issue Framing Material by:
Eileen L. Daniel, *SUNY College at Brockport*

ISSUE

Is the Cost of Treating Cancer Unsustainable?

YES: Lee N. Newcomer, from "Myths and Realities in Cancer Care: Another Point of View," *Health Affairs* (2014)

NO: Dana P. Goldman and Tomas Philipson, from "Five Myths About Cancer Care in America," *Health Affairs* (2014)

Learning Outcomes

After reading this issue, you will be able to:

- Understand the complex nature of cancer.
- Discuss the reasons why the disease has been so difficult to eradicate.
- Discuss cancer treatments, costs, and their side effects.
- Discuss why the cost of cancer treatments has risen so sharply.

ISSUE SUMMARY

YES: UnitedHealthcare's vice president for oncology, physician Lee Newcomer believes that the cost to treat cancer will be unsustainable in the near future and will undermine the progress made in cancer treatment.

NO: Professor of public policy Dana Goldman and professor of health economics Tomas Philipson maintain that it's a myth that treatment costs are unsustainable and that restricting patients' treatments is socially wasteful and will likely discourage research innovations.

According to the National Cancer Institute, there will be 18.1 million cancer survivors in 2020, 30 percent more than in 2010, and the cost to treat their disease was $157 billion in 2010 dollars. This is expected to rise as the U.S. population ages and more and more cancers are treated. Cancer is a group of diseases characterized by uncontrolled cellular growth, invasion that intrudes upon and destroys nearby tissues, and may metastasize or spread to other locations in the body via blood or lymph. The malignant characteristics of cancers differentiate them from benign growths or tumors which do not invade or metastasize. Fortunately, most cancers can be treated with drug or chemotherapy, surgery, and/or radiation. The outcome of the disease is based on the type of cancer, for example, lung or breast cancer, and the extent of disease. While cancer affects people of all ages, and a few types of cancer are actually more common in children, most cancer risks increase with age. Cancer rates are increasing as more people live longer and lifestyles change, such as increased smoking occurring in the developing world.

Most cancers have an environmental link, with 90–95 percent of cases attributed to environmental factors and 5–10 percent due to heredity. Typical environmental factors that contribute to cancer deaths include diet and obesity (30–35 percent), smoking and tobacco use (25–30 percent), infectious agents (15–20 percent), and ionizing and nonionizing radiation (up to 10 percent). The remaining may be caused by stress, lack of exercise, and some environmental pollutants. Cancer prevention is related to those active measures that decrease the incidence of the disease. Since the vast majority of cancer risk factors are environmental or lifestyle-related, cancer is largely a preventable disease. Individuals who avoid tobacco, maintain a healthy weight, eat a diet rich in fruits and vegetables, exercise, use alcohol in moderation, take measures to prevent the transmission of sexually transmitted diseases, and avoid exposure to air pollution are likely to significantly reduce their risks of the disease.

Cancer's reputation is a deadly one. In reality about half of patients receiving treatment for invasive cancer will not survive the disease or the treatment. And the cost of these treatments continues to rise and the population in the developed world continues to age. The survival rate, however, can vary significantly by the type of cancer, ranging from basically all patients surviving to almost no patients surviving. Predicting either short-term or long-term survival is challenging and depends on a variety of factors. The most important factors are the type of cancer and the patient's age and overall health. Medically frail patients suffering simultaneously from other illnesses have lower survival rates than otherwise healthy patients. Despite strong social pressure to maintain an upbeat, optimistic attitude or act like a determined "fighter" to "win the battle," research has not shown that personality traits have a connection to survival.

In 1971 then President Richard Nixon signed the National Cancer Act of 1971. The goal of the Act was to find a cure for cancer by increased research to improve the understanding of cancer biology and the development of more effective treatments such as targeted drug therapies, all requiring extensive research costs. The Act is also viewed as the beginning of the war on cancer and the vow to end the disease for good. Despite significant progress in the treatment of certain forms of cancer, the disease in general remains a major cause of death 40 years after this effort began leading to a perceived lack of progress and to new legislation aimed at augmenting the original National Cancer Act of 1971. New research directions, in part based on the results of the Human Genome Project, hold promise for a better understanding of the heredity factors underlying cancer, and the development of new diagnostics, treatments, preventive measures, and early detection ability. The question raised by Lee Newcomer is whether or not the cost to treat cancer will be sustainable in the near future. He asks whether or not these costs will actually undermine the progress made in cancer treatment. Dana Goldman and Tomas Philipson disagree and maintain that restricting patients' treatments based on cost is socially wasteful and will likely discourage research innovations.

YES ↵

Lee N. Newcomer

Myths and Realities in Cancer Care: Another Point of View

Based on current trends, economists predict that in less than three years a family's typical health insurance premium and out-of-pocket costs will equal 50 percent of the average US-household income.[1] The same study notes that fourteen years later the cost of health care coverage will equal 100 percent of household income. As costs continue to rise, health care providers and researchers must discover methods to reduce the cost of care while advancing the progress that has been made against cancer. In this commentary I take the same five myths that Dana Goldman and Tomas Philipson have sought to debunk[2] and, in reverse order, offer additional considerations that policy makers should take into account.

Myth 5: Supportive Care Is Overused

Goldman and Philipson are correct: It is a myth that supportive care is overused. However, supportive care is undermined by misuse. A study of 1,849 lung and colon cancer patients treated at multiple centers demonstrated underuse of supportive care, with only 17 percent of patients with high-risk chemotherapy regimens receiving granulocyte colony stimulating factors (G-CSFs) to prevent low blood counts.[4] The same study also showed significant overuse. Overall, for these patients, 97 percent of the G-CSFs that were administered were not recommended by evidence-based guidelines.

Palliative care offers one pathway to the discussions of patient goals that are critical for assuring the appropriate use of supportive care. A trial of all lung cancer patients in an academic oncology clinic randomized patients to standard oncology care or to standard oncology care with a palliative care consultation. The palliative care group had better quality-of-life scores, lived 2.7 months longer, used less chemotherapy, and had less aggressive end-of-life care.[4] The palliative care patients established clear goals for their therapy at the beginning of treatment. Without that vital discussion, assigning value to supportive care is either flawed or impossible.

Myth 4: Cancer Treatment at the End of Life Is of Low Value

Goldman and Philipson argue that patients are willing to pay more for hopeful therapy—especially for cancer treatments. The papers supporting this assertion use hypothetical estimates of a patient's willingness to pay. Yet real-world data suggest that patients are less willing to reach into their own pockets for cancer therapies with limited values. An analysis of a large payer data set examined the compliance of oncology patients with specialty pharmacy support-including twenty-four-hour access to oncology pharmacists for side-effect management and compliance encouragement-compared to oncology patients with less comprehensive support from retail pharmacies. Each group paid a $50 copayment for drugs costing about $5,000 per prescription. The mean possession ratio, a measure of compliance based on prescription filled, was 66 percent in the specialty pharmacy group and 58 percent in the retail group.[5] Presumably, the additional support enjoyed by the first group eliminated medical reasons for noncompliance, explaining its 12 percent higher rate of compliance. The remaining 34 percent rate of noncompliance is, therefore, probably the effect of cost. If $50 keeps a patient from purchasing an oncology drug at the end of life, it is hard to believe the melanoma study[6] cited by Goldman and Philipson showing that patients are willing to pay $54,000 for a hypothetical treatment. The difference between these two studies is that one highlights patients' willingness to spend their own money, and the other shows patients' willingness to spend someone else's money.

Myth 3: Treatment Costs Are Unsustainable

As already stated, the US health care system cannot continue to spend at its current trend. The average household cannot be expected to spend its entire income on health care. Because of their high prices, new drugs are attracting the most attention, but cancer therapy involves more than just drugs. Chemotherapy drugs represent 24 percent of total care costs, inpatient and outpatient facility services account for 54 percent, and physician services constitute the remaining 22 percent of total costs for commercially insured cancer patients at UnitedHealthcare.[7] A recent study demonstrated that by finding savings elsewhere, five medical oncology groups could reduce the total cost of cancer care by 34 percent in a cohort of 810 patients, even as they increased cancer drug spending by 179 percent.[7]

Cancer patients are widely portrayed by patient advocates as having an extraordinary financial burden for their illness. Goldman and Philipson, for example, cite examples of patients paying 50 percent of the cost of newer cancer agents.[8] But that is not always the case. Such enormous out-of-pocket expenses are typically associated with low-cost insurance that offers fewer benefits. Patients in these frequently cited examples are almost always taking high-cost oral cancer medications or other specialty medications like them—such as treatment of multiple sclerosis, for example—under low-premium pharmacy plans. Higher-premium plans offer more reasonable patient cost sharing such as the $50 copayment example described earlier. Furthermore, most oncology drugs are given under the medical benefit of an insurance plan, in which drugs are usually subject to the same coverage benefits as the intensive care unit visit mentioned by Goldman and Philipson. Under the medical benefit, out-of-pocket expenses are almost always capped, and once the cap is met, claims are covered completely. Members who purchase insurance with good benefits will pay a higher premium, but their coverage will make their individual cost sustainable.

I agree with many of the points made by Goldman and Philipson debunking Myth 3 that treatment costs are unsustainable. First, treatments that have little or no health benefit should be challenged for reimbursement. Second, cancer patients should not bear more burden than other severely ill patients simply because they have cancer. Hospitals often use this tactic when they purchase oncology practices: On average, according to internal UnitedHealthcare data, medical oncologists in private practice are paid 22 percent more than Medicare rates for providing chemotherapy. However, hospitals that own oncology practices or employ medical oncologists can use their contracting leverage to earn reimbursement for the same service at an average of 146 percent more than Medicare, also according to internal UnitedHealthcare data. It is not right that cancer patients are bearing this heavier burden.

Myth 2: Detection, Not Treatment, Accounts for Most of the Survival Gains

As Goldman and Philipson argue, the number of adult cancers with significant improvement in survival due to treatment breakthroughs is impressive; breast cancer, colon cancer, multiple myeloma, and chronic myelogenous leukemia are good examples. Even more impressive is the progress in pediatric cancer largely as a result of rigorous enrollment of nearly every child into clinical trials. In stark contrast, only about 3 percent of adult cancer patients are enrolled in clinical trials. The US medical care system is missing a great opportunity to quickly learn about new therapies. Enrolling more adults in cancer clinical trials will accelerate the pace of new cancer drug approvals.

Unfortunately, the number of trials being offered is diminishing because of decreased funding and lengthy approval processes. But many organizations have begun to take new approaches. The lung cancer master protocol, the Multiple Myeloma Research Foundation, and the I-SPY adaptive breast cancer trials have shown what is possible when the principles of collaboration, speed, and access are given priority. These programs are proof that the US research system can improve its performance.

Myth 1: The War on Cancer Has Been a Failure

The term "failure" is relative and, I agree with Goldman and Philipson, misguided. When one compares the improvement in survival with heart disease versus cancer—the nation's two largest killers—it is clear that cardiac survival has improved far more than cancer survival.[9] More importantly, both diseases are causing less mortality. To use the metaphor of war, many battles have been won in cancer, but the theater of operations is much larger because there are scores of cancer types. Progress, even at a slower rate, is not failure.

Researchers, patient advocates, and policy makers should, nevertheless, push harder to improve the rate of progress. Finding ways to make cancer care affordable must be an important part of that effort.

Conclusion

A myth is a story, usually without basis in fact, that one tells to explain some practice or event. As Goldman and Philipson have shown, solid facts demonstrate that the cancer community is producing better treatments and outcomes. Yet these advances, though encouraging, can be better. The same cancer community that has achieved such important progress still faces another big challenge: to produce these treatments faster and for less cost.

References

1 Young RA, DeVoe JE. Who will have health insurance in the future? An updated projection. Am Fam Med. 2012;10(12) :156–62.

2 Goldman DP, Philipson T. Five myths about cancer care in America. Health Aff (Millwood). 2014;33(10):1801–04.

3 Temel JS, Greer JA, Muzikansky A, Gallagher ER, Admane S, Jackson VA, et al. Early palliative care for patients with metastatic non-smallcell lung cancer. N Engl J Med. 2010;363(8):733–42.

4 Potosky AL, Malin JL, Kim B, Chrischilles EA, Makgoeng SB, Howlander N, et al. Use of colonystimulating factors with chemotherapy: opportunities for cost savings and improved outcomes. J Natl Cancer Inst. 2011;103(12):979–82.

5 Tschida SJ, Aslam S, Lal LS, Khan TT, Shrank WH, Bhattarai GR, et al. Outcomes of a specialty pharmacy program for oral oncology medications. Am J Pharm Benefits. 2012;4(4):165–74.

6 Lakdawalla DN, Romley JA, Sanchez Y, Maclean JR, Penrod JR, Philipson T. How cancer patients value hope and the implications for cost-effectiveness assessments of high-cost cancer therapies. Health Aff (Millwood). 2012;31(4):676–82.

7 Newcomer LN, Gould B, Page RD, Donelan SA, Perkins M. Changing physician incentives for affordable, quality cancer care: results of an episode payment model. J Oncol Pract. 2014 Jul. [Epub ahead of print].

8 Fenn KM, Evans SB, McCorkle R, DiGiovanna MP, Pustzai L, Sanft T, et al. Impact of financial burden of cancer on survivors' quality of life. J Oncol Pract. 2014 May. [Epub ahead of print].

9 Murphy SL, Xu J, Kochanek KD. Deaths: final data for 2010. National Vital Statistics Reports. 2013;61(4):1–17.

LEE N. NEWCOMER is an oncology physician and vice president of UnitedHealthcare.

Dana P. Goldman and Tomas Philipson ➜ **NO**

Five Myths About Cancer Care in America

Much has been made recently about the cost of cancer treatment, often played out in editorials in cancer journals or on the opinion pages of major newspapers.[1,2] Some of the concern reflects beliefs that arose years ago when the illness was not as well understood. In this commentary we present some of the more common myths in America and the much more nuanced reality of today.

Myth 1: The War on Cancer Has Been a Failure

Perhaps no myth is so pervasive and yet so misguided than the one that declares that the war on cancer has been a failure.[3] Today cancer patients live longer, healthier, and happier lives than those in prior decades. Survival rates for all cancers increased by almost four years during the period 1988–2000,[4] creating twenty-three million additional life-years and generating $1.9 trillion in additional value to society, once the health gains are tallied.[5] Survival rates have continued to improve in recent years. A rough comparison of these health benefits with spending on research and development—both private and public—suggests a substantial social return on investment.

Furthermore, progress is being made in dealing with the extreme toxicity of chemotherapy and radiation regimens. Newer therapies often allow better quality of life. For example, long-term breast cancer survivors see an overall improvement in the two years following diagnosis,[6] and delays in chemotherapy have been shown to negatively affect patients' quality of life in some instances.[7] So, while cancer still remains a pernicious disease, there is hope that it can be managed as a chronic illness, with modest side effects.

Myth 2: Detection, Not Treatment, Accounts for Most of the Survival Gains

The public's attention often is drawn to the benefits of early detection. If a tumor is found earlier, it can be treated before metastasis and dramatically improve survival.

Celebrities such as Katie Couric and events such as National Breast Cancer Awareness Month encourage screening, and new technologies have made detection more accurate and less invasive.[8] The result has been that screening for some of the most common cancers has increased steadily.[9]

Thus, it comes as a surprise to many that treatment, not detection, has driven the majority of survival gains over the last few decades. During 1988–2000 almost 80 percent of the aforementioned survival gains were attributable to improvements in treatment, with the remaining 20 percent attributable to better detection. By some estimates, early detection accounted for only 3 percent of the increase in all cancer survival.[4]

Furthermore, better detection has no value if effective treatment is not available. A diagnosis of multiple myeloma in the 1960s meant a median survival rate of less than one year,[10] compared to more than six years today.[11] Patients diagnosed with metastatic colorectal cancer could expect an eight-month median overall survival rate two decades ago, compared to thirty months today.[12] These make detection far more valuable. Thus, perhaps ironically, the best way to encourage more screening may be to identify better, earlier-stage treatments.

Myth 3: Treatment Costs Are Unsustainable

As noted earlier, the rising cost of overall cancer treatment—especially the contribution of highprice therapies—has drawn a lot of attention recently.[1] However, this debate avoids a fundamental issue that is broader than cancer care—namely, that the focus should be on the price of health, not the price of health care services.

An analogy with highly active antiretroviral therapy (HAART) to treat HIV is instructive. HAART, which was introduced in the 1990s, dramatically increased longevity for HIV-positive patients,[13] although at a significant financial cost to these patients.[14] Prior to the introduction of HAART, an HIV-positive patient could not buy a longer life at any price. The advent of HAART thus lowered the price of a longer life, although the price of treatment rose.

Goldman, Dana P.; Philipson, Tomas. From *Health Affairs*, vol. 33, no. 10, pp. 1801–1804. Copyright © 2014 by Project HOPE. Used with permission.

Ultimately, more than 93 percent of the benefits of developing the new treatment accrued to patients in the form of longer lives, rather than to manufacturers.[15]

Similar declines were seen in the price of health for cancer patients, as measured by the price of each quality-adjusted life-year (QALY). Just over a decade ago, patients suffering from chronic myeloid leukemia faced grim prospects for survival. With the introduction of tyrosinekinase inhibitors (TKIs) in 2002, life expectancy increased by 5.5 QALYs, at a cost of $57,000 per QALY saved.[16] Given that the value of a life-year in the United States falls in the range of $200,000–$300,000,[17] TKIs seem like a good deal. Thus, society secured good value, even at brand-name prices. Next year, one of the first TKIs will lose its patent, and the price could fall dramatically as a generic enters the market.

Of course, not all cancer treatments have had such dramatic improvements on life expectancy, and some drugs may not be worth the cost. However, when the cost of innovative drugs is viewed over their branded and generic lifetime, it seems that a good deal is being obtained for the cancer dollars expended, with substantial increases in survival at reasonable cost.

So why the uproar about cancer in particular? Many health care services have higher costs than oncology drugs—the cost of a stay in the intensive care unit (ICU) is about $20,000[18]—or provide little value for the money, such as magnetic resonance images (MRIs) for sprained ankles.[19] Yet one does not see such handwringing about ICU costs or MRIs because payers and providers have deemed those costs to be acceptable and appropriately allocated.

In fact, the outrage arises because it is the patient, not the insurer, who has to pay. Among specialty drugs, cancer drugs have the highest out-of-pocket spending burden imposed on patients.[20] Patients may be asked to pay 50 percent of the cost of newer cancer drugs out of pocket,[21] compared with a much smaller fraction of the cost of an ICU stay. This financial burden can be "devastating," according to leading oncologists.[2]

Clearly reimbursement for treatments that have little or no health benefit should be challenged. However, blanket policies that shift the cost burden onto a subset of patients with rare or difficult-to-treat cancers—or that lower all prices together—would discourage future innovation and deprive patients of novel therapies.

Myth 4: Cancer Treatment at the End of Life Is of Low Value

This myth arises from a fundamental misconception about the value of care delivered to the terminally ill.[22] More specifically, policy makers assume that the value

of a life-year remains constant, regardless of a patient's circumstances. Evidence—and consumer behavior—would suggest otherwise.

An anecdote is helpful. In 2008 the *New York Times* published a story on Avastin, a drug that inhibits the growth of new blood vessels, emphasizing the dilemma posed by its modest improvement in survival rates and high cost. A few days later, reader Jana Jett Loeb wrote a Letter to the Editor, poignantly explaining the value of Avastin to treat her father's glioblastoma off-label: "The hope this drug provides our family is just as important to prolonging my father's life as the drug itself."[23]

As Loeb makes clear, there is additional value in treatments that give people hope, despite modest survival benefit. One study estimated that patients with metastatic disease value treatment at levels twenty-three times higher than the cost of the therapy.[24] It is also known that median survival does not capture the right-tail chance of success often associated with the hope of full remission. As a result, coverage decisions based solely on median survival will neglect the great social value for a minority who live long after the trial ends.

This does not mean that insurers should cover all hopeful therapies in the absence of clinical evidence. However, it does mean that the way in which trial results are evaluated should be reconsidered. A recent study demonstrated that 77 percent of cancer patients with melanoma preferred hopeful therapies, even with uncertainty as to where they would fall on the survival curve, and were willing to pay over $54,000 for a hypothetical treatment with the same median survival but a better chance at long-term survival.[25]

Second, behavior demonstrates that life is more precious when less of it remains. Ordinary people recognize this point, but current quality-of-life metrics do not. While patients often refuse to take their ordinary medications when copayments increase just a few dollars, cancer drugs are different. Patients are willing to pay substantial amounts out-of-pocket, indicating tremendous consumer value.[20,24]

Third, society as a whole places higher value on treatments for those who are sicker. Surveys show that people are reluctant to forgo care for the elderly, even if resources devoted to that care could more effectively improve population health if used elsewhere.[26] The same survey suggests that people would rather society choose interventions that make the lives of a few much better off than interventions that make the lives of many only slightly better off. In the United Kingdom, growing complaints about denials of effective but costly treatments for life-threatening diseases have prompted a compassionate care exception to the cost-effectiveness threshold for patients with poor prognoses.

Finally, recent evidence suggests that healthy people are willing to pay higher premiums for access to treatments analysts often deem of no value. By some estimates, adults in the United States are willing to pay on average an extra $2.60 in insurance premiums for every dollar of cancer drug coverage.[27] Bottom line, the QALY-based approach to decide necessity is inconsistent with patients' and society's value of cancer care.

Myth 5: Supportive Care is Overused

Many of the most effective cancer treatments have significant side effects, including pain, nausea, fatigue, anemia, and susceptibility to infection. Supportive care therapies, such as colony stimulating factors and anti-emetics, address one or more of these side effects. Nevertheless, many view them as a cost with little benefit.[22]

In reality, supportive care enables the administration of more aggressive chemotherapy regimens by avoiding or managing the debilitating effects of the toxicity. Aggressive regimens, facilitated by supportive care, slow disease progression and improve overall survival.

Indeed, some of the best clinical trials include supportive care as part of the protocols.[28] However, the incidence of neutropenia and the use of supportive care therapies are underreported in clinical trial publications, underrepresenting the value to society of supportive care.[29,30] As treatments evolve over time, supportive care regimens will remain an integral part of innovation and patient care.

Conclusion

Cancer has always been the "Emperor of All Maladies."[31] But any illness with such a majestic designation is bound to be surrounded by myths, many of which arose years ago when the illness was much less understood. The reality of cancer today is of a disease far more nuanced, reflecting systematic progress in treating the disease. New paradigms have led to the development of groundbreaking biologic therapies, with a lower risk of adverse events and side effects—but also with a commensurate cost.

It is now known that cancer is actually hundreds of diseases, many of which are rare. Scientific discovery will likely not allow for the development of "common cancer" treatments that will be effective in all cases. Rather, identified cancer subtypes that can be targeted by drugs are ultimately costly to develop, particularly when the treated population is small. Coverage policies that place undue burden on patients may discourage further innovation of treatments targeting rare genetic mutations and tumor subtypes. The call to artificially lower drug prices may address immediate affordability problems but—if done incorrectly—will come at too high a cost for future cancer patients' health.

Notes

1 Experts in Chronic Myeloid Leukemia. The price of drugs for chronic myeloid leukemia (CML) is a reflection of the unsustainable prices of cancer drugs: from the perspective of a large group of CML experts. Blood. 2013;121(22) :4439–42.

2 Bach PB, Saltz LB, Wittes RE. In cancer care, cost matters. New York Times. 2012 Oct 15;Sect. A:25.

3 Faguet GB. The war on cancer: an anatomy of failure, a blueprint for the future. New York (NY): Springer; 2005.

4 Sun E, Jena AB, Lakdawalla D, Reyes C, Philipson TJ, Goldman DP. The contributions of improved therapy and early detection to cancer survival gains, 1988–2000. Forum for Health Economics and Policy. 2010;13 (2): Article 1.

5 Lakdawalla DN, Sun EC, Jena AB, Reyes CM, Goldman DP, Philipson TJ . An economic evaluation of the war on cancer. J Health Econ. 2010;29(3): 333–46.

6 Hsu T, Ennis M, Hood N, Graham M, Goodwin PJ. Quality of life in longterm breast cancer survivors. J Clin Oncol. 2013;31(28):3540–8.

7 Calhoun EA, Chang C-H, Welshman EE, Cella D. The impact of chemotherapy delays on quality of life in patients with cancer. J Support Oncol. 2004;2(2):64–65.

8 Whitlock EP, Lin JS, Liles E, Beil TL, Fu R. Screening for colorectal cancer: a targeted, updated systematic review for the U.S. Preventive Services Task Force. Ann Intern Med. 2008;149(9) :638–58.

9 Clarke TC, Soler-Vila H, Fleming LE, Christ SL, Lee DJ, Arheart KL. Trends in adherence to recommended cancer screening: the US population and working cancer survivors. Front Oncol. 2012 ;2:190.

10 Kumar SK, Rajkumar SV, Dispenzieri A, Lacy MQ, Hayman SR, Buadi FK, et al. Improved survival in multiple myeloma and the impact of novel therapies. Blood. 2008;111(5):2516–20.

11 Kumar SK, Dispenzieri A, Lacy MQ, Gertz MA, Buadi FK, Pandey S, et al. Continued improvement in survival in multiple myeloma: changes in early mortality and outcomes in older patients. Leukemia. 2014;28(5):1122–8.

12 Kopetz S, Chang GJ, Overman MJ, Eng C, Sargent DJ, Larson DW, et al. Improved survival in metastatic colorectal cancer is associated with adoption of hepatic resection and improved chemotherapy. J Clin Oncol. 2009;27(22):3677–83.

13 Sansone GR, Frengley JD. Impact of HAART on causes of death of persons with late-stage AIDS. J Urban Health. 2000;77(2):166–75.

14 Goldman DP, Bhattacharya J, Leibowitz AA, Joyce GF, Shapiro MF, Bozzette SA. The impact of state policy on the costs of HIV infection. Med Care Res Rev. 2001;58(1):31–53; discussion 54–9.

15 Philipson TJ, Jena AB. Surplus appropriation from R&D and health care technology assessment procedures. Cambridge (MA): National Bureau of Economic Research; 2006 Feb. (NBER Working Paper No. 12016).

16 Reed SD, Anstrom KJ, Li Y, Schulman KA. Updated estimates of survival and cost effectiveness for imatinib versus interferon-alpha plus low-dose cytarabine for newly diagnosed chronic-phase chronic myeloid leukaemia. Pharmacoeconomics. 2008;26(5):435–46.

17 Aldy JE, Viscusi WK. Adjusting the value of a statistical life for age and cohort effects. Rev Econ Stat. 2008;90(3):573–81.

18 Dasta JF, McLaughlin TP, Mody SH, Piech CT. Daily cost of an intensive care unit day: the contribution of mechanical ventilation. Crit Care Med. 2005;33(6):1266–71.

19 American Academy of Orthopaedic Surgeons. Sprained ankle [Internet]. Rosemont (IL): AAOS; 2012 Sep [cited 2014 Aug 26] . Available from: http://orthoinfo.aaos.org/topic.cfm?topic=a00150

20 Goldman DP, Joyce GF, Lawless G, Crown WH, Willey V. Benefit design and specialty drug use. Health Aff (Millwood). 2006;25(5):1319–31.

21 Smith TJ, Hillner BE. Bending the cost curve in cancer care. N Engl J Med. 2011;364(21):2060–5.

22 Schnipper LE, Smith TJ, Raghavan D, Blayney DW, Ganz PA, Mulvey TM, et al. American Society of Clinical Oncology identifies five key opportunities to improve care and reduce costs: the top five list for oncology. J Clin Oncol. 2012; 30(1 4):1715–24.

23 Letter to the editor. The high price for a drug, and hope. New York Times. 2008 Jul 12.

24 Seabury SA, Goldman DP, Maclean JR, Penrod JR, Lakdawalla DN. Patients value metastatic cancer therapy more highly than is typically shown through traditional estimates. Health Aff (Millwood). 2012;31(4):691–9.

25 Lakdawalla DN, Romley JA. Sanchez Y, Maclean JR, Penrod JR, Philipson T. How cancer patients value hope and the implications for cost-effectiveness assessments of high-cost cancer therapies. Health Aff (Millwood). 2012;31(4):676–82 .

26 Nord E, Richardson J, Street A, Kuhse H, Singer P. Maximizing health benefits vs egalitarianism: an Australian survey of health issues. Soc Sci Med. 1995;41(10):1429–37.

27 Romley JA, Sanchez Y, Penrod JR, Goldman DP. Survey results show that adults are willing to pay higher insurance premiums for generous coverage of specialty drugs. Health Aff (Millwood). 2012;31(4):683–90.

28 National Cancer Institute. Prospective phase 2 trial of cabazitaxel in patients with temozolomide refractory glioblastoma multiforme [Internet]. Bethesda (MD): National Cancer Institute; 2013 [cited 2014 Aug 26]. Available from: http://www.cancer.gov/clinicaltrials/search/view?cdrid=750138&version=HealthProfessional&protocolsearchid=9363709

29 Dale DC, McCarter GC, Crawford J, Lyman GH. Myelotoxicity and dose intensity of chemotherapy: reporting practices from randomized clinical trials. J Natl Compr Canc Netw. 2003;1(3):440–54.

30 Duff JM, Leather H, Walden EO, LaPlant KD, George TJ Jr. Adequacy of published oncology randomized controlled trials to provide therapeutic details needed for clinical application. J Natl Cancer Inst. 2010;102(10):702–5.

31 Mukherjee S. The emperor of all maladies: a biography of cancer. New York (NY): Simon and Schuster; 2011.

Dana P. Goldman is the Leonard D. Schaeffer Chair and director of the University of Southern California Leonard D. Schaeffer Center for Health Policy and Economics and professor of public policy, pharmacy, and economics at the USC Sol Price School of Public Policy and USC School of Pharmacy.

Tomas Philipson is a professor of health economics at the University of Chicago with posts in the Harris School of Public Policy Studies, Department of Economics, and the University of Chicago Law School.

EXPLORING THE ISSUE

Is the Cost of Treating Cancer Unsustainable?

Critical Thinking and Reflection

1. Why are some cancers so difficult to successfully treat?
2. What are effective ways to reduce the risk of developing cancer?
3. Describe what factors are involved in predicting short- and long-term cancer survival rates.
4. Discuss why increasing costs may undermine the progress made in cancer treatment.

Is There Common Ground?

While many diseases have similar or worse outcomes, cancer is generally more feared than heart disease or diabetes. Cancer is regarded as a disease that must be "battled" and a "war" on cancer has been declared. Fighting or military-like descriptions are often used to address cancer's human effects, and they emphasize the need for the patient to take immediate, decisive actions himself or herself, rather than to delay, to ignore, or to rely on others caring for him or her. This fight is fought with a full array of treatments including surgery, radiation, and chemotherapy. Newer and more targeted therapies are coming, though the cost of this research continues to climb.

Why have costs escalated so much? On some levels, it's the price of success. Cancer deaths have been declining in the United States since the early 1990s. Two out of three people now live at least 5 years after a cancer diagnosis, up from one out of two in the 1970s, according to the American Society of Clinical Oncology doctors who treat the disease. Nine out of 10 women with early-stage breast cancer are alive 5 years after their diagnosis and are likely cured. Modern treatments have fewer side effects and allow patients to have a greater quality of life than chemotherapy did in the past. But they are far more toxic financially.

Of the nation's 10 most expensive medical conditions, cancer has the highest per-person price. The total cost of treating cancer in the United States rose from about $95.5 billion in 2000 to $124.6 billion in 2010, the National Cancer Institute estimated. The true tab is higher—the agency bases its estimates on average costs from 2001 to 2006, before many expensive treatments were available. Cancer costs are projected to reach $158 billion, in 2010 dollars, by the year 2020, because of a growing population of older people who are more likely to develop cancer. That's the societal cost. For individual patients, costs can vary widely even for the same drug. And cost can still be a concern long after initial treatment. Although all cancer patients want and deserve the best possible treatment, the reality of the cost of treatment is an unfortunate part of the disease.

Additional Resources

Langton, J. M., Blanch, B., Drew, A. K., Haas, M., Ingham, J. M., & Pearson, S. (2014). Retrospective studies of end-of-life resource utilization and costs in cancer care using health administrative data: A systematic review. *Palliative Medicine*, *28*(10), 1167–1196

Makary, M. (2014). The cost of chasing cancer. *Time*, *183*(9), 24.

New cancer drugs bring benefits but increase costs. (2015). *PharmacoEconomics & Outcomes News*, *722*(1), 20.

The elephant in the room: The high cost of progress in oncology. (2014). *PharmacoEconomics & Outcomes News*, *698*(1), 9.

Internet References . . .

American Cancer Society

www.cancer.org

American Medical Association (AMA)

www.ama-assn.org

Centers for Disease Control and Prevention

www.cdc.gov/

MedScape: The Online Resource for Better Patient Care

www.medscape.com

U.S. National Institutes of Health (NIH)

www.nih.gov

Selected, Edited, and with Issue Framing Material by:
Eileen L. Daniel, *SUNY College at Brockport*

ISSUE

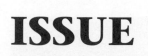

Should Marijuana Be Legalized for Medicinal Purposes?

YES: **Kevin Drum**, from "The Patriot's Guide to Legalization," *Mother Jones* (2009)

NO: **Abigail Sullivan Moore**, from "This Is Your Brain on Drugs," *New York Times* (2014)

Learning Outcomes
After reading this issue, you will be able to: • Discuss the physical risks associated with marijuana use.   • Assess the cognitive, social, behavioral, and legal issues associated with the use of marijuana.   • Assess the viability of legalization of marijuana.   • Discuss marijuana's medicinal purposes.

ISSUE SUMMARY

YES: Political columnist and blogger Kevin Drum contends that medical marijuana is now legal in more than a dozen states without any serious problems or increased usage.

NO: Journalist Abigail Sullivan Moore counters that young people who smoke marijuana frequently are more likely to have mental health problems and learning difficulties.

At one time there were no laws in the United States regulating the use or sale of drugs, including marijuana. Rather than by legislation, their use was regulated by religious teaching and social custom. As society grew more complex and more heterogeneous, the need for more formal regulation of drug sales, production, and use developed.

Attempts at regulating patent medications through legislation began in the early 1900s. In 1920 Congress, under pressure from temperance organizations, passed an amendment prohibiting the manufacture and sale of all alcoholic beverages. From 1920 until 1933, the demand for alcohol was met by organized crime, who either manufactured it illicitly or smuggled it into the United States. The government's inability to enforce the law, as well as increasing violence, finally led to the repeal of Prohibition in 1933.

Many years later, in the 1960s, drug usage again began to worry many Americans. Heroin abuse had become

epidemic in urban areas, and many middle-class young adults had begun to experiment with marijuana and LSD by the end of the decade. Cocaine also became popular first among the middle class and later among inner-city residents. More recently, crack houses, babies born with drug addictions, and drug-related crimes and shootings are the images of a new epidemic of drug abuse.

Many of those who believe illicit drugs are a major problem in America, however, are usually referring to hard drugs, such as cocaine and heroin. Soft drugs like marijuana, though not legal, are not often perceived as a major threat to the safety and well-being of citizens. Millions of Americans have tried marijuana and did not become addicted. The drug has also been used illegally by those suffering from AIDS, glaucoma, and cancer to alleviate their symptoms and to stimulate their appetites. Should marijuana be legalized as a medicine, or is it too addictive and dangerous? In California, Proposition 215 passed in the November 1996 ballot. A similar measure passed in

Arizona. These initiatives convinced voters to relax current laws against marijuana use for medical and humane reasons. Several other states followed and legalized marijuana for medicinal purposes.

Opponents of these recent measures argue that marijuana use has been steadily rising among teenagers and that this may lead to experimentation with hard drugs. There is concern that if marijuana is legal via a doctor's prescription, the drug will be more readily available. There is also concern that the health benefits of smoking marijuana are overrated. For instance, among glaucoma sufferers, in order to achieve benefits from the drug, patients would literally have to be stoned all the time. Unfortunately, the efficacy of marijuana is unclear because, as an illicit drug, studies to adequately test it have been thwarted by drug control agencies.

Although marijuana's effectiveness in treating the symptoms of disease is unclear, is it actually dangerous and addictive? Scientists contend that the drug can negatively affect cognition and motor function. It can also have an impact on short-term memory and can interfere with perception and learning. Physical health effects include lung damage. Until recently, scientists had little evidence that marijuana was actually addictive. Whereas heavy users did not seem to experience actual withdrawal symptoms, studies with laboratory animals given large doses of THC, the active ingredient in marijuana, suffered withdrawal symptoms similar to those of rodents withdrawing from opiates.

Not all researchers agree, however, that marijuana is dangerous and addictive. The absence of well-designed, long-term studies on the effects of marijuana use further complicates the issue, as does the current potency of the drug. Growers have become more skilled about developing strains of marijuana with high concentrations of THC. Today's varieties may be three to five times more potent than the pot used in the 1960s. Much of the data are unclear, but what is known is that young users of the drug are likely to have problems learning. In addition, some users are at risk for developing dependence.

In the following selections, Kevin Drum states that there are no proven studies to support the view that marijuana prohibition is justified. Abigail Sullivan Moore argues that marijuana causes many physical and psychological effects, and is particularly harmful to adolescents.

YES ↵

Kevin Drum

The Patriot's Guide to Legalization

Have you ever looked at our marijuana policy? I mean really looked at it?

When we think of the drug war, it's the heavy-duty narcotics like heroin and cocaine that get most of the attention. And why not? That's where the action is. It's not marijuana that is sustaining the Taliban in Afghanistan, after all. When Crips and Bloods descend into gun battles in the streets of Los Angeles, they're not usually fighting over pot. The junkie who breaks into your house and steals your Blu-ray player isn't doing it so he can score a couple of spliffs.

No, the marijuana trade is more genteel than that. At least, I used to think it was. Then, like a lot of people, I started reading about the open warfare that has erupted among the narcotraffickers in Mexico and is now spilling across the American border. Stories of drugs coming north and arsenals of guns going south. Thousands of people brutally murdered. Entire towns terrorized. And this was a war not just over cocaine and meth, but marijuana as well.

And I began to wonder: Maybe the war against pot is about to get a lot uglier. After all, in the 1920s, Prohibition gave us Al Capone and the St. Valentine's Day Massacre, and that was over plain old whiskey and rum. Are we about to start paying the same price for marijuana?

If so, it might eventually start to affect me, too. Indirectly, sure, but that's more than it ever has before. I've never smoked a joint in my life. I've only seen one once, and that was 30 years ago. I barely drink, I don't smoke, and I don't like coffee. When it comes to mood altering substances, I live the life of a monk. I never really cared much if marijuana was legal or not.

But if a war is breaking out over the stuff, I figured maybe I should start looking at the evidence on whether marijuana prohibition is worth it. Not the spin from the drug czar at one end or the hemp hucksters at the other. Just the facts, as best as I could figure them out. So I did. Here's what I found.

In 1972, the report of the National Commission on Marihuana and Drug Abuse urged that possession of marijuana for personal use be decriminalized. A small wave of states followed this recommendation, but most refused; in Washington, President Carter called for eliminating penalties for small-time possession, but Congress stonewalled. And that's the way things have stayed since the late '70s. Some states have decriminalized, most haven't, and possession is still a criminal offense under federal law. So how has that worked out?

I won't give away the ending just yet, but one thing to know is this: On virtually every subject related to cannabis (an inclusive term that refers to both the sativa and indica varieties of the marijuana plant, as well as hashish, bhang, and other derivatives), the evidence is ambiguous. Sometimes even mysterious. So let's start with the obvious question.

Does decriminalizing cannabis have any effect at all? It's remarkably hard to tell—in part because drug use is faddish. Cannabis use among teens in the United States, for example, went down sharply in the '80s, bounced back in the early '90s, and has declined moderately since. Nobody really knows why.

We do, however, have studies that compare rates of cannabis use in states that have decriminalized vs. states that haven't. And the somewhat surprising conclusion, in the words of Robert MacCoun, a professor of law and public policy at the University of California-Berkeley, is simple: "Most of the evidence suggests that decriminalization has no effect."

But decriminalization is not legalization. In places that have decriminalized, simple possession is still illegal; it's just treated as an administrative offense, like a traffic ticket. And production and distribution remain felonies. What would happen if cannabis use were fully legalized?

No country has ever done this, so we don't know. The closest example is the Netherlands, where possession and sale of small amounts of marijuana is de facto legal in the famous coffeehouses. MacCoun and a colleague, Peter Reuter of the University of Maryland, have studied the Dutch experience and concluded that while legalization at first had little effect, once the coffeehouses began advertising and promoting themselves more aggressively in the 1980s, cannabis use more than doubled in a decade.

Then again, cannabis use in Europe has gone up and down in waves, and some of the Dutch increase (as well as a later decrease, which followed a tightening of the coffeehouse laws in the mid-'90s) may have simply been part of those larger waves.

The most likely conclusion from the overall data is that if you fully legalized cannabis, use would almost certainly go up, but probably not enormously. MacCoun guesses that it might rise by half—say, from around 15 percent of the population to a little more than 20 percent. "It's not going to triple," he says. "Most people who want to use marijuana are already finding a way to use marijuana."

Still, there would be a cost. For one thing, a much higher increase isn't out of the question if companies like Philip Morris or R.J. Reynolds set their finest minds on the promotion of dope. And much of the increase would likely come among the heaviest users. "One person smoking eight joints a day is worth more to the industry than fifty people each smoking a joint a week," says Mark Kleiman, a drug policy expert at UCLA. "If the cannabis industry were to expand greatly, it couldn't do so by increasing the number of casual users. It would have to create and maintain more chronic zonkers." And that's a problem. Chronic use can lead to dependence and even long-term cognitive impairment. Heavy cannabis users are more likely to be in auto accidents. There have been scattered reports of respiratory and fetal development problems. Still, sensible regulation can limit the commercialization of pot, and compared to other illicit drugs (and alcohol), its health effects are fairly mild. Even a 50 percent increase in cannabis use might be a net benefit if it led to lower rates of use of other drugs.

So would people just smoke more and drink less? Maybe. The generic term for this effect in the economics literature is "substitute goods," and it simply means that some things replace other things. If the total demand for transportation is generally steady, an increase in sales of SUVs will lead to a decrease in the sales of sedans. Likewise, if the total demand for intoxicants is steady, an increase in the use of one drug should lead to a decrease in others.

Several years ago, John DiNardo, an economist now at the University of Michigan, found a clever way to test this via a natural experiment. Back in the 1980s, the Reagan administration pushed states to raise the drinking age to 21. Some states did this early in the decade, some later, and this gave DiNardo the idea of comparing data from the various states to see if the Reagan policy worked.

He found that raising the drinking age did lead to lower alcohol consumption; the effect was modest but real. But then DiNardo hit on another analysis—comparing cannabis use in states that raised the drinking age early with those that did it later. And he found that indeed, there seemed to be a substitution effect. On average, among high school seniors, a 4.5 percent decrease in drinking produced a 2.4 percent increase in getting high.

But what we really want to know is whether the effect works in the other direction: Would increased marijuana use lead to less drinking? "What goes up should go down," DiNardo told me cheerfully, but he admits that in the absence of empirical evidence this hypothesis depends on your faith in basic economic models.

Some other studies are less encouraging than DiNardo's, but even if the substitute goods effect is smaller than his research suggests—if, say, a 30 percent increase in cannabis use led to a 5 or 10 percent drop in drinking—it would still be a strong argument in favor of legalization. After all, excessive drinking causes nearly 80,000 deaths per year in the United States, compared to virtually none for pot. Trading alcohol consumption for cannabis rise might be a pretty attractive deal.

But what about the gateway effect? This has been a perennial bogeyman of the drug warriors. Kids who use pot, the TV ads tell us, will graduate to ecstasy, then coke, then meth, and then—who knows? Maybe even talk radio.

Is there anything to this? There are two plausible pathways for the gateway theory. The first is that drug use of any kind creates an affinity for increasingly intense narcotic experiences. The second is that when cannabis is illegal, the only place to get it is from dealers who also sell other stuff.

The evidence for the first pathway is mixed. Research in New Zealand, for example, suggests that regular cannabis use is correlated with higher rates of other illicit drug use, especially in teenagers. A Norwegian study comes to similar conclusions, but only for a small segment of "troubled" teenagers. Other research, however, suggests that these correlations aren't caused by gateway effects at all, but by the simple fact that kids who like drugs do drugs. All kinds of drugs.

The second pathway was deliberately targeted by the Dutch when they began their coffeehouse experiment in the '70s in part to sever the connection of cannabis with the illicit drug market. The evidence suggests that it worked: Even with cannabis freely available, Dutch cannabis use is currently about average among developed countries and use of other illicit drugs is about average, too. Easy access to marijuana, outside the dealer network for harder drugs, doesn't seem to have led to greater use of cocaine or heroin.

So, to recap: Decriminalization of simple possession appears to have little effect on cannabis consumption. Full legalization would likely increase use only moderately as long as heavy commercialization is prohibited, although the effect on chronic users might be more substantial. It would increase heroin and cocaine use only slightly if at all, and it might decrease alcohol consumption by a small amount. Which leads to the question:

Can we still afford prohibition? The consequences of legalization, after all, must be compared to the cost of the status quo. Unsurprisingly, this too is hard to quantify. The worst effects of the drug war, including property crime and gang warfare, are mostly associated with cocaine, heroin, and meth. Likewise, most drug-law enforcement is aimed at harder drugs, not cannabis; contrary to conventional wisdom, only about 44,000 people are currently serving prison time on cannabis charges—and most of those are there for dealing and distribution, not possession.

Still, the University of Maryland's Reuter points out that about 800,000 people are arrested for cannabis possession every year in the United States. And even though very few end up being sentenced to prison, a study of three counties in Maryland following a recent marijuana crackdown suggests that a third spend at least one pretrial night in jail and a sixth spend more than ten days. That takes a substantial human toll. Overall, Harvard economist Jeffrey Miron estimates the cost of cannabis prohibition in the United States at $13 billion annually and the lost tax revenue at nearly $7 billion.

So what are the odds of legalization? Slim. For starters, the United States, along with virtually every other country in the world, is a signatory to the 1961 Single Convention on Narcotic Drugs (and its 1988 successor), which flatly prohibits legalization of cannabis. The only way around this is to unilaterally withdraw from the treaties or to withdraw and then reenter with reservations. That's not going to happen.

At the federal level, there's virtually no appetite for legalizing cannabis either. Though public opinion has made steady strides, increasing from around 20 percent favoring marijuana legalization in the Reagan era to nearly 40 percent favoring it today, the only policy change in Washington has been Attorney General Eric Holder's announcement in March that the Obama administration planned to end raids on distributors of medical marijuana. (Applications for pot dispensaries promptly surged in Los Angeles County.)

The real action in cannabis legalization is at the state level. More than a dozen states now have effective medical marijuana laws, most notably California. Medical marijuana dispensaries are dotted all over the state, and it's common knowledge that the "medical" part is in many cases a thin fiction. Like the Dutch coffeehouses, California's dispensaries are now a de facto legal distribution network that severs the link between cannabis and other illicit drugs for a significant number of adults (albeit still only a fraction of total users). And the result? Nothing. "We've had this experiment for a decade and the sky hasn't fallen," says Paul Armentano, deputy director of the National Organization for the Reform of Marijuana Laws. California Assemblyman Tom Ammiano has even introduced a bill that would legalize, tax, and regulate marijuana; it has gained the endorsement of the head of the state's tax collection agency, which informally estimates it could collect $1.3 billion a year from cannabis sales. Still, the legislation hasn't found a single cosponsor, and isn't scheduled for so much as a hearing.

Which is too bad. Going into this assignment, I didn't care much personally about cannabis legalization. I just had a vague sense that if other people wanted to do it, why not let them? But the evidence suggests pretty clearly that we ought to significantly soften our laws on marijuana. Too many lives have been mined and too much money spent for a social benefit that, if not zero, certainly isn't very high.

And it may actually happen. If attitudes continue to soften; if the Obama administration turns down the volume on anti-pot propaganda; if medical dispensaries avoid heavy commercialization; if drug use remains stable; and if emergency rooms don't start filling up with drug-related traumas while all this is happening, California's experience could go a long way toward destigmatizing cannabis use. That's a lot of ifs.

Still, things are changing. Even GOP icon Arnold Schwarzenegger now says, "I think it's time for a debate." That doesn't mean he's in favor of legalizing pot fight this minute, but it might mean we're getting close to a tipping point. Ten years from now, as the flower power generation enters its 70s, you might finally be able to smoke a fully legal, taxed, and regulated joint.

Kevin Drum is a political columnist and blogger.

Abigail Sullivan Moore

➡ **NO**

This Is Your Brain on Drugs

The gray matter of the nucleus accumbens, the walnut-shaped pleasure center of the brain, was glowing like a flame, showing a notable increase in density. "It could mean that there's some sort of drug learning taking place," speculated Jodi Gilman, at her computer screen at the Massachusetts General Hospital–Harvard Center for Addiction Medicine. Was the brain adapting to marijuana exposure, rewiring the reward system to demand the drug?

Dr. Gilman was reviewing a composite scan of the brains of 20 pot smokers, ages 18 to 25. What she and fellow researchers at Harvard and Northwestern University found within those scans surprised them. Even in the seven participants who smoked only once or twice a week, there was evidence of structural differences in two significant regions of the brain. The more the subjects smoked, the greater the differences.

Moderate marijuana use by healthy adults seems to pose little risk, and there are potential medical benefits, including easing nausea and pain. But it has long been known that, with the brain developing into the mid-20s, young people who smoke early and often are more likely to have learning and mental health problems. Now researchers suggest existing studies are no longer sufficient. Much of what's known is based on studies conducted years ago with much less powerful pot.

Marijuana samples seized by the federal Drug Enforcement Agency show the concentration of THC, the drug's psychoactive compound, rising from a mean of 3.75 percent in 1995 to 13 percent in 2013. Potency seesaws depending on the strain and form. Fresh Baked, which sells recreational marijuana in Boulder, Colo., offers "Green Crack," with a THC content of about 21 percent, and "Phnom Penh," with about 8 percent. The level in a concentrate called "Bubble Hash" is about 70 percent; cartridges for vaporizers, much like e-cigarettes, range from 15 to 30 percent THC.

High-THC marijuana is associated with paranoia and psychosis, according to a June article in *The New England Journal of Medicine*. "We have seen very, very significant increases in emergency room admissions associated with marijuana use that can't be accounted for solely on the basis of changes in prevalence rates," said Nora D. Volkow, director of the National Institute on Drug Abuse and a co-author of the THC study. "It can only be explained by the fact that current marijuana has higher potency associated with much greater risk for adverse effects." Emergency room visits related to marijuana have nearly doubled, from 66,000 in 2004 to 129,000 in 2011, according to the Substance Abuse and Mental Health Services Administration.

Higher potency may also accelerate addiction. "You don't have to work so hard to get high," said Alan J. Budney, a researcher and professor at Dartmouth's medical school. "As you make it easier to get high, it makes a person more vulnerable to addiction." Among adults, the rate is one of 11; for teenagers, one of six.

Concerns over increasing potency, and rising usage among the young, is giving new urgency to research.

For the Harvard-Northwestern study, published in the April issue of *The Journal of Neuroscience*, the team scanned the brains of 40 young adults, most from Boston-area colleges. Half were nonusers; half reported smoking for one to six years and showed no signs of dependence. Besides the seven light smokers, nine used three to five days a week and four used, on average, daily. All smokers showed abnormalities in the shape, density and volume of the nucleus accumbens, which "is at the core of motivation, the core of pleasure and pain, and every decision that you make," explained Dr. Hans Breiter, a co-author of the study and professor of psychiatry and behavioral sciences at Northwestern's medical school.

Similar changes affected the amygdala, which is fundamental in processing emotions, memories and fear responses.

What is already known is that in casual users, THC can disrupt focus, working memory, decision making and motivation for about 24 hours. "The fact that we can see these structural effects in the brain could indicate that the effects of THC are longer lasting than we previously thought," said Dr. Gilman, an instructor in psychology at Harvard's medical school.

The study was preliminary and small, and attempts to replicate it are underway. Meanwhile, Dr. Gilman is trying to figure out how the findings relate to brain function and behavior.

One day in September, she was assessing Emma, a student who said her smoking—almost every day—didn't interfere with school, work or other obligations. For $100 to go toward study-abroad plans, Emma politely plowed through nearly three hours of tests on cognitive functions that are or might be affected by THC, like the ability to delay gratification (would it be better to have $30 tonight or $45 in 15 days?) and motivation (a choice between computer games, the harder one offering a bigger payoff). For memory, Emma listened to lists of words, repeating back those she recalled. Next came risk. Would she bungee jump? Eat high-cholesterol food? ("These kids tend to be risk takers, particularly with their own health and safety," Dr. Gilman said.)

A final test: Did Emma crave a joint? Her response: somewhat.

Dr. Gilman is concerned about pot's impact on the college population. "This is when they are making some major life decisions," she said, "choosing a major, making long-lasting friendships."

Dr. Volkow noted another problem: Partying on a Saturday night may hinder studying for a test or writing a paper due on Monday. "Maybe you won't have the motivation to study, because there's no reward, no incentive," she said.

Evidence of long-term effects is also building. A study released in 2012 showed that teenagers who were found to be dependent on pot before age 18 and who continued using it into adulthood lost an average of eight I.Q. points by age 38. And last year at Northwestern, Dr. Breiter and colleagues also saw changes in the nucleus accumbens among adults in their early 20s who had smoked daily for three years but had stopped for at least two years.

They had impaired working memories as well. "Working memory is key for learning," Dr. Breiter said. "If I were to design a substance that is bad for college students, it would be marijuana."

ABIGAIL SULLIVAN MOORE is a freelance journalist.

EXPLORING THE ISSUE

Should Marijuana Be Legalized for Medicinal Purposes?

Critical Thinking and Reflection

1. What are the pros and cons of legalization of marijuana for medicinal purposes?
2. Would legalization of marijuana offer a major benefit to individuals with cancer and other diseases?
3. Describe the impact legalization would have on marijuana usage.
4. Why is marijuana particularly harmful to adolescents?

Is There Common Ground?

Recent laws in several states legalizing marijuana for medicinal purposes make many people nervous. The majority of Americans are against making marijuana completely legal even if prescribed to individuals who have legitimate medicinal need for the drug. A compromise might be to decriminalize marijuana, making it neither strictly legal nor illegal. If decriminalized, there would be no penalty for personal or medical use or possession, although there would continue to be criminal penalties for sale and distribution to minors. Marijuana has been decriminalized in a few states, but it is illegal in most of the country.

While decriminalization appeals to many, in early 1992 the Drug Enforcement Administration published a document stating that the federal government was justified in its continued prohibition of marijuana for medicinal purposes. The report indicated that too many questions surrounded the effectiveness of medicinal marijuana. See "Medical Marijuana on Trial," *The New York Times* (March 29, 2005), and "The Right Not to Be in Pain: Using Marijuana for Pain Management," *The Nation* (February 3, 2003). The effectiveness of marijuana as therapy for cancer patients and AIDS patients continues to be debated, but the Center on Addiction and Substance Abuse of Columbia University maintains that recent research suggests that the drug is addictive and can wreck the lives of users, particularly teenagers. They argue that legalizing marijuana would undermine the impact of drug education and increase usage.

Additional Resources

Cerdá, M., Wall, M., Keyes, K. M., Galea, S., & Hasin, D. (2012). Medical marijuana laws in 50 states: Investigating the relationship between state legalization of medical marijuana and marijuana use, abuse and dependence. *Drug & Alcohol Dependence, 120*(1/3), 22–27.

Dickinson, T. (2015). The war on drugs is burning out. *Rolling Stone, 1226*, 33–37.

Friese, B., & Grube, J. W. (2013). Legalization of medical marijuana and marijuana use among youths. *Drugs: Education, Prevention & Policy, 20*(1), 33–39.

Monte, A. A., Zane, R. D., & Heard, K. J. (2015). The implications of marijuana legalization in Colorado. *Journal of the American Medical Association, 313*(3), 241–242.

Noonan, D. (2015). Marijuana's medical future. *Scientific American, 312*(2), 32–34.

Internet References . . .

Food and Drug Administration (FDA)

www.fda.gov

National Institute on Drug Abuse (NIDA)

www.nida.nih.gov

National Institutes on Health: National Institute on Drug Abuse

www.drugabuse.gov/nidahome.html

National Organization for the Reform of Marijuana Laws (NORML)

http://norml.org/

Web of Addictions

www.well.com/user/woa

Selected, Edited, and with Issue Framing Material by:
Eileen L. Daniel, *SUNY College at Brockport*

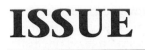

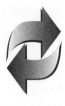

Is the Use of "Smart" Pills for Cognitive Enhancement Dangerous?

YES: Alan Schwarz, from "Drowned in a Stream of Prescriptions," *The New York Times* (2013)

NO: Joshua Gowin, from "How 'Smart Drugs' Enhance Us," *Psychology Today* (2009)

Learning Outcomes
After reading this issue, you will be able to:
• Discuss the legitimate uses for drugs such as Ritalin and Adderall.
• Understand the addictive qualities of these drugs.
• Understand how people without ADHD are able to acquire prescriptions for the drugs.
• Understand the consequences of abusing these drugs.
• Assess why illicit use of stimulant drugs has increased dramatically over the past 10 years.

ISSUE SUMMARY

YES: Pulitzer Prize-nominated reporter Alan Schwarz maintains that "smart pills" such as Adderall can significantly improve the lives of children and others with ADHD but that too many young adults who do not have the condition fake the symptoms and get prescriptions for the highly addictive and dangerous drugs.

NO: Psychologist Joshua Gowin argues that these drugs aren't much different from a cup of coffee and should be treated accordingly.

Medication therapy is a major part of treating attention deficit hyperactive disorder (ADHD), a common condition that affects children and adolescents and can continue into adulthood for some. Individuals with ADHD generally have difficulty paying attention, focusing, or concentrating. They seem to be unable to follow directions and are easily bored or frustrated with tasks. They also are likely to continuously move and tend to display impulsive behaviors. Overall, these behaviors are generally common in children without ADHD, but they occur more frequently than usual and are more severe in a child with ADHD.

For the past several decades, multiple types of stimulant drugs have been prescribed to treat the symptoms of ADHD. These medications enable individuals with ADHD to better focus their thoughts and overlook distractions and are effective for the majority of patients who take them.

Stimulant medications used to treat ADHD can have side effects, but these tend to happen early in treatment and are usually mild and short-lived, especially when monitored by a physician. The most common side effects include insomnia, weight loss and decreased appetite, and jitteriness. Occasionally, drugs to treat ADHD can cause more serious side effects such as an increased risk of cardiovascular problems. They may also exacerbate psychiatric conditions like depression, psychosis, or anxiety. ADHD medications are illegal to take without a prescription as they can produce serious side effects and are potentially addictive.

Despite the potential for addiction, prescription stimulant abuse has dramatically increased over the past decade. About 30 percent of stimulant drug use may be diverted to nonmedical usage. College students and young adults take them with the belief that these medications help with mental abilities including studying, memorizing, and test taking. Most people think of ADHD as a difficulty with controlling thought, hence the belief that ADHD medications help with thought control. Interestingly, evidence suggests that when people are given rote learning tasks such as memorizing items on a list, their performance *is* improved by ADHD stimulants. These effects are strongest when people learn the items on the list and have to remember them at least a day after learning. This effect does seem to come from the learning process, because the participants do not need to be on the medication during the test in order to see the effect.

Few research studies, however, have studied memory for complex kinds of information that demand genuine in-depth understanding of the material. So it is not possible to determine whether ADHD stimulants are simply assisting with learning the kinds of random items that typically appear on memory tests or whether they would also help with the types of complex knowledge important in high school and college classes.

Another area where ADHD stimulants seem to have impact is with *working memory*, the amount of information that people can hold in their mind at the same time. Many research investigations suggest that these medications have limited or no effect on working memory, but a few studies show otherwise. Improvement is most likely to be seen in individuals whose normal working memory capacity is the smallest. While the research is inconclusive on the overall advantages of taking stimulant drugs on cognitive enhancement, the risks are clear. Over time, continued use of ADHD medications can make users less effective intellectually due to poor mental functioning mostly caused by insomnia, addiction, or malnutrition. Other side effects that can impair performance include paranoia, aggression, and irritability that can accompany these drugs. Individuals taking the drugs prescribed by physicians are regularly monitored for these side effects as well as disturbances in heart rate, sleep, mood, and appetite.

In the YES and NO selections, Pulitzer Prize nominated reporter Alan Schwarz maintains that "smart pills" such as Adderall can significantly improve the lives of children and others with ADHD but that too many young adults who do not have the condition fake the symptoms and get prescriptions for the highly addictive and dangerous drugs. They take the drugs with the belief that their ability to study, learn, and take tests will be enhanced, though the research is mostly not supportive. Psychologist Joshua Gowin argues that these drugs aren't much different from a cup of coffee and should be treated accordingly.

YES ↵   Alan Schwarz

Drowned in a Stream of Prescriptions

Before his addiction, Richard Fee was a popular college class president and aspiring medical student. "You keep giving Adderall to my son, you're going to kill him," said Rick Fee, Richard's father, to one of his son's doctors.

Virginia Beach—Every morning on her way to work, Kathy Fee holds her breath as she drives past the squat brick building that houses Dominion Psychiatric Associates.

It was there that her son, Richard, visited a doctor and received prescriptions for Adderall, an amphetamine-based medication for attention deficit hyperactivity disorder. It was in the parking lot that she insisted to Richard that he did not have A.D.H.D., not as a child and not now as a 24-year-old college graduate, and that he was getting dangerously addicted to the medication. It was inside the building that her husband, Rick, implored Richard's doctor to stop prescribing him Adderall, warning, "You're going to kill him."

It was where, after becoming violently delusional and spending a week in a psychiatric hospital in 2011, Richard met with his doctor and received prescriptions for 90 more days of Adderall. He hanged himself in his bedroom closet two weeks after they expired.

The story of Richard Fee, an athletic, personable college class president and aspiring medical student, highlights widespread failings in the system through which five million Americans take medication for A.D.H.D., doctors and other experts said.

Medications like Adderall can markedly improve the lives of children and others with the disorder. But the tunnel-like focus the medicines provide has led growing numbers of teenagers and young adults to fake symptoms to obtain steady prescriptions for highly addictive medications that carry serious psychological dangers. These efforts are facilitated by a segment of doctors who skip established diagnostic procedures, renew prescriptions reflexively and spend too little time with patients to accurately monitor side effects.

Richard Fee's experience included it all. Conversations with friends and family members and a review of detailed medical records depict an intelligent and articulate young man lying to doctor after doctor, physicians issuing hasty diagnoses, and psychiatrists continuing to prescribe medication—even increasing dosages—despite evidence of his growing addiction and psychiatric breakdown.

Very few people who misuse stimulants devolve into psychotic or suicidal addicts. But even one of Richard's own physicians, Dr. Charles Parker, characterized his case as a virtual textbook for ways that A.D.H.D. practices can fail patients, particularly young adults. "We have a significant travesty being done in this country with how the diagnosis is being made and the meds are being administered," said Dr. Parker, a psychiatrist in Virginia Beach. "I think it's an abnegation of trust. The public needs to say this is totally unacceptable and walk out."

Young adults are by far the fastest-growing segment of people taking A.D.H.D. medications. Nearly 14 million monthly prescriptions for the condition were written for Americans ages 20 to 39 in 2011, two and a half times the 5.6 million just four years before, according to the data company I.M.S. Health. While this rise is generally attributed to the maturing of adolescents who have A.D.H.D. into young adults—combined with a greater recognition of adult A.D.H.D. in general—many experts caution that savvy college graduates, freed of parental oversight, can legally and easily obtain stimulant prescriptions from obliging doctors.

"Any step along the way, someone could have helped him—they were just handing out drugs," said Richard's father. Emphasizing that he had no intention of bringing legal action against any of the doctors involved, Mr. Fee said: "People have to know that kids are out there getting these drugs and getting addicted to them. And doctors are helping them do it."

•

". . . when he was in elementary school he fidgeted, daydreamed and got A's. he has been an A-B student until mid college when he became scattered and he wandered while reading. He never had to study. Presently without medication, his mind thinks most of the time, he procrastinated, he multitasks not finishing in a timely manner."

Dr. Waldo M. Ellison
Richard Fee initial evaluation
Feb. 5, 2010

•

Richard began acting strangely soon after moving back home in late 2009, his parents said. He stayed up for days at a time, went from gregarious to grumpy and back, and scrawled compulsively in notebooks. His father, while trying to add Richard to his health insurance policy, learned that he was taking Vyvanse for A.D.H.D.

Richard explained to him that he had been having trouble concentrating while studying for medical school entrance exams the previous year and that he had seen a doctor and received a diagnosis. His father reacted with surprise. Richard had never shown any A.D.H.D. symptoms his entire life, from nursery school through high school, when he was awarded a full academic scholarship to Greensboro College in North Carolina. Mr. Fee also expressed concerns about the safety of his son's taking daily amphetamines for a condition he might not have.

"The doctor wouldn't give me anything that's bad for me," Mr. Fee recalled his son saying that day. "I'm not buying it on the street corner."

Richard's first experience with A.D.H.D. pills, like so many others', had come in college. Friends said he was a typical undergraduate user—when he needed to finish a paper or cram for exams, one Adderall capsule would jolt him with focus and purpose for six to eight hours, repeat as necessary.

So many fellow students had prescriptions or stashes to share, friends of Richard recalled in interviews, that guessing where he got his was futile. He was popular enough on campus—he was sophomore class president and played first base on the baseball team—that they doubted he even had to pay the typical $5 or $10 per pill.

"He would just procrastinate, wait till the last minute and then take a pill to study for tests," said Ryan Sykes, a friend. "It got to the point where he'd say he couldn't get anything done if he didn't have the Adderall."

Various studies have estimated that 8 percent to 35 percent of college students take stimulant pills to enhance school performance. Few students realize that giving or accepting even one Adderall pill from a friend

with a prescription is a federal crime. Adderall and its stimulant siblings are classified by the Drug Enforcement Administration as Schedule II drugs, in the same category as cocaine, because of their highly addictive properties.

"It's incredibly nonchalant," Chris Hewitt, a friend of Richard, said of students' attitudes to the drug. "It's: 'Anyone have any Adderall? I want to study tonight,'" said Mr. Hewitt, now an elementary school teacher in Greensboro.

After graduating with honors in 2008 with a degree in biology, Richard planned to apply to medical schools and stayed in Greensboro to study for the entrance exams. He remembered how Adderall had helped him concentrate so well as an undergraduate, friends said, and he made an appointment at the nearby Triad Psychiatric and Counseling Center.

According to records obtained by Richard's parents after his death, a nurse practitioner at Triad detailed his unremarkable medical and psychiatric history before recording his complaints about "organization, memory, attention to detail." She characterized his speech as "clear," his thought process "goal directed" and his concentration "attentive."

Richard filled out an 18-question survey on which he rated various symptoms on a 0-to-3 scale. His total score of 29 led the nurse practitioner to make a diagnosis of "A.D.H.D., inattentive-type"—a type of A.D.H.D. without hyperactivity. She recommended Vyvanse, 30 milligrams a day, for three weeks.

Phone and fax requests to Triad officials for comment were not returned.

Some doctors worry that A.D.H.D. questionnaires, designed to assist and standardize the gathering of a patient's symptoms, are being used as a shortcut to diagnosis. C. Keith Conners, a longtime child psychologist who developed a popular scale similar to the one used with Richard, said in an interview that scales like his "have reinforced this tendency for quick and dirty practice."

Dr. Conners, an emeritus professor of psychiatry and behavioral sciences at Duke University Medical Center, emphasized that a detailed life history must be taken and other sources of information—such as a parent, teacher, or friend—must be pursued to learn the nuances of a patient's difficulties and to rule out other maladies before making a proper diagnosis of A.D.H.D. Other doctors interviewed said they would not prescribe medications on a patient's first visit, specifically to deter the faking of symptoms.

According to his parents, Richard had no psychiatric history, or even suspicion of problems, through college. None of his dozen high school and college acquaintances interviewed for this article said he had ever shown or mentioned behaviors related to A.D.H.D.—certainly not the "losing things" and "difficulty awaiting turn" he reported on the Triad questionnaire—suggesting that he probably faked or at least exaggerated his symptoms to get his diagnosis.

That is neither uncommon nor difficult, said David Berry, a professor and researcher at the University of Kentucky. He is a co-author of a 2010 study that compared two groups of college students—those with diagnoses of A.D.H.D. and others who were asked to fake symptoms—to see whether standard symptom questionnaires could tell them apart. They were indistinguishable.

"With college students," Dr. Berry said in an interview, "it's clear that it doesn't take much information for someone who wants to feign A.D.H.D. to do so."

Richard Fee filled his prescription for Vyvanse within hours at a local Rite Aid. He returned to see the nurse three weeks later and reported excellent concentration: "reading books—read 10!" her notes indicate. She increased his dose to 50 milligrams a day. Three weeks later, after Richard left a message for her asking for the dose to go up to 60, which is on the high end of normal adult doses, she wrote on his chart, "Okay rewrite."

Richard filled that prescription later that afternoon. It was his third month's worth of medication in 43 days.

•

"The patient is a 23-year-old Caucasian male who presents for refill of vyvanse—recently started on this while in NC b/c of lack of motivation/loss of drive. Has moved here and wants refill."

Dr. Robert M. Woodard
Notes on Richard Fee
Nov. 11, 2009

•

Richard scored too low on the MCAT in 2009 to qualify for a top medical school. Although he had started taking Vyvanse for its jolts of focus and purpose, their side effects began to take hold. His sleep patterns increasingly scrambled and his mood darkening, he moved back in with his parents in Virginia Beach and sought a local physician to renew his prescriptions.

A friend recommended a family physician, Dr. Robert M. Woodard. Dr. Woodard heard Richard describe how well Vyvanse was working for his A.D.H.D., made a diagnosis of "other malaise and fatigue" and renewed his prescription for one month. He suggested that Richard thereafter see a trained psychiatrist at Dominion Psychiatric Associates—only a five-minute walk from the Fees' house.

With eight psychiatrists and almost 20 therapists on staff, Dominion Psychiatric is one of the better-known

practices in Virginia Beach, residents said. One of its better-known doctors is Dr. Waldo M. Ellison, a practicing psychiatrist since 1974.

In interviews, some patients and parents of patients of Dr. Ellison's described him as very quick to identify A.D.H.D. and prescribe medication for it. Sandy Paxson of nearby Norfolk said she took her 15-year-old son to see Dr. Ellison for anxiety in 2008; within a few minutes, Mrs. Paxson recalled, Dr. Ellison said her son had A.D.H.D. and prescribed him Adderall.

"My son said: 'I love the way this makes me feel. It helps me focus for school, but it's not getting rid of my anxiety, and that's what I need,'" Mrs. Paxson recalled. "So we went back to Dr. Ellison and told him that it wasn't working properly, what else could he give us, and he basically told me that I was wrong. He basically told me that I was incorrect."

Dr. Ellison met with Richard in his office for the first time on Feb. 5, 2010. He took a medical history, heard Richard's complaints regarding concentration, noted how he was drumming his fingers and made a diagnosis of A.D.H.D. with "moderate symptoms or difficulty functioning." Dominion Psychiatric records of that visit do not mention the use of any A.D.H.D. symptom questionnaire to identify particular areas of difficulty or strategies for treatment.

As the 47-minute session ended, Dr. Ellison prescribed a common starting dose of Adderall: 30 milligrams daily for 21 days. Eight days later, while Richard still had 13 pills remaining, his prescription was renewed for 30 more days at 50 milligrams.

Through the remainder of 2010, in appointments with Dr. Ellison that usually lasted under five minutes, Richard returned for refills of Adderall. Records indicate that he received only what was consistently coded as "pharmacologic management"—the official term for quick appraisals of medication effects—and none of the more conventional talk-based therapy that experts generally consider an important component of A.D.H.D. treatment.

His Adderall prescriptions were always for the fast-acting variety, rather than the extended-release formula that is less prone to abuse.

•

"PATIENT DOING WELL WITH THE MEDICATION, IS CALM, FOCUSED AND ON TASK, AND WILL RETURN TO OFFICE IN 3 MONTHS"

Dr. Waldo M. Ellison
Notes on Richard Fee
Dec. 11, 2010

•

Regardless of what he might have told his doctor, Richard Fee was anything but well or calm during his first year back home, his father said.

Blowing through a month's worth of Adderall in a few weeks, Richard stayed up all night reading and scribbling in notebooks, occasionally climbing out of his bedroom window and on to the roof to converse with the moon and stars. When the pills ran out, he would sleep for 48 hours straight and not leave his room for 72. He got so hot during the day that he walked around the house with ice packs around his neck—and in frigid weather, he would cool off by jumping into the 52-degree backyard pool.

As Richard lost a series of jobs and tensions in the house ran higher—particularly when talk turned to his Adderall—Rick and Kathy Fee continued to research the side effects of A.D.H.D. medication. They learned that stimulants are exceptionally successful at mollifying the impulsivity and distractibility that characterize classic A.D.H.D., but that they can cause insomnia, increased blood pressure and elevated body temperature. Food and Drug Administration warnings on packaging also note "high potential for abuse," as well as psychiatric side effects such as aggression, hallucinations and paranoia.

A 2006 study in the journal *Drug and Alcohol Dependence* claimed that about 10 percent of adolescents and young adults who misused A.D.H.D. stimulants became addicted to them. Even proper, doctor-supervised use of the medications can trigger psychotic behavior or suicidal thoughts in about 1 in 400 patients, according to a 2006 study in *The American Journal of Psychiatry*. So while a vast majority of stimulant users will not experience psychosis—and a doctor may never encounter it in decades of careful practice—the sheer volume of prescriptions leads to thousands of cases every year, experts acknowledged.

When Mrs. Fee noticed Richard putting tape over his computer's camera, he told her that people were spying on him. (He put tape on his fingers, too, to avoid leaving fingerprints.) He cut himself out of family pictures, talked to the television and became increasingly violent when agitated.

In late December, Mr. Fee drove to Dominion Psychiatric and asked to see Dr. Ellison, who explained that federal privacy laws forbade any discussion of an adult patient, even with the patient's father. Mr. Fee said he had tried unsuccessfully to detail Richard's bizarre behavior, assuming that Richard had not shared such details with his doctor.

"I can't talk to you," Mr. Fee recalled Dr. Ellison telling him. "I did this one time with another family, sat down and talked with them, and I ended up getting sued. I can't talk with you unless your son comes with you."

Mr. Fee said he had turned to leave but distinctly recalls warning Dr. Ellison, "You keep giving Adderall to my son, you're going to kill him."

Dr. Ellison declined repeated requests for comment on Richard Fee's case. His office records, like those of other doctors involved, were obtained by Mr. Fee under Virginia and federal law, which allow the legal representative of a deceased patient to obtain medical records as if he were the patient himself.

As 2011 began, the Fees persuaded Richard to see a psychologist, Scott W. Sautter, whose records note Richard's delusions, paranoia and "severe and pervasive mental disorder." Dr. Sautter recommended that Adderall either be stopped or be paired with a sleep aid "if not medically contraindicated."

Mr. Fee did not trust his son to share this report with Dr. Ellison, so he drove back to Dominion Psychiatric and, he recalled, was told by a receptionist that he could leave the information with her. Mr. Fee said he had demanded to put it in Dr. Ellison's hands himself and threatened to break down his door in order to do so.

Mr. Fee said that Dr. Ellison had then come out, read the report and, appreciating the gravity of the situation, spoken with him about Richard for 45 minutes. They scheduled an appointment for the entire family.

•

"meeting with parents—concern with 'metaphoric' speaking that appears to be outside the realm of appropriated one to one conversation. Richard says he does it on purpose—to me some of it sounds like pre-psychotic thinking."

Dr. Waldo M. Ellison
Notes on Richard Fee
Feb. 23, 2011

•

Dr. Ellison stopped Richard Fee's prescription—he wrote "no Adderall for now" on his chart and the next day refused Richard's phone request for more. Instead he prescribed Abilify and Seroquel, antipsychotics for schizophrenia that do not provide the bursts of focus and purpose that stimulants do. Richard became enraged, his parents recalled. He tried to back up over his father in the Dominion Psychiatric parking lot and threatened to burn the house down. At home, he took a baseball bat from the garage, smashed flower pots and screamed, "You're taking my medicine!"

Richard disappeared for a few weeks. He returned to the house when he learned of his grandmother's death, the Fees said.

The morning after the funeral, Richard walked down Potters Road to what became a nine-minute visit with Dr. Ellison. He left with two prescriptions: one for Abilify, and another for 50 milligrams a day of Adderall.

According to Mr. Fee, Richard later told him that he had lied to Dr. Ellison—he told the doctor he was feeling great, life was back on track and he had found a job in Greensboro that he would lose without Adderall. Dr. Ellison's notes do not say why he agreed to start Adderall again.

Richard's delusions and mood swings only got worse, his parents said. They would lock their bedroom door when they went to sleep because of his unpredictable rages. "We were scared of our own son," Mr. Fee said. Richard would blow through his monthly prescriptions in 10 to 15 days and then go through hideous withdrawals. A friend said that he would occasionally get Richard some extra pills during the worst of it, but that "it wasn't enough because he would take four or five at a time."

One night during an argument, after Richard became particularly threatening and pushed him over a chair, Mr. Fee called the police. They arrested Richard for domestic violence. The episode persuaded Richard to see another local psychiatrist, Dr. Charles Parker.

Mrs. Fee said she attended Richard's initial consultation on June 3 with Dr. Parker's clinician, Renee Strelitz, and emphasized his abuse of Adderall. Richard "kept giving me dirty looks," Mrs. Fee recalled. She said she had later left a detailed message on Ms. Strelitz's voice mail, urging her and Dr. Parker not to prescribe stimulants under any circumstances when Richard came in the next day.

Dr. Parker met with Richard alone. The doctor noted depression, anxiety and suicidal ideas. He wrote "no meds" with a box around it—an indication, he explained later, that he was aware of the parents' concerns regarding A.D.H.D. stimulants.

Dr. Parker wrote three 30-day prescriptions: Clonidine (a sleep aid), Venlafaxine (an antidepressant) and Adderall, 60 milligrams a day.

In an interview last November, Dr. Parker said he did not recall the details of Richard's case but reviewed his notes and tried to recreate his mind-set during that appointment. He said he must have trusted Richard's assertions that medication was not an issue, and must have figured that his parents were just philosophically anti-medication. Dr. Parker recalled that he had been reassured by Richard's intelligent discussions of the ins and outs of stimulants and his desire to pursue medicine himself.

"He was smart and he was quick and he had A's and B's and wanted to go to medical school—and he had all the deportment of a guy that had the potential to do that," Dr. Parker said. "He didn't seem like he was a drug person at all, but rather a person that was misunderstood, really desirous of becoming a physician. He was very slick and smooth. He convinced me there was a benefit."

Mrs. Fee was outraged. Over the next several days, she recalled, she repeatedly spoke with Ms. Strelitz over the phone to detail Richard's continued abuse of the medication (she found nine pills gone after 48 hours) and hand-delivered Dr. Sautter's appraisal of his recent psychosis. Dr. Parker confirmed that he had received this information.

Richard next saw Dr. Parker on June 27. Mrs. Fee drove him to the clinic and waited in the parking lot. Soon afterward, Richard returned and asked to head to the pharmacy to fill a prescription. Dr. Parker had raised his Adderall to 80 milligrams a day.

Dr. Parker recalled that the appointment had been a 15-minute "med check" that left little time for careful assessment of any Adderall addiction. Once again, Dr. Parker said, he must have believed Richard's assertions that he needed additional medicine more than the family's pleas that it be stopped.

"He was pitching me very well—I was asking him very specific questions, and he was very good at telling me the answers in a very specific way," Dr. Parker recalled. He added later, "I do feel partially responsible for what happened to this kid."

•

"Paranoid and psychotic . . . thinking that the computer is spying on him. He has also been receiving messages from stars at night and he is unable to be talked to in a reasonable fashion . . . The patient denies any mental health problems . . . fairly high risk for suicide."

Dr. John Riedler
Admission note for Richard Fee
Virginia Beach Psychiatric Center
July 8, 2011

•

The 911 operator answered the call and heard a young man screaming on the other end. His parents would not give him his pills. With the man's language scattered and increasingly threatening, the police were sent to the home of Rick and Kathy Fee.

The Fees told officers that Richard was addicted to Adderall, and that after he had received his most recent prescription, they allowed him to fill it through his mother's insurance plan on the condition that they hold it and dispense it appropriately. Richard was now demanding his next day's pills early.

Richard denied his addiction and threats. So the police, noting that Richard was an adult, instructed the Fees to give him the bottle. They said they would comply only if he left the house for good. Officers escorted Richard off the property.

A few hours later Richard called his parents, threatening to stab himself in the head with a knife. The police found him and took him to the Virginia Beach Psychiatric Center.

Described as "paranoid and psychotic" by the admitting physician, Dr. John Riedler, Richard spent one week in the hospital denying that he had any psychiatric or addiction issues. He was placed on two medications: Seroquel and the antidepressant Wellbutrin, no stimulants. In his discharge report, Dr. Riedler noted that Richard had stabilized but remained severely depressed and dependent on both amphetamines and marijuana, which he would smoke in part to counter the buzz of Adderall and the depression from withdrawal.

(Marijuana is known to increase the risk for schizophrenia, psychosis and memory problems, but Richard had smoked pot in high school and college with no such effects, several friends recalled. If that was the case, "in all likelihood the stimulants were the primary issue here," said Dr. Wesley Boyd, a psychiatrist at Children's Hospital Boston and Cambridge Health Alliance who specializes in adolescent substance abuse.)

Unwelcome at home after his discharge from the psychiatric hospital, Richard stayed in cheap motels for a few weeks. His Adderall prescription from Dr. Parker expired on July 26, leaving him eligible for a renewal. He phoned the office of Dr. Ellison, who had not seen him in four months.

•

"moved out of the house—doesn't feel paranoid or delusional. Hasn't been on meds for a while—working with a friend wiring houses for 3 months—doesn't feel he needs the abilify or seroquel for sleep."

Dr. Waldo M. Ellison
Notes on Richard Fee
July 25, 2011

•

The 2:15 p.m. appointment went better than Richard could have hoped. He told Dr. Ellison that the pre-psychotic and metaphoric thinking back in March had receded, and that all that remained was his A.D.H.D. He said nothing of his visits to Dr. Parker, his recent prescriptions or his week in the psychiatric hospital.

At 2:21 p.m., according to Dr. Ellison's records, he prescribed Richard 30 days' worth of Adderall at 50 milligrams a day. He also gave him prescriptions postdated for Aug. 23 and Sept. 21, presumably to allow him to get pills into late October without the need for followup appointments. (Virginia state law forbids the dispensation of 90 days of a controlled substance at one time, but does allow doctors to write two 30-day prescriptions in advance.)

Virginia is one of 43 states with a formal Prescription Drug Monitoring Program, an online database that lets doctors check a patient's one-year prescription history, partly to see if he or she is getting medication elsewhere. Although pharmacies are required to enter all prescriptions for controlled substances into the system, Virginia law does not require doctors to consult it.

Dr. Ellison's notes suggest that he did not check the program before issuing the three prescriptions to Richard, who filled the first within hours.

The next morning, during a scheduled appointment at Dr. Parker's clinic, Ms. Strelitz wrote in her notes: "Richard is progressing. He reported staying off of the Adderall and on no meds currently. Focusing on staying healthy, eating well and exercising."

About a week later, Richard called his father with more good news: a job he had found overseeing storm cleanup crews was going well. He was feeling much better.

But Mr. Fee noticed that the more calm and measured speech that Richard had regained during his hospital stay was gone. He jumped from one subject to the next, sounding anxious and rushed. When the call ended, Mr. Fee recalled, he went straight to his wife.

"Call your insurance company," he said, "and find out if they've filled any prescriptions for Adderall."

•

"spoke to father—richard was in VBPC [Virginia Beach Psychiatric Center] and OD on adderall—NO STIMULANTS—HE WAS ALSO SEEING DR. PARKER"

Dr. Waldo M. Ellison
Interoffice e-mail
Aug. 5, 2011

•

An insurance representative confirmed that Richard had filled a prescription for Adderall on July 25. Mr. Fee confronted Dr. Ellison in the Dominion Psychiatric parking lot.

Mr. Fee told him that Richard had been in the psychiatric hospital, had been suicidal and had been taking Adderall through June and July. Dr. Ellison confirmed that he had written not only another prescription but two others for later in August and September.

"He told me it was normal procedure and not 90 days at one time," Mr. Fee recalled. "I flipped out on him: 'You gave my son 90 days of Adderall? You're going to kill him!'"

Mr. Fee said he and Dr. Ellison had discussed voiding the two outstanding scripts. Mr. Fee said he had been told that it was possible, but that should Richard need emergency medical attention, it could keep him from getting what would otherwise be proper care or medication. Mr. Fee confirmed that with a pharmacist and decided to drive to Richard's apartment and try to persuade him to rip up the prescriptions.

"I know that you've got these other prescriptions to get pills," Mr. Fee recalled telling Richard. "You're doing so good. You've got a job. You're working. Things with us are better. If you get them filled, I'm worried about what will happen."

"You're right," Mr. Fee said Richard had replied. "I tore them up and threw them away."

Mr. Fee spent two more hours with Richard making relative small talk—increasingly gnawed, he recalled later, by the sense that this was no ordinary conversation. As he looked at Richard he saw two images flickering on top of each other—the boy he had raised to love school and baseball, and the desperate addict he feared that boy had become.

Before he left, Mr. Fee made as loving a demand as he could muster.

"Please. Give them to me," Mr. Fee said.

Richard looked his father dead in the eye.

"I destroyed them," he said. "I don't have them. Don't worry."

•

"Richard said that he has stopped Adderall and wants to work on continuing to progress."

Renee Strelitz
Session notes
Sept. 13, 2011

•

Richard generally filled his prescriptions at a CVS on Laskin Road, less than three miles from his parents' home. But on Aug. 23, he went to a different CVS about 11 miles away, closer to Norfolk and farther from the locations that his father might have called to alert them to the situation. For his Sept. 21 prescription he traveled even farther, into Norfolk, to get his pills.

On Oct. 3, Richard visited Dr. Ellison for an appointment lasting 17 minutes. The doctor prescribed two weeks

of Strattera, a medication for A.D.H.D. that contains no amphetamines and, therefore, is neither a controlled substance nor particularly prone to abuse. His records make no mention of the Adderall prescription Richard filled on Sept. 21; they do note, however, "Father says that he is crazy and abusive of the Adderall—has made directives with regard to giving Richard anymore stimulants—bringing up charges—I explained this to Richard."

Prescription records indicate that Richard did not fill the Strattera prescription before returning to Dr. Ellison's office two weeks later to ask for more stimulants.

"Patient took only a few days of Strattera 40 mg—it calmed him but not focusing," the doctor's notes read. "I had told him not to look for much initially—He would like a list of MD who could rx adderall."

Dr. Ellison never saw Richard again. Given his patterns of abuse, friends said, Richard probably took his last Adderall pill in early October. Because he abruptly stopped without the slow and delicate reduction of medication that is recommended to minimize major psychological risks, especially for instant-release stimulants, he crashed harder than ever.

Richard's lifelong friend Ryan Sykes was one of the few people in contact with him during his final weeks. He said that despite Richard's addiction to Adderall and the ease with which it could be obtained on college campuses nearby, he had never pursued it outside the doctors' prescriptions.

"He had it in his mind that because it came from a doctor, it was O.K.," Mr. Sykes recalled.

On Nov. 7, after arriving home from a weekend away, Mrs. Fee heard a message on the family answering machine from Richard, asking his parents to call him. She phoned back at 10 that night and left a message herself.

Not hearing back by the next afternoon, Mrs. Fee checked Richard's cellphone records—he was on her plan—and saw no calls or texts. At 9 p.m. the Fees drove to Richard's apartment in Norfolk to check on him. The lights were on; his car was in the driveway. He did not answer. Beginning to panic, Mr. Fee found the kitchen window ajar and climbed in through it.

He searched the apartment and found nothing amiss.

"He isn't here," Mr. Fee said he had told his wife.

"Oh, thank God," she replied. "Maybe he's walking on the beach or something."

They got ready to leave before Mr. Fee stopped.

"Wait a minute," he said. "I didn't check the closet."

•

"Spoke with Richard's mother, Kathy Fee, today. She reported that Richard took his life last November. Family is devasted and having a difficult time. Offered assistance for family."

Renee Strelitz
Last page of Richard Fee file
June 21, 2012

•

Friends and former baseball teammates flocked to Richard Fee's memorial service in Virginia Beach. Most remembered only the funny and gregarious guy they knew in high school and college; many knew absolutely nothing of his last two years. He left no note explaining his suicide.

At a gathering at the Fees' house afterward, Mr. Fee told them about Richard's addiction to Adderall. Many recalled how they, too, had blithely abused the drug in college—to cram, just as Richard had—and could not help but wonder if they had played the same game of Russian roulette.

"I guarantee you a good number of them had used it for studying—that shock was definitely there in that room," said a Greensboro baseball teammate, Danny Michael, adding that he was among the few who had not. "It's so prevalent and widely used. People had no idea it could be abused to the point of no return."

Almost every one of more than 40 A.D.H.D. experts interviewed for this article said that worst-case scenarios like Richard Fee's can occur with any medication—and that people who do have A.D.H.D., or parents of children with the disorder, should not be dissuaded from considering the proven benefits of stimulant medication when supervised by a responsible physician.

Other experts, however, cautioned that Richard Fee's experience is instructive less in its ending than its evolution—that it underscores aspects of A.D.H.D. treatment that are mishandled every day with countless patients, many of them children.

"You don't have everything that happened with this kid, but his experience is not that unusual," said DeAnsin Parker, a clinical neuropsychologist in New York who specializes in young adults. "Diagnoses are made just this quickly, and medication is filled just this quickly. And the lack of therapy is really sad. Doctors are saying, 'Just take the meds to see if they help,' and if they help, 'You must have A.D.H.D.'"

Dr. Parker added: "Stimulants will help anyone focus better. And a lot of young people like or value that feeling, especially those who are driven and have ambitions. We have to realize that these are potential addicts—drug addicts don't look like they used to."

The Fees decided to go. The event was sponsored by the local chapter of Children and Adults with Attention Deficit Disorder (Chadd), the nation's primary advocacy group for A.D.H.D. patients. They wanted to attend the question-and-answer session afterward with local doctors and community college officials.

The evening opened with the local Chadd coordinator thanking the drug company Shire—the manufacturer of several A.D.H.D. drugs, including Vyvanse and extended-release Adderall—for partly underwriting the event. An hourlong film directed and narrated by two men with A.D.H.D. closed by examining some "myths" about stimulant medications, with several doctors praising their efficacy and safety. One said they were "safer than aspirin," while another added, "It's O.K.—there's nothing that's going to happen."

Sitting in the fourth row, Mr. Fee raised his hand to pose a question to the panel, which was moderated by Jeffrey Katz, a local clinical psychologist and a national board member of Chadd. "What are some of the drawbacks or some of the dangers of a misdiagnosis in somebody," Mr. Fee asked, "and then the subsequent medication that goes along with that?"

Dr. Katz looked straight at the Fees as he answered, "Not much."

Adding that "the medication itself is pretty innocuous," Dr. Katz continued that someone without A.D.H.D. might feel more awake with stimulants but would not consider it "something that they need."

"If you misdiagnose it and you give somebody medication, it's not going to do anything for them," Dr. Katz concluded. "Why would they continue to take it?"

Mr. Fee slowly sat down, trembling. Mrs. Fee placed her hand on his knee as the panel continued.

ALAN SCHWARZ is a Pulitzer Prize-nominated reporter for *The New York Times*.

Joshua Gowin

➜ **NO**

How "Smart Drugs" Enhance Us

If I only had a (better) brain.

The French Revolution was largely conceived in Parisian coffee houses such as Café Procope, where the radical journalist Jean-Paul Marat sipped java during his energetic diatribes and Robespierre's habitual consumption only increased his rebellious fervor. Voltaire reportedly guzzled over ten cups each day. Although they didn't know about caffeine at the time (it wasn't discovered until 1819, 30 years after the French Revolution), they certainly didn't overlook the stimulating effects of consuming a cup of perk. Some coffee-enthusiasts might suggest that imbibing the early-morning helper contributed to the monarchy's demise and the rise of the new Republic.

Our understanding of pharmacology has come a long way since the Reign of Terror. Recently, 'smart drugs' have been touted as a remedy to an array of problems, from bad moods to failing economies. What have we gained with the advent of modern cognitive enhancers?

A cup of coffee is a far cry from the sophisticated stimulants used by many on a daily basis. For example, Adderall and Ritalin, prescribed for the treatment of Attention-Deficit Hyperactivity Disorder (ADHD), work by helping individuals focus their attention without being easily distracted. For a child diagnosed with ADHD, these drugs can greatly improve both behavior and school performance. Adderall, composed of mixed amphetamine salts, and Ritalin, an amphetamine derivative, are also two of the drugs most widely used by healthy adults as purported brain boosters. Surveys at some universities have shown that up to 35% of students have obtained these drugs for use as a study aid, though most of them do not have ADHD (ADHD affects only 3–4% of people). For students without prescriptions, they usually have little trouble acquiring Ritalin or Adderall from friends or schoolmates. Students with prescriptions sometimes even sell their unneeded doses.

Given the dramatic rise in use for studying, ethicists have debated whether cognitive-enhancing drugs are unfair.

Those who take them may have an advantage on tests versus students who attempt to study using their wits alone. If taking drugs could provide a cognitive edge, you might expect that these students would outperform their classmates. Some wonder if parents might begin forcing their children to take smart-drugs in order to maintain competitive grades.

In order to address this issue, The College Life Study began periodically surveying university students a few years ago to better understand how health-related behaviors, including all varieties of drug use, affect school performance and career development. At a recent conference, Amelia Arria, the lead researcher, presented data about the use of Ritalin and Adderall as study drugs. The students who used these drugs more often also tended to skip more classes and smoke more pot. In terms of performance, they tended to have lower GPAs, in the 2.0–3.0 range, not higher ones. It seems, rather than as a tool to get ahead, students used stimulants while cramming to catch up for lost study time. Students earning As were mostly doing so by steady work throughout the semester, without the assistance of modern medicine.

Of course, this finding merits some caveats. Maybe the students using cognitive-enhancers did better than they would have otherwise. Just because most students (without ADHD) who use pharmacological aids don't perform better, some users may see a dramatic improvement. Nonetheless, so far it appears that Ritalin and Adderall offer the greatest assistance to the people they're prescribed to, those diagnosed with ADHD. As for the rest of students, Adderall may not be an unequivocal performance enhancer. The results of this study suggest that if a gap exists, the students who don't take study drugs are edging out those who do.

Arria reminds that evidence has been inconclusive so far about whether the enhancement for studying is real or perceived in healthy adults. In another study, students were given pills labeled either 'Ritalin' or 'placebo' and asked to take a mock SAT examination. The students given pills labeled 'Ritalin' reported feeling greater focus and mental clarity but their scores weren't any better—perhaps because the labels were misleading: both groups actually received a placebo.

A third common cognitive-enhancer, modafinil, first entered the market to help people with narcolepsy stay awake. A great deal of research has since looked at the potential benefits of modafinil for a variety of purposes. In healthy adults who are sleep-deprived, modafinil can improve mood, provide 10–12 hours of wakeful, focused productivity and improve cognition to a similar extent as caffeine, but without the jitteriness—and the effects last longer. After working overnight in the emergency room, doctors who took a single dose of modafinil kept their eyes open more easily than doctors who didn't take modafinil during morning lectures. However, they were just as weary on the drive home, and they had more difficulty falling asleep once they finally made it to bed. For patients with traumatic brain injury, major depressive disorder or schizophrenia, modafinil had a substantial effect on reducing fatigue, excessive sleepiness and depression, but it did not provide any benefit greater than placebo. For well-rested, healthy adults, the benefits remain controversial. While some studies have demonstrated that well-rested individuals can show modest improvement on memory tasks with modafinil, there may be a ceiling effect. High-functioning, healthy adults with adequate sleep may not receive any noticeable benefit because they are already performing optimally.

What is the difference between cognitive-enhancers like modafinil or Adderall and predecessors like caffeine? The chemical compounds differ, and they have unique mechanisms of action. Pharmaceutical packaging gives them elegance and refinement. Most people believe they'll work, so they offer at minimum a placebo effect. Even if, at heart, they're simply newer, prettier double-shots of espresso, there may still be some advantages to taking these drugs, such as longer-lasting effects and no jitteriness.

Do these drugs make you smarter? More likely, they allow you to productively use your pre-existing intelligence, even if you didn't get a great night of rest beforehand. After ingesting one of these pills, an average person won't suddenly discover a cure for cancer or write a symphony that would make Beethoven envious. If someone is seeking a miraculous transformation, they're better off booking a room at a Holiday Inn Express or going about it the old-fashioned way—by signing a deal with the devil.

Joshua Gowin is a psychologist and former intern at *Psychology Today.*

EXPLORING THE ISSUE

Is the Use of "Smart" Pills for Cognitive Enhancement Dangerous?

Critical Thinking and Reflection

1. Why do so many young people fake symptoms in order to acquire "smart drugs"?
2. Describe the side effects of stimulant drugs such as Ritalin and Adderall. What are the effects that appeal to users?
3. What are the legitimate uses for stimulant drugs such as Ritalin and Adderall?

Is There Common Ground?

On some elite college campuses, up to 25 percent of students admit to nonmedical use of stimulant drugs. "Smart" drugs are also widely used off campus by business executives and others who wish to gain a competitive edge and to better meet deadlines. The drugs are becoming common and many people believe they have much to offer individuals and society and should be made more available. The benefits of enhancement drugs include increased alertness and focus and improvement in some types of memory. Among those who do not have ADHD, research has shown that stimulants consistently and significantly enhance learning of material recalled days later, an obvious advantage when studying for an exam. The drugs may even positively affect certain types of judgment. Improvements in memory and cognitive control have been reported in multiple studies, mainly using the drug Ritalin.

While the drugs may offer the benefit of cognitive enhancement, there is question as to whether their use is both cheating and drug abuse. Will there be pressure among students to take drugs just to keep up with their peers? One of the biggest concerns, however, is that cognitive enhancement may be wrong not because it is so physically risky or because it creates an unleveled playing field but because it redefines the nature of human achievement itself. The obvious parallel to performance-enhancing drug use among professional and amateur athletes is often made. While ethicists ponder this, the reality is that there are also health risks since the effects of chronic unregulated doses of stimulant drugs can be toxic. The drugs can also cause psychosis, actual cognitive deficits, and addiction.

Additional Resources

Bagot, K. S., & Kaminer, Y. (2014). Efficacy of stimulants for cognitive enhancement in non-attention deficit hyperactivity disorder youth: A systematic review. *Addiction, 109*(4), 547–557.

Franke, A. G., Lieb, K., & Hildt, E. (2012). What users think about the differences between caffeine and illicit/prescription stimulants for cognitive enhancement. *PLoS One, 7*, 1–7.

Varga, M. D. (2012). Adderall abuse on college campuses: A comprehensive literature review. *Journal of Evidence-Based Social Work, 9*(3), 293–313.

Vrecki, S. A. (2013). Just how cognitive is "cognitive enhancement"? On the significance of emotions in university students' experiences with study drugs. *AJOB Neuroscience, 4*, 4–12.

Webb, J. R., Valased, M. R., & North, C. S. (2013). Prevalence of stimulant use in a sample of US medical students. *Annals of Clinical Psychiatry, 25*, 27–32.

Internet References . . .

Food and Drug Administration

www.fda.gov

National Institute on Drug Abuse (NIDA)

www.nida.nih.gov

National Institute of Mental Health (NIMH). Attention Deficit Hyperactivity Disorder (ADHD)

www.nimh.nih.gov/health/publications/index.shtml

Selected, Edited, and with issue Framing Material by:
Eileen L. Daniel, *SUNY College at Brockport*

ISSUE

Should Embryonic Stem Cell Research Be Permitted?

YES: Jeffrey Hart, from "NR on Stem Cells: The Magazine Is Wrong," *National Review* (2004)

NO: Ramesh Ponnuru, from "NR on Stem Cells: The Magazine Is Right," *National Review* (2004)

Learning Outcomes

After reading this issue, you will be able to:

- Discuss the basic characteristics of stem cells.
- Understand the potential benefits of stem cell therapy.
- Assess the difference between adult and embryonic stem cells.

ISSUE SUMMARY

YES: Professor Jeffrey Hart contends there are many benefits to stem cell research and that a ban on funded cloning research is unjustified.

NO: Writer Ramesh Ponnuru argues that a single-celled human embryo is a living organism, which directs its own development and should not be used for experimentation.

Research using human stem cells could one day lead to cures for diabetes, could restore mobility to paralyzed individuals, and may offer treatment for diseases such as Alzheimer's and Parkinson's. It may be possible for humans to regenerate body parts, or create new cells to treat disease. Stem cells, which have the potential to develop into many different cell types, serve as a type of repair system for the body. They can theoretically divide without limit to replenish other cells as long as the person or animal still lives. When a stem cell divides, each new cell has the potential to either remain a stem cell or become another type of cell with a more specialized function, such as a brain or blood cell.

There are two important characteristics of stem cells, which differentiate them from other types of cells. First, they are unspecialized cells that renew themselves for long periods through cell division. Second, under certain conditions, they can be become cells with special functions such as heart cells or the insulin-producing cells of

the pancreas. Researchers mainly work with two kinds of stem cells from animals and humans: embryonic stem cells and adult stem cells, which have different functions and characteristics. Scientists learned different ways to get or derive stem cells from early rodent embryos over 20 years ago.

Detailed study of the biology of mouse stem cells led to the discovery, in 1998, of how to isolate stem cells from human embryos and grow the cells in the lab. The embryos used in these studies were created for infertility purposes through *in vitro* fertilization procedures and when no longer needed for that purpose, they were donated for research with the informed consent of the donor.

Researchers have hypothesized that embryonic stem cells may, at some point in the future, become the basis for treating diseases such as Parkinson's disease, diabetes, and heart disease. Scientists need to study stem cells to learn about their important properties and what makes them different from specialized cell types. As researchers discover more about stem cells, it may become possible to use the cells not just in cell-based therapies but also for screening new drugs and preventing birth defects.

Researching stem cells will allow scientists to understand how they transform into the array of specialized cells that make us human. Some of the most serious medical conditions, such as cancer and birth defects, are due to events that occur somewhere in this process. A better understanding of normal cell development will allow scientists to understand and possibly correct the errors that cause these conditions. Another potential application of stem cells is making cells and tissues for medical therapies. A type of stem cell, pluripotents, offers the possibility of a renewable source of replacement cells and tissues to treat a myriad of diseases, conditions, and disabilities including Parkinson's and Alzheimer's diseases, spinal cord injury, stroke, burns, heart disease, diabetes, and arthritis.

The Bush Administration did not support embryonic stem cell research, which they believed is experimentation on potential human life. As a result, researchers must rely on funding from business, private foundations, and other sources. While the potential for stem cells is great, there is not universal support for this research. In the YES and NO selections, Jeffrey Hart, a senior editor at *National Review*, contends that there are many benefits to stem cell research and that a federal ban on funded experimentation is unjustified. Ramesh Ponnuru argues that stem cell research is amoral since it involves the use of human embryos.

YES ↵

Jeffrey Hart

NR on Stem Cells: The Magazine Is Wrong

National Review has consistently taken a position on stem-cell research that requires some discussion here. Three editorials early this year were based on the assertion that a single fertilized cell is a "human being." This premise—and the conclusions drawn from it—require challenge on conservative grounds, as they have never been approved by American law or accepted as common convention.

The first 2004 editorial appeared in the January 26 issue, and made a series of assertions about recent legislation in New Jersey. It included the notion that it is now "possible" to create a human embryo there—through cloning—that, at age eight months, could be sold for research. But this dystopian fantasy could become fact in no American jurisdiction.

In the March 8 NR we read another editorial; this one achieved greater seriousness. Still, it called for a "new law" that "would say that human beings, however small and young, may not be treated instrumentally and may not be deliberately destroyed."

In all of the editorials, we are asked to accept the insistent dogma that a single fertilized cell is a "human being, however small and young," and is not to be "deliberately destroyed."

This demand grates—because such "human beings" are deliberately destroyed all the time, and such "mass homicide" arouses no public outcry. In fact, there are about 100,000 fertilized cells now frozen in maternity clinics. These are the inevitable, and so deliberate, by-products of in vitro fertilization, accepted by women who cannot conceive children naturally. No wonder there has been no outcry: Where reality shows medical waste that would otherwise lie useless, NR's characterization of these frozen embryos as "small and young" makes one think of the Gerber baby.

The entire NR case against stem-cell research rests, like a great inverted pyramid, on the single assertion that these cells are "human beings"—a claim that is not self-evidently true. Even when the naked eye is aided by a microscope, these cells—"zygotes," to use the proper terminology—do not look like human beings. That resemblance does not emerge even as the zygote grows into the hundred-cell organism, about the size of a pinhead, called a "blastocyst." This is the level of development at which stem cells are produced: The researcher is not interested in larger embryos, much less full-blown, for-sale fetuses.

I myself have never met anyone who bites into an apple, gazes upon the seeds there, and sees a grove of apple trees. I think we must conclude, if we are to use language precisely, that the single fertilized cell is a *developing* or *potential* human being—many of which are destroyed during in vitro fertilization, and even in the course of natural fertilization. But just as a seed—a *potential* apple tree—is no orchard, a *potential* child is not yet a human being.

There is more to this matter than biology: In question is NR's very theory of—and approach to—politics. Classic and valuable arguments in this magazine have often taken the form of Idea (or paradigm) versus Actuality. Here are a few such debates that have shaped the magazine, a point of interest especially to new readers.

Very early in NR's history, the demand for indisputably conservative candidates gave way to William F. Buckley Jr.'s decisive formulation that NR should prefer "the most conservative electable candidate." WFB thus corrected his refusal to vote for Eisenhower, who was at least more conservative than Stevenson. Senior editor James Burnham, a realist, also voted for Ike; in his decision, Actuality won out.

In the 1956 crisis in Hungary, Burnham's profoundly held Idea about the necessity for Liberation in Europe contrasted with Eisenhower's refusal, based on Actuality, to intervene in a landlocked nation where Soviet ground and air superiority was decisive. But later on, Burnham, choosing Actuality over the Idea, saw much sooner than most conservatives that Nixon's containment and "Vietnamization" could not work in South Vietnam, which was a sieve. The "peace" that was "at hand" in 1972 was the peace of the grave.

A final example: In the late 1960s, senior editor Brent Bozell's theoretical demand for perfect Catholic morality—

argued in a very fine exchange with another senior editor, Frank Meyer—was rejected by NR.

Thus the tension between Idea and Actuality has a long tradition at NR, revived by this question of stem cells. Ultimately, American constitutional decision-making rests upon the "deliberate consent" of a self-governing people. Such decision-making by consensus usually accords no participant everything he desires, and thus is non-utopian. Just try an absolute, ideological ban on in vitro fertilization, for example, and observe the public response.

In fact, an editorial (NR, August 6, 2001) has held that even in vitro fertilization is hard to justify morally. Understandably, NR has soft-pedaled this opinion: The magazine's view that a single cell is a "human being" has never been expressed in or embraced by American law. It represents an absolutization of the "human being" claim for a single cell. It stands in contradiction to the "deliberate sense" theory NR has heretofore espoused. And, at this very moment, it is being contradicted in the Actual world of research practice.

Recently, for instance, a Harvard researcher produced 17 stem-cell "lines" from the aforementioned leftover frozen cells. The researcher's goal is not homicide, of course, but the possible cure of dreadful diseases. It seems to me that the prospect of eliminating horrible, disabling ailments justifies, morally, using cells that are otherwise doomed. Morality requires the weighing of results, and the claim to a "right to life" applies in both directions. Those lifting that phrase from the Declaration of Independence do not often add "liberty and the pursuit of happiness," there given equal standing as "rights"—rights that might be more widely enjoyed in the wake of stem-cell advances.

As I said earlier, the evolution of NR as a magazine that matters has involved continuing arguments between Idea and Actuality. Here, the Idea that a single fertilized cell is a human being, and that destroying one is a homicide, is not sustainable. That is the basis—the only basis—for NR's position thus far on stem-cell research. Therefore NR's position on the whole issue is unsustainable.

Buckley has defined conservatism as the "politics of reality." That is the strength of conservatism, a Burkean strength, and an anti-utopian one. I have never heard a single cytologist affirming the proposition that a single

cell is a "human being"; here, Actuality will prevail, as usual.

In recommending against federal funding for most stem-cell research, President Bush stated that 60 lines of stem cells that already exist are adequate for current research. The National Institutes of Health has said that this is incorrect. There are in fact 15 lines, and these are not adequate even for current research. The president was misinformed. But Actuality is gaining ground nonetheless: Harvard University has recently announced the formation of a $100 million Harvard Stem Cell Institute. And Harvard physicians are conducting community-education programs to counter misinformation (Reuters, March 3): "Scientists at Harvard University announced on Wednesday that they had created 17 batches of stem cells from human embryos in defiance of efforts by President Bush to limit such research. 'What we have done is to make use of previously frozen human fertilized eggs that otherwise were going to be discarded,' [Dr. Douglas] Melton told reporters in a telephone briefing."

Not unexpectedly, and after losing one of its top scientists in the field to Cambridge (England), the University of California, Berkeley, announced that it was pursuing stem-cell research. Other UCs also made such announcements, and California state funding has been promised. It is easy to see that major research universities across the nation—and in any nation that can afford them—will either follow or lose their top scientists in this field. Experience shows that it is folly to reject medical investigation, a folly the universities and private-sector researchers will be sure to avoid.

Weak in theory, and irrelevant in practice, opposition to stem-cell research is now an irrelevance across the board; on this matter, even the president has made himself irrelevant. All this was to be expected: The only surprise has been the speed with which American research is going forward. It is pleasant to have the private sector intervene, as at Harvard, not to mention the initiatives of the states. In practical terms, this argument is over. *National Review* should not make itself irrelevant by trying to continue it.

JEFFREY HART is a senior editor of the *National Review*.

Ramesh Ponnuru

→ **NO**

NR on Stem Cells: The Magazine Is Right

National Review does not oppose stem-cell research. It approves of research on stem cells taken from adult somatic cells, or from umbilical cords. It opposes stem-cell research only when obtaining those cells destroys embryonic human beings, whether these beings are created through cloning, in vitro fertilization, or the old-fashioned way. Jeff Hart challenges NR's stance for three reasons: He disputes the idea that single-celled human embryos are human beings, he questions the prudence of advancing that idea, and he thinks the humanitarian goal of the research justifies the means.

Professor Hart starts his argument by noting that American law has never treated the single-celled embryo as a human being. This is true. But it never treated it as anything else, either. What would American law have had to say about the embryo in 1826, or, for that matter, in 1952?

The single-celled human embryo is neither dead nor inanimate. It is a living organism, not a functional part of another organism, and it directs its own development, according to its genetic template, through the embryonic, fetal, infant, and subsequent stages of development. (The terms "blastocyst," "adolescent," and "newborn" denote stages of development in a being of the same type, not different types of beings.) It is a *Homo sapiens,* not a member of some other species—which is why it is valuable to scientists in the first place. Strictly speaking, it is not even an "it": It has a sex.

"Even when the naked eye is aided by a microscope," writes Professor Hart, early embryos "do not look like human beings." Actually, they look *exactly* like human beings—the way human beings look at that particular stage of development. We all looked like that, at that age. Professor Hart believes that science can open up whole worlds of knowledge and possibility to us. He should be willing to entertain the possibility that among the insights we have gained is the revelation that human beings at their beginnings look like nothing we have ever seen before.

Professor Hart notes that many embryos die naturally. And so? Infant mortality rates have been very high in some societies; old people die all the time. That does not mean it is permissible to kill infants or old people.

I should also comment about the New Jersey law that makes it legally possible to create a human embryo through cloning, develop it through the fetal stage, and sell it for research purposes at eight months. Professor Hart writes that "this dystopian fantasy could become fact in no American jurisdiction." Sadly, this is untrue: In most American jurisdictions, no law on the books would prevent this scenario from taking place.

In the past, scientists have been quite interested in doing research on aborted fetuses. Right now, the early embryo is a hotter research subject. But neither Professor Hart nor I can rule out the possibility that research on cloned fetuses will be thought, in a few years, to hold great promise. If scientists want to conduct such research, the only legal obstacles will be the statutes of those states that have banned human cloning—the very laws that NR favors. New Jersey has brought this dystopia one step closer.

It would be possible for Professor Hart to concede that the history of a body begins with its conception—that we were all once one-celled organisms, in the sense that "we" were never a sperm cell and an egg cell—while still claiming that it would have been morally defensible to destroy us at that time. Our intrinsic moral worth came later, he might argue: when we developed sentience, abstract reasoning, relationships with others, or some other distinguishing attribute. According to this viewpoint, human beings as such have no intrinsic right to life; many human beings enjoy that right only by virtue of qualities they happen to possess.

The implications of this theory, however, extend beyond the womb. Infants typically lack the immediately exercisable capacity for abstract mental reasoning, too—which is how Peter Singer and others have justified infanticide. It is impossible to identify a non-arbitrary point at which there is "enough" sentience or meaningful interaction to confer a right to life. It is also impossible to explain why some people do not have basic rights more or less than other people depending on how much of the accidental quality they possess. In other words, the foundation of human equality is destroyed as soon as we suggest that private actors may treat some members of the human species as though they were mere things. The claim in the Declaration of Independence that "all men are created equal" becomes a self-evident lie.

Life comes before liberty and the pursuit of happiness in that declaration, and at no point is it suggested that liberty includes a right to kill, or that happiness may be pursued through homicide. Morality often "requires the weighing of results," as Professor Hart writes. But we would not kill one five-year-old child for the certain prospect of curing cancer, let alone the mere possibility—because the act would be intrinsically immoral. Or would we? Professor Hart writes that it is "folly to reject medical investigation." So much for restrictions on human experimentation.

Apple seeds are not a grove of trees. An infant is not an adult, either, just a potential adult, but that doesn't mean you can kill it. Professor Hart objects to the use of the words "young" and "small" to characterize the entities whose destruction we are debating. Since the argument for terminating them turns precisely on their having 100 cells or fewer (they're small), and on their not yet having advanced to later stages of human development (they're young), it's hard to see his point.

Let me turn now to the question of the politics of Actuality. NR is, in principle, against the intentional destruction of human embryos. But we have been quite mindful of political circumstances. As Professor Hart notes, we have not said much about regulating the practices of fertility clinics. (He faults us for both running wild with ideas and prudently declining to do so; also, freezing something is not the same as destroying it.) Prudence has kept us from urging the president to fight for a ban on all research that destroys human embryos. We have principally asked for two things: a ban on governmental funding of such research, and a ban on human cloning—even suggesting a simple moratorium on cloning as a compromise. We are not calling, to pursue one of Professor Hart's analogies, for an invasion of Hungary here. But neither are we suggesting that we are indifferent to the Soviet domination of Eastern Europe.

Our position on cloning is not that of some political fringe: It is the position of President Bush. It is the position of the House of Representatives, which has twice voted to ban human cloning. It is a position that, depending on the wording of the poll question, somewhere between one-third and two-thirds of the public shares. It is the position of the governments of Canada and Germany. NR has fought lonelier battles.

We are sometimes told that, in a pluralistic society in which many people have different views about such matters as the moral status of the human embryo, we cannot impose public policies that assume the correctness of some views over others. I cannot agree. Some people will not accept the justice of a ban on cloning for research; few policies command the full assent of all people of good will. But disagreement about the requirements of justice is no excuse for failing to do it.

Ramesh Ponnuru is a senior editor at the *National Review*.

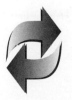

EXPLORING THE ISSUE

Should Embryonic Stem Cell Research Be Permitted?

Critical Thinking and Reflection

1. What are the differences between adult and embryonic stem cells?
2. Why are many individuals opposed to stem cell research?
3. Why did the government under the Bush Administration deny funding for stem cell research?

Is There Common Ground?

Many scientists believe that human embryonic stem cell research could one day lead to a cure for a variety of diseases that plague humans. While a cure for diabetes, cancer, Parkinson's, and other diseases would greatly benefit humanity, there are many who believe that it is amoral to use human embryos for this purpose. These individuals believe that every human being begins as a single-cell zygote, and develops into an embryo, fetus, and then is born. To destroy the embryonic stem cell is to destroy a potential life, which many cannot justify. The Bush Administration supported these beliefs and enacted a moratorium on U.S. federal funding for embryonic stem cell research. When Barack Obama became president, he issued an executive order that lifted restrictions on U.S. federal funding for research on human embryonic stem cells (ESCs). The advocates of stem cell research celebrated the issuance of the order. However, the order is sparsely worded and leaves the details to be worked out by the National Institutes of Health.

In "Distinctly Human: The When, Where and How of Life's Beginnings," John Collins Harvey (*Commonweal*, February 8, 2002) asserts that the human embryo is a living human being from the moment of conception. As such, it should never be used as an object or considered as a means to an end. It should not be killed so that parts of it can be used for the benefit of another person. That sentiment is echoed by William Sanders in "Embryology: Inconvenient Facts," *First Things* (December 2004), who believes that adult human stems cells have been proven to have great value in the invention of new and better medical treatments, but the value of ESCs is theoretical and cannot justify killing an embryo. In "Many Say Adult Stem Cell Reports Overplayed," *Journal of the American Medical Association* (2001), the value of adult stem cells is debated.

Additional Resources

Baggaley, K. (2015). Stem cells help mend brain damage. *Science News, 187*(6), 13.

Begley, S. (2014). The stem cell solution. *The Saturday Evening Post, 286*(6), 52–55.

Kolios, G. & Moodley, Y. (2012). Introduction to stem cells and regenerative medicine. *Respiration, 85*(1), 3–10.

Mukhopadhyay, C. S., Tokas, J., & Mathur, P. D. (2011). Prospects and ethical concerns of embryonic stem cells research—a review. *Veterinary World, 4*(6), 281–286.

Robertson, J. A. (2010). Embryo stem cell research: Ten years of controversy. *Journal of Law, Medicine & Ethics, 38*(2), 191–203.

Internet References . . .

International Society for Stem Cell Research

www.isscr.org/

National Bioethics Advisory Commission: Publications

www.bioethics.gov/pubs.html

U.S. National Institutes of Health (NIH)

www.nih.gov

Unit 3

UNIT

Mind–Body Relationships

Humans have long sought to extend life, eliminate disease, and prevent sickness. In modern times, people depend on technology to develop creative and innovative ways to improve health, extend life, and treat disease. However, as true cures for diseases such as AIDS, cancer, drug addiction, and heart disease continue to elude scientists and doctors, many people question whether or not modern medicine has reached a plateau in improving health. As a result, over the last decade, an emphasis has been placed on prevention as a way to maintain wellness. Prevention includes maintaining a healthy mind, body, and spirit. In addition, the theme of healing prayer is very common in the history of spirituality.

Selected, Edited, and with Issue Framing Material by:
Eileen L. Daniel, *SUNY College at Brockport*

ISSUE

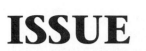

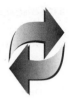

Should Addiction to Drugs Be Labeled a Brain Disease?

YES: Alan I. Leshner, from "Addiction Is a Brain Disease," *Issues in Science and Technology* (2001)

NO: Alva Noë, from "Addiction Is Not a Disease of the Brain," *National Public Radio* (2011)

Learning Outcomes

After reading this issue, you will be able to:

- Discuss the causes of drug addiction.
- Discuss the argument that addiction is a disease and not a behavioral issue.
- Understand the various types of treatment for drug and alcohol addiction.

ISSUE SUMMARY

YES: Alan I. Leshner, director of the National Institute on Drug Abuse at the National Institutes of Health, believes that addiction to drugs and alcohol is not a behavioral condition but a treatable disease.

NO: Professor Alva Noë counters that addiction is a phenomenon that can only be understood in terms of the life choices, needs, and understanding of the whole person.

There are many different theories as to why some individuals become addicted to alcohol or other drugs. Historically, drug and alcohol dependency has been viewed as either a disease or a moral failing. In more recent years, other theories of addiction have been developed, including behavioral, genetic, socio-cultural, and psychological theories.

The view that drug addiction and alcoholism are moral failings maintains that abusing drugs is voluntary behavior that the user chooses to do. Users choose to overindulge in such a way that they create suffering for themselves and others. American history is marked by repeated and failed government efforts to control this abuse by eliminating drug and alcohol use with legal sanctions, such as the enactment of Prohibition in the late 1920s and the punishment of alcoholics and drug users via jail sentences and fines. However, there seem to be several contradictions to this behavioral model of addiction. Addiction may be a complex condition that is caused by multiple factors, including environment, biology, and others. It is not totally clear that addiction is a voluntary behavior. And from a historical perspective, punishing alcoholics and drug addicts has been ineffective.

In the United States today, the primary theory for understanding the causes of addiction is the disease model rather than the moral model. Borrowing from the modern mental health movement, addiction as a disease has been promoted by mental health advocates who tried to change the public's perception of severe mental illness. Diseases like bipolar disorder and schizophrenia were defined as the result of brain abnormalities rather than environmental factors or poor parenting. Likewise, addiction was not a moral weakness but a brain disorder that could be treated. In 1995 the National Institute on Drug Addiction (NIDA) supported the idea that drug addiction was a type of brain disorder. Following NIDA's support, the concept of addiction as a brain disease has become more widely accepted.

This model has been advocated by the medical and alcohol treatment communities as well as self-help groups such as Alcoholics Anonymous and Narcotics Anonymous.

The disease model implies that addiction is not the result of voluntary behavior or lack of self-control; it is caused by biological factors, which are treatable. While there are somewhat different interpretations of this theory, it generally refers to addiction as an organic brain syndrome with biological and genetic origins rather than voluntary and behavioral origins.

Alan Leshner believes that taking drugs causes changes in neurons in the central nervous system that compel the individual to use drugs. These neurological changes, which are not reversible, force addicts to continue to take drugs. Professor Alva Noë disagrees. He believes that most addicts are not innocent victims of chronic disease but individuals who are responsible for their illness and recovery.

YES ↵

Alan I. Leshner

Addiction Is a Brain Disease

The United States is stuck in its drug abuse metaphors and in polarized arguments about them. Everyone has an opinion. One side insists that we must control supply, the other that we must reduce demand. People see addiction as either a disease or as a failure of will. None of this bumpersticker analysis moves us forward. The truth is that we will make progress in dealing with drug issues only when our national discourse and our strategies are as complex and comprehensive as the problem itself.

A core concept that has been evolving with scientific advances over the past decade is that drug addiction is a brain disease that develops over time as a result of the initially voluntary behavior of using drugs. The consequence is virtually uncontrollable compulsive drug craving, seeking, and use that interferes with, if not destroys, an individual's functioning in the family and in society. This medical condition demands formal treatment.

We now know in great detail the brain mechanisms through which drugs acutely modify mood, memory, perception, and emotional states. Using drugs repeatedly over time changes brain structure and function in fundamental and long-lasting ways that can persist long after the individual stops using them. Addiction comes about through an array of neuroadaptive changes and the laying down and strengthening of new memory connections in various circuits in the brain. We do not yet know all the relevant mechanisms, but the evidence suggests that those long-lasting brain changes are responsible for the distortions of cognitive and emotional functioning that characterize addicts, particularly including the compulsion to use drugs that is the essence of addiction. It is as if drugs have highjacked the brain's natural motivational control circuits, resulting in drug use becoming the sole, or at least the top, motivational priority for the individual. Thus, the majority of the biomedical community now considers addiction, in its essence, to be a brain disease: a condition caused by persistent changes in brain structure and function.

This brain-based view of addiction has generated substantial controversy, particularly among people who seem able to think only in polarized ways. Many people erroneously still believe that biological and behavioral explanations are alternative or competing ways to understand phenomena, when in fact they are complementary and integratable. Modern science has taught that it is much too simplistic to set biology in opposition to behavior or to pit willpower against brain chemistry. Addiction involves inseparable biological and behavioral components. It is the quintessential biobehavioral disorder.

Many people also erroneously still believe that drug addiction is simply a failure of will or of strength of character. Research contradicts that position. However, the recognition that addiction is a brain disease does not mean that the addict is simply a hapless victim. Addiction begins with the voluntary behavior of using drugs, and addicts must participate in and take some significant responsibility for their recovery. Thus, having this brain disease does not absolve the addict of responsibility for his or her behavior, but it does explain why an addict cannot simply stop using drugs by sheer force of will alone. It also dictates a much more sophisticated approach to dealing with the array of problems surrounding drug abuse and addiction in our society.

The Essence of Addiction

The entire concept of addiction has suffered greatly from imprecision and misconception. In fact, if it were possible, it would be best to start all over with some new, more neutral term. The confusion comes about in part because of a now archaic distinction between whether specific drugs are "physically" or "psychologically" addicting. The distinction historically revolved around whether or not dramatic physical withdrawal symptoms occur when an individual stops taking a drug; what we in the field now call "physical dependence."

However, 20 years of scientific research has taught that focusing on this physical versus psychological distinction is off the mark and a distraction from the real issues. From both clinical and policy perspectives, it

Leshner, Alan I.. "Addiction Is a Brain Disease, and It Matters", *SCIENCE* 278:45–47 (1997).

actually does not matter very much what physical withdrawal symptoms occur. Physical dependence is not that important, because even the dramatic withdrawal symptoms of heroin and alcohol addiction can now be easily managed with appropriate medications. Even more important, many of the most dangerous and addicting drugs, including methamphetamine and crack cocaine, do not produce very severe physical dependence symptoms upon withdrawal.

What really matters most is whether or not a drug causes what we now know to be the essence of addiction: uncontrollable, compulsive drug craving, seeking, and use, even in the face of negative health and social consequences. This is the crux of how the Institute of Medicine, the American Psychiatric Association, and the American Medical Association define addiction and how we all should use the term. It is really only this compulsive quality of addiction that matters in the long run to the addict and to his or her family and that should matter to society as a whole. Compulsive craving that overwhelms all other motivations is the root cause of the massive health and social problems associated with drug addiction. In updating our national discourse on drug abuse, we should keep in mind this simple definition: Addiction is a brain disease expressed in the form of compulsive behavior. Both developing and recovering from it depend on biology, behavior, and social context.

It is also important to correct the common misimpression that drug use, abuse, and addiction are points on a single continuum along which one slides back and forth over time, moving from user to addict, then back to occasional user, then back to addict. Clinical observation and more formal research studies support the view that, once addicted, the individual has moved into a different state of being. It is as if a threshold has been crossed. Very few people appear able to successfully return to occasional use after having been truly addicted. Unfortunately, we do not yet have a clear biological or behavioral marker of that transition from voluntary drug use to addiction. However, a body of scientific evidence is rapidly developing that points to an array of cellular and molecular changes in specific brain circuits. Moreover, many of these brain changes are common to all chemical addictions, and some also are typical of other compulsive behaviors such as pathological overeating.

Addiction should be understood as a chronic recurring illness. Although some addicts do gain full control over their drug use after a single treatment episode, many have relapses. Repeated treatments become necessary to increase the intervals between and diminish the intensity of relapses, until the individual achieves abstinence.

The complexity of this brain disease is not atypical, because virtually no brain diseases are simply biological in nature and expression. All, including stroke, Alzheimer's disease, schizophrenia, and clinical depression, include some behavioral and social aspects. What may make addiction seem unique among brain diseases, however, is that it does begin with a clearly voluntary behavior—the initial decision to use drugs. Moreover, not everyone who ever uses drugs goes on to become addicted. Individuals differ substantially in how easily and quickly they become addicted and in their preferences for particular substances. Consistent with the biobehavioral nature of addiction, these individual differences result from a combination of environmental and biological, particularly genetic, factors. In fact, estimates are that between 50 and 70 percent of the variability in susceptibility to becoming addicted can be accounted for by genetic factors.

Over time the addict loses substantial control over his or her initially voluntary behavior, and it becomes compulsive. For many people these behaviors are truly uncontrollable, just like the behavioral expression of any other brain disease. Schizophrenics cannot control their hallucinations and delusions. Parkinson's patients cannot control their trembling. Clinically depressed patients cannot voluntarily control their moods. Thus, once one is addicted, the characteristics of the illness—and the treatment approaches—are not that different from most other brain diseases. No matter how one develops an illness, once one has it, one is in the diseased state and needs treatment.

Moreover, voluntary behavior patterns are, of course, involved in the etiology and progression of many other illnesses, albeit not all brain diseases. Examples abound, including hypertension, arteriosclerosis and other cardiovascular diseases, diabetes, and forms of cancer in which the onset is heavily influenced by the individual's eating, exercise, smoking, and other behaviors.

Addictive behaviors do have special characteristics related to the social contexts in which they originate. All of the environmental cues surrounding initial drug use and development of the addiction actually become "conditioned" to that drug use and are thus critical to the development and expression of addiction. Environmental cues are paired in time with an individual's initial drug use experiences and, through classical conditioning, take on conditioned stimulus properties. When those cues are present at a later time, they elicit anticipation of a drug experience and thus generate tremendous drug craving. Cue-induced craving is one of the most frequent causes of drug use relapses, even after long periods of abstinence, independently of whether drugs are available.

The salience of environmental or contextual cues helps explain why reentry to one's community can be so difficult for addicts leaving the controlled environments of treatment or correctional settings and why aftercare is so essential to successful recovery. The person who became addicted in the home environment is constantly exposed to the cues conditioned to his or her initial drug use, such as the neighborhood where he or she hung out, drug-using buddies, or the lamppost where he or she bought drugs. Simple exposure to those cues automatically triggers craving and can lead rapidly to relapses. This is one reason why someone who apparently overcame drug cravings while in prison or residential treatment could quickly revert to drug use upon returning home. In fact, one of the major goals of drug addiction treatment is to teach addicts how to deal with the cravings caused by inevitable exposure to these conditioned cues.

Implications

Understanding addiction as a brain disease has broad and significant implications for the public perception of addicts and their families, for addiction treatment practice, and for some aspects of public policy. On the other hand, this biomedical view of addiction does not speak directly to and is unlikely to bear significantly on many other issues, including specific strategies for controlling the supply of drugs and whether initial drug use should be legal or not. Moreover, the brain disease model of addiction does not address the question of whether specific drugs of abuse can also be potential medicines. Examples abound of drugs that can be both highly addicting and extremely effective medicines. The best-known example is the appropriate use of morphine as a treatment for pain. Nevertheless, a number of practical lessons can be drawn from the scientific understanding of addiction.

It is no wonder addicts cannot simply quit on their own. They have an illness that requires biomedical treatment. People often assume that because addiction begins with a voluntary behavior and is expressed in the form of excess behavior, people should just be able to quit by force of will alone. However, it is essential to understand when dealing with addicts that we are dealing with individuals whose brains have been altered by drug use. They need drug addiction treatment. We know that, contrary to common belief, very few addicts actually do just stop on their own. Observing that there are very few heroin addicts in their 50s or 60s, people frequently ask what happened to those who were heroin addicts 30 years ago, assuming that they must have quit on their own. However, longitudinal

studies find that only a very small fraction actually quit on their own. The rest have either been successfully treated, are currently in maintenance treatment, or (for about half) are dead. Consider the example of smoking cigarettes: Various studies have found that between 3 and 7 percent of people who try to quit on their own each year actually succeed. Science has at last convinced the public that depression is not just a lot of sadness; that depressed individuals are in a different brain state and thus require treatment to get their symptoms under control. The same is true for schizophrenic patients. It is time to recognize that this is also the case for addicts.

The role of personal responsibility is undiminished but clarified. Does having a brain disease mean that people who are addicted no longer have any responsibility for their behavior or that they are simply victims of their own genetics and brain chemistry? Of course not. Addiction begins with the voluntary behavior of drug use, and although genetic characteristics may predispose individuals to be more or less susceptible to becoming addicted, genes do not doom one to become an addict. This is one major reason why efforts to prevent drug use are so vital to any comprehensive strategy to deal with the nation's drug problems. Initial drug use is a voluntary, and therefore preventable, behavior.

Moreover, as with any illness, behavior becomes a critical part of recovery. At a minimum, one must comply with the treatment regimen, which is harder than it sounds. Treatment compliance is the biggest cause of relapses for all chronic illnesses, including asthma, diabetes, hypertension, and addiction. Moreover, treatment compliance rates are no worse for addiction than for these other illnesses, ranging from 30 to 50 percent. Thus, for drug addiction as well as for other chronic diseases, the individual's motivation and behavior are clearly important parts of success in treatment and recovery.

Implications for treatment approaches and treatment expectations. Maintaining this comprehensive biobehavioral understanding of addiction also speaks to what needs to be provided in drug treatment programs. Again, we must be careful not to pit biology against behavior. The National Institute on Drug Abuse's recently published Principles of Effective Drug Addiction Treatment provides a detailed discussion of how we must treat all aspects of the individual, not just the biological component or the behavioral component. As with other brain diseases such as schizophrenia and depression, the data show that the best drug addiction treatment approaches attend to the entire individual, combining the use of medications, behavioral therapies, and attention to necessary social services and rehabilitation. These might include such services as family therapy to enable the patient to return to successful family life, mental health services, education and vocational training, and housing services.

That does not mean, of course, that all individuals need all components of treatment and all rehabilitation services. Another principle of effective addiction treatment is that the array of services included in an individual's treatment plan must be matched to his or her particular set of needs. Moreover, since those needs will surely change over the course of recovery, the array of services provided will need to be continually reassessed and adjusted.

What to do with addicted criminal offenders. One obvious conclusion is that we need to stop simplistically viewing criminal justice and health approaches as incompatible opposites. The practical reality is that crime and drug addiction often occur in tandem: Between 50 and 70 percent of arrestees are addicted to illegal drugs. Few citizens would be willing to relinquish criminal justice system control over individuals, whether they are addicted or not, who have committed crimes against others. Moreover, extensive real-life experience shows that if we simply incarcerate addicted offenders without treating them, their return to both drug use and criminality is virtually guaranteed.

A growing body of scientific evidence points to a much more rational and effective blended public health/ public safety approach to dealing with the addicted offender. Simply summarized, the data show that if addicted offenders are provided with well-structured drug treatment while under criminal justice control, their recidivism rates can be reduced by 50 to 60 percent for subsequent drug use and by more than 40 percent for further criminal behavior. Moreover, entry into drug treatment need not be completely voluntary in order for it to work. In fact, studies suggest that increased pressure to stay in treatment—whether from the legal system or from family members or employers—actually increases the amount of time patients remain in treatment and improves their treatment outcomes.

Findings such as these are the underpinning of a very important trend in drug control strategies now being implemented in the United States and many foreign countries. For example, some 40 percent of prisons and jails in this country now claim to provide some form of drug treatment to their addicted inmates, although we do not know the quality of the treatment provided. Diversion to drug treatment programs as an alternative to incarceration is gaining popularity across the United States. The widely applauded growth in drug treatment courts over the past five years—to more than 400—is another successful example of the blending of public health and public safety approaches. These drug courts use a combination of criminal justice sanctions and drug use monitoring and treatment tools to manage addicted offenders.

Updating the Discussion

Understanding drug abuse and addiction in all their complexity demands that we rise above simplistic polarized thinking about drug issues. Addiction is both a public health and a public safety issue, not one or the other. We must deal with both the supply and the demand issues with equal vigor. Drug abuse and addiction are about both biology and behavior. One can have a disease and not be a hapless victim of it.

We also need to abandon our attraction to simplistic metaphors that only distract us from developing appropriate strategies. I, for one, will be in some ways sorry to see the War on Drugs metaphor go away, but go away it must. At some level, the notion of waging war is as appropriate for the illness of addiction as it is for our War on Cancer, which simply means bringing all forces to bear on the problem in a focused and energized way. But, sadly, this concept has been badly distorted and misused over time, and the War on Drugs never became what it should have been: the War on Drug Abuse and Addiction. Moreover, worrying about whether we are winning or losing this war has deteriorated to using simplistic and inappropriate measures such as counting drug addicts. In the end, it has only fueled discord. The War on Drugs metaphor has done nothing to advance the real conceptual challenges that need to be worked through.

I hope, though, that we will all resist the temptation to replace it with another catchy phrase that inevitably will devolve into a search for quick or easy-seeming solutions to our drug problems. We do not rely on simple metaphors or strategies to deal with our other major national problems such as education, health care, or national security. We are, after all, trying to solve truly monumental, multidimensional problems on a national or even international scale. To devalue them to the level of slogans does our public an injustice and dooms us to failure.

Understanding the health aspects of addiction is in no way incompatible with the need to control the supply of drugs. In fact, a public health approach to stemming an epidemic or spread of a disease always focuses comprehensively on the agent, the vector, and the host. In the case of drugs of abuse, the agent is the drug, the host is the abuser or addict, and the vector for transmitting the illness is clearly the drug suppliers and dealers that keep the agent flowing so readily. Prevention and treatment are the strategies to help protect the host. But just as we must deal with the flies and mosquitoes that spread infectious diseases, we must directly address all the vectors in the drug-supply system.

In order to be truly effective, the blended public health/public safety approaches advocated here must be implemented at all levels of society—local, state, and national. All drug problems are ultimately local in character and impact, since they differ so much across geographic settings and cultural contexts, and the most effective solutions are implemented at the local level. Each community must work through its own locally appropriate antidrug implementation strategies, and those strategies must be just as comprehensive and science-based as those instituted at the state or national level.

The message from the now very broad and deep array of scientific evidence is absolutely clear. If we as a society ever hope to make any real progress in dealing with our drug problems, we are going to have to rise above moral outrage that addicts have "done it to themselves" and develop strategies that are as sophisticated and as complex as the problem itself. Whether addicts are "victims" or not, once addicted they must be seen as "brain disease patients."

Moreover, although our national traditions do argue for compassion for those who are sick, no matter how they contracted their illnesses, I recognize that many addicts have disrupted not only their own lives but those of their families and their broader communities, and thus do not easily generate compassion. However, no matter how one may feel about addicts and their behavioral histories, an extensive body of scientific evidence shows that approaching addiction as a treatable illness is extremely cost-effective, both financially and in terms of broader societal impacts such as family violence, crime, and other forms of social upheaval. Thus, it is clearly in everyone's interest to get past the hurt and indignation and slow the drain of drugs on society by enhancing drug use prevention efforts and providing treatment to all who need it.

ALAN I. LESHNER is the director of the National Institute on Drug Abuse.

Alva Noë   ➜ **NO**

Addiction Is Not a Disease of the Brain

Addiction has been moralized, medicalized, politicized, and criminalized.

And, of course, many of us are addicts, have been addicts or have been close to addicts. Addiction runs very hot as a theme.

Part of what makes addiction so compelling is that it forms a kind of conceptual/political crossroads for thinking about human nature. After all, to make sense of addiction we need to make sense of what it is to be an agent who acts, with values, in the face of consequences, under pressure, with compulsion, out of need and desire. One needs a whole philosophy to understand addiction.

Today I want to respond to readers who were outraged by my willingness even to question whether addiction is a disease of the brain.

Let us first ask: what makes something—a substance or an activity—addictive? Is there a property shared by all the things to which we can get addicted?

Unlikely. Addictive substances such as alcohol, heroin and nicotine are chemically distinct. Moreover, activities such as gambling, eating, sex—activities that are widely believed to be addictive—have no ingredients.

And yet it is remarkable—as Gene Heyman notes in his excellent book on addiction—that there are only 20 or so distinct activities and substances that produce addiction. There must be something in virtue of which these things, and these things alone, give rise to the distinctive pattern of use and abuse in the face of the medical, personal and legal perils that we know can stem from addiction.

What do gambling, sex, heroin and cocaine—and the other things that can addict us—have in common?

One strategy is to look not to the substances and activities themselves, but to the effects that they produce in addicts. And here neuroscience has delivered important insights.

If you feed an electrical wire through a rat's skull and onto to a short dopamine release circuit that connects the VTA (ventral tegmental area) and the nucleus accumbens, and if you attach that wire to a lever-press, the rat will self-stimulate—press the lever to produce the increase in dopamine—and it will do so basically forever, forgoing food, sex, water and exercise. Addiction, it would seem, is produced by direct action on the brain!

And indeed, there is now a substantial body of evidence supporting the claim that all drugs or activities of abuse (as we can call them) have precisely this kind of effect on this dopamine neurochemical circuit.

When the American Society of Addiction Medicine recently declared addiction to be a brain disease their conclusion was based on findings like this. Addiction is an effect brought about in a neurochemical circuit in the brain. If true, this is important, for it means that if you want to treat addiction, you need to find ways to act on this neural substrate.

All the rest—the actual gambling or drug taking, the highs and lows, the stealing, lying and covering up, the indifference to work and incompetence in the workplace, the self-loathing and anxiety about getting high, or getting discovered, or about trying to stop, and the loss of friends and family, the life stories and personal and social pressures—all these are merely symptoms of the underlying neurological disease.

But not so fast. Consider:

All addictive drugs and activities elevate the dopamine release system. Such activation, we may say, is a necessary condition of addiction. But it is very doubtful that it is sufficient. Neuroscientists refer to the system in question as the "reward-reinforcement pathway" precisely because all rewarding activities, including nonaddictive ones like reading the comics on Sunday morning or fixing the leaky pipe in the basement, modulate its activity. Elevated activity in the reward-reinforcement pathway is a normal concomitant of healthy, nonaddictive, engaged life.

Neuroscientists like to say that addictive drugs and activities, but not the nonaddictive ones, "highjack" the reward-reinforcement pathway, they don't merely activate it. This is the real upshot of the rat example. The rat preferred lever-pressing to everything; it dis-valued everything in comparison with lever-pressing. And not because

Noë, Alva. From 13.7: Cosmos & Culture, September 9, 2011. Copyright © 2011 by Alva Noë. Reprinted by permission of Alva Noë and NPR. www.npr.org/blogs/13.7/2010/05/21/127029133/about-13-7-cosmos-and-culture

of the intrinsic value of lever-pressing, but because of the link artificially established between the lever-pressing and the dopamine release.

If this is right, then we haven't discovered, in the reward reinforcement system, a neurochemical signature of addiction. We haven't discovered the place where addiction happens in the brain. After all, the so-called high-jacking of the reward system is not itself a neurochemical process; it is a process whereby neurochemical events get entrained within in a larger pattern of action and decision making.

Is addiction a disease of the brain? That's a bit like saying that eating is a phenomenon of the stomach. The stomach is an important part of the story. But don't forget the mouth, the intestines, the blood, and don't forget the hunger, and also the whole socially-sustained practice of producing, shopping for and cooking food.

And so with addiction. The neural events in VTA clearly belong to the underlying mechanisms of addiction. They are necessary, but not sufficient; they are only part of the story.

Remember: normally there is a dynamic quality to our actions and preferences, just as there is with those of rats. We enjoy exercising, but we soon get tired or bored. But rest, too, soon loses its appeal. We eat, and then we are sated. And then we are ready for the treadmill again. And so on. Things have gradually changing and complementary values. In addiction, this dynamic goes rigid. The addict's goal assumes a fixed value, and the value of everything shrinks to zero, and with terrible costs.

Our strategy was to look for systematic effects that all and only the addictive drugs and activities have on addicts. And we've found what we were looking for. The effects are behavioral and experiential. The things that addict us all produce a very distinctive breakdown in the organization of our preferences, actions and choices.

Is addiction a disease of the brain? This strikes me as a dubious falsification of what is, really, a phenomenon that can only be understood in terms of the life choices, needs and understanding of the whole person.

ALVA NOË is a professor of philosophy at the University of California, Berkeley. The main focus of his work is the theory of perception and consciousness. He earned a PhD from Harvard University.

EXPLORING THE ISSUE

Should Addiction to Drugs Be Labeled a Brain Disease?

Critical Thinking and Reflection

1. What are the root causes of drug and alcohol addiction?
2. What are the benefits to labeling addiction a brain disease?
3. Why could it be harmful to label addiction a brain disease?
4. Describe the types of treatment for alcohol and drug addiction.

Is There Common Ground?

One of the most valuable aspects of labeling addiction a disease is that it removes alcohol and drugs from the moral realm. It is proposed that addiction sufferers should be treated and helped, rather than scorned and punished. Though the moral model of addiction has by no means disappeared in the United States, today more resources are directed toward rehabilitation than punishment. Increasingly, it is being recognized and understood that fines, victim-blaming, and imprisonment do little to curb alcohol and drug addiction in society.

An article, "New Insights into the Genetics of Addiction" (*Nature Reviews Genetics*, April 2009) indicates that genetics contributes significantly to susceptibility to this disorder, but identification of vulnerable genes has lagged. In "It's Time for Addiction Science to Supersede Stigma" (*Science News*, November 8, 2009), the author discusses advances made in the scientific community in studying *addictions*, and says that people should regard drug addicts the same they regard other people with *brain diseases*. To do this, it should be recognized that *addictions* are a form of *brain disease*, and rather than blaming people for becoming addicted, energy should be spent on finding solutions.

Critics argue, however, that this belief either under-emphasizes or ignores the impact of self-control, learned behaviors, and many other factors which lead to alcohol and drug abuse. Furthermore, most treatment programs in the United States are based on the concept of addiction as a brain disease, and most are considered to be generally ineffective when judged by their high relapse rates. Many researchers claim that advances in neuroscience are changing the way mental health issues such as addiction are understood and addressed as brain diseases. While calling addiction a brain disease and medical condition legitimizes it, many scientists do not completely support this model.

It appears that the causes of addiction are complex and that brain, mind, and behavioral specialists are rethinking the whole notion of addiction. With input from neuroscience, biology, pharmacology, psychology, and genetics, they're questioning assumptions and identifying some common characteristics among addicts, which will, it is hoped, improve treatment outcomes and even prevent people from using drugs in the first place.

Additional Resources

Alavi, S., Ferdosi, M., Jannatifard, F., Eslami, M., Alaghemandan, H., & Setare, M. (2012). Behavioral addiction versus substance addiction: Correspondence of psychiatric and psychological views. *International Journal of Preventive Medicine, 3*(4), 290–294.

Campbell, M. (2015). Ten ethical failings in addiction treatment. *Alcoholism & Drug Abuse Weekly, 27*(10), 5–6.

Elam, M. (2015). How the brain disease paradigm remoralizes addictive behaviour. *Science as Culture, 24*(1), 46–64.

Karim, R., & Chaudhri, P. (2012). Behavioral addictions: An overview. *Journal of Psychoactive Drugs, 44*(1), 5–17.

Vrecko, S. (2010). Birth of a brain disease: Science, the state and addiction neuropolitics. *History of the Human Sciences, 23*(4), 52–67.

Internet References . . .

American Psychological Association (APA)

www.apa.org

National Institutes of Health: National Institute on Drug Abuse

www.drugabuse.gov/nidahome.html

Web of Addictions

www.well.com/user/woa

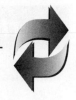

Selected, Edited, and with Issue Framing Material by:
Eileen L. Daniel, *SUNY College at Brockport*

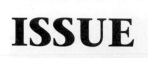

ISSUE

Do Religion and Prayer Benefit Health?

YES: **Thomas J. Cottle**, from "Our Thoughts and Our Prayers," *The Antioch Review* (2006)

NO: **Michael Shermer**, from "Prayer and Healing: The Verdict Is In and the Results Are Null," *Skeptic* (2006)

Learning Outcomes
After reading this issue, you will be able to:
• Discuss the benefits of prayer for those suffering from an illness.   • Discuss the argument that the relationship between prayer and health cannot adequately be measured.   • Discuss the ways in which prayer could be used as part of a treatment program.

ISSUE SUMMARY

YES: Psychologist and educator Thomas J. Cottle believes that prayer can fill patients with a spirit of security when confronted with illness.

NO: Author Michael Shermer contends that intercessory prayer offered by strangers on the health and recovery of patients undergoing coronary bypass surgery is ineffective. He also addresses flaws in studies showing a relationship between prayer and health.

Practitioners of holistic medicine believe that people must take responsibility for their own health by practicing healthy behaviors and maintaining positive attitudes instead of relying on health providers. They also believe that physical disease has behavioral, psychological, and spiritual components. These spiritual components can be explained by the relationship between beliefs, mental attitude, and the immune system. Until recently, few studies existed to prove a relationship between religion and health.

Much of modern medicine has spent the past century ridding itself of mysticism and relying on science. Twenty years ago, no legitimate physician would have dared to study the effects of religion on disease. Recently, however, at the California Pacific Medical Center in San Francisco, California, Elisabeth Targ, clinical director of psychosocial oncology research, has recruited 20 faith healers to determine if prayer can affect the outcome of disease. Targ states that her preliminary results are encouraging. In addition to Targ's study, other research has shown that religion and spirituality can help determine health and well-being. According to a 1995 investigation at Dartmouth College, one of the strongest predictors of success after open-heart surgery was the level of comfort patients derived from religion and spirituality. Other recent studies have linked health with church attendance, religious commitment, and spirituality. There are, however, other studies that have not been as successful; a recent one involving the effects of prayer on alcoholics found no relationship.

Can spirituality or prayer in relation to health and healing be explained scientifically? Prayer or a sense of spirituality may function in a similar manner as stress management or relaxation. Spirituality or prayer may cause the release of hormones that help lower blood pressure or produce other benefits. Although science may never be able to exactly determine the benefits of spirituality, it does appear to help some people.

In the YES and NO selections, Thomas J. Cottle states that prayer can have a significant influence over the body. Michael Shermer argues that religious prayer does not heal the sick and the studies showing the relationship between religion and healing are flawed.

YES ↩

Thomas J. Cottle

Our Thoughts and Our Prayers

Little grates on me as much as the clichés hurled again and again on television. Families in mourning have to hear about this closure business, whatever it means. Or those ubiquitous questions, When you heard that your parents had died, what was going through your mind? When the flood destroyed your community, what was that like?

Another one that has always rankled me is the predictable statement following the announcement of a death: "Our thoughts and prayers go out to the families." One would think that intelligent people could come up with something more thoughtful, sensitive, caring. But then the words were addressed to me.

I felt obliged to tell a patient of mine that I would have to call him regarding our next appointment as I was about to undergo surgery and didn't know how long a recuperation period I was facing. Seemingly without thinking, he looked at me and said softly, "I'll pray for you, Doc." His words had no sooner filled the air than I felt the tears. Apparently, the prayers of this man were exactly what I wanted. A devout Catholic tells me, a Jew, he will pray for me, and at once I am filled with some peculiar spirit of security, or is it a release from something? A release, perhaps, from a lifetime void of the spiritual? Normally I will think, pray what you wish, my friend, but just don't mention the name of your Lord. But this time that thought never emerged, and it was not because he was my patient; I had no desire to censure a single word, a single holy name. I felt filled up, somehow, with the mere statement that he would pray for me. And I have no idea what praying actually means, much less whether there really is something called a power that emanates from this activity.

In the hospital, on the morning following surgery, I obeyed orders and walked the floor. Around and around the nurses' station, pitiful laps in corridors that remind one of anything but a walking track. But it is here that one meets the other lap walkers, the other post-surgery folks. And the talk goes right to the heart of the medical matter, names rarely exchanged. This one has cells dying in his prostate, each cellular death causing exquisite pain. I ask about his PSA readings and hear a number that astonishes me; it is in the high fifties. I have a macabre urge to tell him if it gets to sixty he might want to sell. And this one, a strong looking man pushing an IV stand in front of him, was doing so well, even with a blood thinner issue from a previous cardiac condition threatening his surgery and recovery that the doctors sent him home. Three hours later he couldn't eliminate fluids and here he was back on the same floor, walking the track.

Then I met Sammy, a man in his early sixties who told me he had survived prostate cancer, colon cancer, and was living with diabetes. He had just been operated on yet again for another problem. Sammy is an educator, a father of six, a truly good man, and a man of God. "God is good," he said, seemingly a hundred times during our laps together. "He looks out for us; He has shaped the whole thing." Prostate cancer, colon cancer, diabetes, another operation, God is good. God was still good when later that first post-operative day Sammy suddenly couldn't eliminate fluids and had to be catheterized. Of course God was still good. The words are intended merely as a pronouncement of healing.

My assurance to Sammy that he was going to be fine paled next to his spiritually founded assurances. "God doesn't want me yet. Nor you. He wants you," Sammy said, "to keep educating people." And do you know, when he said those words, I believed him. I believed him not in the spirit of, well, you have to have faith in something and I don't see any rabbi with an enlarged prostate walking the corridor. I believed him as if a scientist had recited unalloyed scientific facts to me. Fact One: God doesn't want you. Fact Two: Water is two parts hydrogen, one part oxygen.

Sammy grew tired and I walked him to his room where slowly, laboriously, he climbed onto his bed. He knew I was there watching him. "I will come to you later," he whispered. "We'll pray together." Once again, I felt comforted. I wanted that praying together moment more than I wanted a sumptuous meal. I hoped he would remember his promise.

Americans, I have learned recently, pray a great deal. Seventy-seven percent of people pray outside of any religious service. Even people who don't believe in God pray. They may even pray all the time. Inexact, the numbers coming from a national poll, it is strange to think that so many people call themselves spiritual, not necessarily religious.

Two-thirds of the people in the poll said they pray because it makes them feel secure, comforted, hopeful. Whereas twenty-one percent reported that they pray they might possess material things, seventy-two percent pray for the well-being of others. Fewer people, actually, are attending religious services now that they are caught up in a strangling recession, but still they pray. "Our thoughts and prayers go out to the families."

The little I have read offers mixed reviews on the subject of whether praying for another actually makes a difference. Some research alleges that prayer is so powerful it affects even those who have no knowledge anyone is praying for them. Other research suggests that if you think it works then it works. And still other research cannot find a shred of evidence that prayer does anything other than gratify the person praying. I don't know what to think. No, that's not true; I do know one thing. I know my patient and Sammy prayed for me, believed in their prayers, and believed, moreover, that their prayers would help me, not just them. "I'll pray for you, Doc," and "I will come to your room and we will pray together," I choose to believe, were proffered as gifts, pure, simple gifts, one human to another. There wasn't a single shard of selfishness, I choose to believe, in either of these utterances.

Prayer, evidently, is about contemplation, philosophical, theological, personal. It is not about conversation. In some corners of the theological world, as, for example, in the mysticism of the Kabbalah, reality itself is meant to be altered, restructured by prayer. And if the universe, the very fabric of creation, is to be repaired by prayer, then why not the single self?

It is written by philosophers and psychologists that identity, whatever is meant by that term, is the *sine qua non* of human nature. Our subjective experiencing of the world, our so-called experiential knowledge, our ability to genuinely understand our own selves, much less have empathy for the selves of others, all are part of this identity business. Can we recognize our selves, psychologists ask, and is there some sub-set of experiences that makes us feel as though we are acting genuinely, or authentically?

Many people actually are able to describe that event or moment when they truly felt they had become the person they were meant to be. As Karl Jaspers wrote, these must be moments when they have a stake in what

is happening. It is not too different from the great drama that inevitably finds characters with huge stakes in the outcome of the plot. Perhaps it is in periods of illness, or recovery, when we beg—or is it pray?—to transform situations, transform reality, when we are most likely to turn to prayer. Perhaps we feel we are losing something, something appears to be slipping away from us, and all that is left is to redefine reality or turn to some activity that convinces us that we still maintain ownership of the situation. Needless to say, our self, or more accurately our sense of self, always remains center stage.

In a sense, the self is little more than a theory, or a narrative, that we constantly construct out of our thoughts and feelings, if in fact we can even separate these two activities. Ceaselessly, we look outside ourselves, often using people as mirrors, as Jacques Lacan wrote, and inside ourselves to formulate this mutable theory that appears to come to us replete with all sorts of assessments and testable hypotheses. Seemingly, we cannot inhibit our urge to make sense of our worlds, and our selves. Rollo May postulated that the notion of repression refers to an inability or unwillingness to become aware of our self, containing as it does our authentic potentials. In a word, if the self represents a mediator between a person and the situation in which he is embedded, like an illness, then perhaps prayer is the method of communication for this mediation.

But prayer seems to require another soul. It evokes in us that sense of needing to speak to someone, or at least know that someone might hear our entreaties. We wonder, perhaps, whether we are even entitled to have our thoughts and feelings if someone is no longer present to hear them. It is often through prayer that we imagine that we can shape some small piece of our reality and thereby regain a sense of worth, competence, or agency. In some instances, and I believe I experienced this, the prayer reminds me that I am still alive; there is still hope upon which to draw life. Dear Someone: Please let my narrative continue. Please let me know that even in illness I may remain somewhat recognizable. Dare I ask to be perceived as distinctive? Is anyone there?

We change, and the landscape changes, and rarely do we experience these changes more vividly than when we enter hospitals. Both our illness and the hospital setting encompass us. Here we are, precisely as Jaspers described, rooted in the world of illness and the treatment, a world that feels simultaneously surreal and infinitely practical. We reflect on it, we pray on it; we cannot deny the utterly real constituents of it. We are defined, in part, by our illness, by our healers, by technology, and by our abilities to draw from what Martha Nussbaum has called our narrative imaginations. Our personal stories, one might say, have taken unpredictable, albeit not wholly unfamiliar turns. We know these stories from others, and we perhaps have always dreaded the moment when these narratives would be about us.

Then suddenly we are members of a new club, a new totality, a new historic unity dominated ironically, not by fellow members, but by ideas. If Jaspers remains a reasonable guide, we have entered the spiritual mode of encompassing; we have entered the realm of the transcendent wherein we exist as beings beyond all objectivity. As I say, it is not unfamiliar territory to us; through art, morality, religion, fantasy, we have been here before. What makes this moment unique is that it has been launched by illness and surgical invasion.

In turning my body over to the surgeon, an act occurring, moreover, during a protracted period of unconsciousness that I shall not remember, I am acknowledging what is labeled the boundary experience. I cannot affect this experience; I cannot influence it. I am left only to suffer, struggle, and pray. I can make it lucid only to myself. No matter the fright, no matter the dread, I feel required to keep my eyes wide open, Sometimes I may achieve transcendence through knowledge, sometimes, as the existentialists write, I can only hope to grasp it through my being, for it forever lies outside my sphere of influence. The meanings are something other than myself, more than mere expressions of myself, more than mere projections of myself. They push me toward meanings outside of myself, like the meaning of death.

But to give life meaning, I must transcend the limits of my physical life, which means my illness and its attendant treatment. I cannot allow myself to once again become the adolescent wondering whether he might live forever. I cannot let myself grapple with that question of whether I will still be, somehow, after life. Or can I? I must recognize, however, that in transcendence, arrived at in part through prayer, I may just have urged my self to reach the core of authentic resilience. I convince myself that I am back creating a trajectory for my life. I am back at work on the narrative that was interrupted by illness, and my fright. Choice and will have been part of my activity, and hence through prayer I feel a certain sense that the power of agency has returned. Or is it that I experience agency as never before?

Thrown into the realm of the spiritual, I pray. One way or another, as Robert Kegan has written, I must make meaning of my illness and treatment, or at least find some context where I imagine, or pray, that a meaning may emerge. When the shallow life doesn't

work, Abraham Maslow taught, there occurs a call to fundamentals. But these fundamentals refer to the experience of being. Said simply, fundamentals make us aware of our very being, if we dare to cease our need to constantly evaluate or criticize, and instead remain vulnerable to the world around us, and within us. Prayer, somehow, aids in this effort.

So now I wonder, do I require these experiences, must I grow ill, must I face death, or the dread of it, merely to encounter the transcendent, and hence my real self? William James was right: these sorts of prayerful contemplations demand supreme mental effort. It isn't at all easy to insist that one's mind attend and hold fast to the boundary situation. It isn't easy to keep one's eyes wide open. How ironic that in some mysterious manner, I feel obliged to close my eyes in prayer in order to achieve a state of mind that will allow me to reopen them. It has become evident that my praying is also a way of offering consent to a particular reality. It is the best I can do, apparently, in wishing to become heroic. Through prayer I imagine that I have launched myself into what Carl Rogers called the stream of life. I have chosen not to surrender, but to become. Which in part means that I am not shaped even by seemingly implacable reality. Prayer, I have convinced myself, is not merely a coping mechanism; it is a mode of being that protects me. It ignites resilience.

The self, Robert Nozick wrote, is in part constituted by its process of change. It is not simply influenced by the world; it changes and ignites changes and then appears to run itself according to these changes. In a word, it dwells in its own capacity to change. Nozick believed that we aim our selves at developing themselves. We long to have our deepest parts connect with, or at least resonate to, what we imagine to be the highest things there are, thereby rendering us the highest things that we can be. This may very well be what we seek through prayer, realizing it is only the medium of prayer that will yield this prize. In fact, we may well be performing at the highest level, and hence feel in touch with our most authentic self precisely when we experience the resiliency of transcendence offered up by prayer. For it is in this act of prayer that we imagine we have reached the highest order of our narratives, and hence confronted the outline of the divine. How precious, therefore, the opportunity provided by adversity.

Sammy did remember. I stopped by his room, the light dim, the ambience antiseptic. He struggled to get out of bed disregarding my protestation. Near the door, he put his arm over my shoulder, held me close, and closed his eyes. I put my arm around his big back, feeling his skin through the opening in his hospital gown. I can't remember, precisely, what he asked of his Lord, but clearly he was urging a power he so trusts to look out for a man he had met, what, three hours before. He was petitioning God, entreating God in my behalf. As he spoke, I wondered how I would react when, ineluctably, he would speak the name of his God. And then I stopped wondering and let his words, how I dread this phrase, flow into me. "I ask this for Tom in the spirit of our Lord Jesus Christ."

We just stood there, the door to the corridor wide open, holding one another. I think I probably was praying, pitiful as it sounds, that his prayers, his acts of interceding, would make a difference. Probably I was praying that I needed his words to heal me as badly as I needed the skills and demonstration of care from the surgeon, residents, and nurses. Count me among the two-thirds of the people in the poll who said they pray because it makes them feel secure, comforted, hopeful. Perhaps I should worship the God Sammy.

But now, as I end, I fear that it can be said that my words here contain clichés as jaded and empty as "Our thoughts and prayers go out to the families." Still, I choose to believe, once again, that both Sammy and my patient clearly considered their prayers to be the most powerful acts they could perform in my behalf. Not because they were founded in religion, nor in ritualistic behavior that has been emulated for centuries, but because, in the same way that blood carries oxygen to the cells, prayers carry love to and from the soul. In fact, merely to open myself to my patient and Sammy was to give permission to entreat my own soul to be acknowledged, then nourished. And yes, I did notice that I commenced a sentence that prayer opens the soul with the words *in fact*.

THOMAS J. COTTLE is a sociologist and licensed clinical psychologist and professor of education at Boston University. He holds a PhD from the University of Chicago.

Michael Shermer

➡ **NO**

Prayer and Healing: The Verdict Is In and the Results Are Null

In a long-awaited comprehensive scientific study on the effects of intercessory prayer on the health and recovery of 1,802 patients undergoing coronary bypass surgery in six different hospitals, prayers offered by strangers had no effect. In fact, contrary to common belief, patients who knew they were being prayed for had a higher rate of post-operative complications such as abnormal heart rhythms, possibly the result of anxiety caused by learning that they were being prayed for and thus their condition was more serious than anticipated.

The study, which cost $2.4 million (most of which came from the John Templeton Foundation), was begun almost a decade ago and was directed by Harvard University Medical School cardiologist Dr. Herbert Benson and published in *The American Heart Journal*. It was by far the most rigorous and comprehensive study on the effects of intercessory prayer on the health and recovery of patients ever conducted. In addition to the numerous methodological flaws in the previous research corrected for in the Benson study, Dr. Richard Sloan, a professor of behavioral medicine at Columbia and author of the forthcoming book, *Blind Faith: The Unholy Alliance of Religion and Medicine*, explained: "The problem with studying religion scientifically is that you do violence to the phenomenon by reducing it to basic elements that can be quantified, and that makes for bad science and bad religion."

The 1,802 patients were divided into three groups, two of which were prayed for by members of three congregations: St. Paul's Monastery in St. Paul, MN; the Community of Teresian Carmelites in Worcester, MA; and Silent Unity, a Missouri prayer ministry near Kansas City, MO. The prayers were allowed to pray in their own manner, but they were instructed to include the following phrase in their prayers: "for a successful surgery with a quick, healthy recovery and no complications." Prayers began the night before the surgery and continued daily for two weeks after. Half the prayer-recipient patients were told that they were being prayed for while the other half were told that they

might or might not receive prayers. The researchers monitored the patients for 30 days after the operations.

Results showed no statistically significant differences between the prayed-for and non-prayed-for groups. Although the following findings were not statistically significant, 59% of patients who knew that they were being prayed for suffered complications, compared with 51% of those who were uncertain whether they were being prayed for or not; and 18% in the uninformed prayer group suffered major complications such as heart attack or stroke, compared with 13% in the group that received no prayers.

This study is particularly significant because Herbert Benson has long been sympathetic to the possibility that intercessory prayer can positively influence the health of patients. His team's rigorous methodologies overcame the numerous flaws that called into question previously published studies. The most commonly cited study in support of the connection between prayer and healing is Randolph C. Byrd's "Positive Therapeutic Effects of Intercessory Prayer in a Coronary Care Unit Population," *Southern Medical Journal* 81 (1998): 826–829. The two best studies on the methodological problems with prayer and healing are the following: Richard Sloan, E. Bagiella, and T. Powell, 1999. "Religion, Spirituality, and Medicine," *The Lancet*, Feb. 20, Vol. 353: 664–667; and: John T. Chibnall, Joseph M. Jeral, Michael Cerullo, 2001. "Experiments on Distant Intercessory Prayer," *Archives of Internal Medicine*, Nov. 26, Vol. 161: 2529–2536. . . .

The Most Significant Flaws in All Such Studies Include the Following:

1. *Fraud.* In 2001, the *Journal of Reproductive Medicine* published a study by three Columbia University researchers claiming that prayer for women undergoing in-vitro fertilization resulted in a pregnancy rate of 50%, double that of women who did not receive prayer. Media

coverage was extensive. ABC News medical correspondent Dr. Timothy Johnson, for example, reported, "A new study on the power of prayer over pregnancy reports surprising results; but many physicians remain skeptical." One of those skeptics was University of California Clinical Professor of Gynecology and Obstetrics Bruce Flamm, who not only found numerous methodological errors in the experiment, but also discovered that one of the study's authors, Daniel Wirth (AKA "John Wayne Truelove"), is not an M.D., but an M.S. in parapsychology who has since been indicted on felony charges for mail fraud and theft, for which he pleaded guilty. The other two authors have refused comment, and after three years of inquiries from Flamm the journal removed the study from its website and Columbia University has launched an investigation.

2. *Lack of Controls.* Many of these studies failed to control for such intervening variables as age, sex, education, ethnicity, socioeconomic status, marital standing, degree of religiosity, and the fact that most religions have sanctions against such behaviors as sexual promiscuity, alcohol and drug abuse, and smoking. When such variables are controlled for, the formerly significant results disappear. One study on recovery from hip surgery in elderly women failed to control for age; another study on church attendance and illness recovery did not consider that people in poorer health are less likely to attend church; a related study failed to control for levels of exercise.

3. *Outcome differences.* In one of the most highly publicized studies of cardiac patients prayed for by born-again Christians, 29 outcome variables were measured but on only six did the prayed-for group show improvement. In related studies, different outcome measures were significant. To be meaningful, the same measures need to be significant across studies, because if enough outcomes are measured some will show significant correlations by chance.

4. *Selective Reporting.* In several studies on the relationship between religiosity and mortality (religious people allegedly live longer), a number of religious variables were used, but only those with significant correlations were reported. Meanwhile, other studies using the same religiosity variables found different correlations and, of course, only reported those. The rest were filed away in the drawer of non-significant findings. When all variables are factored in together, religiosity and mortality show no relationship.

5. *Operational definitions.* When experimenting on the effects of prayer, what, precisely, is being studied? For example, what type of prayer is being employed? (Are Christian, Jewish, Muslim, Buddhist, Wiccan, and Shaman prayers equal?) Who or what is being prayed to? (Are God, Jesus, and a universal life force equivalent?) What is the length and frequency of the prayer? (Are two 10-minute prayers equal to one 20-minute prayer?) How many people are praying and does their status in the religion matter? (Is one priestly prayer identical to ten parishioner prayers?) Most prayer studies either lack such operational definitions, or there is no consistency across studies in such definitions.

6. *Theological implications.* The ultimate flaw in all such studies is theological. If God is omniscient and omnipotent why should he need to be reminded or inveigled that someone needs healing? Scientific prayer makes God a celestial lab rat, leading to bad science and worse religion.

MICHAEL SHERMER is a science writer and the editor-in-chief of *Skeptic*.

EXPLORING THE ISSUE

Do Religion and Prayer Benefit Health?

Critical Thinking and Reflection

1. Why is scientifically measuring the impact of prayer so challenging?
2. Describe possible mechanisms in which prayer and religion may benefit health.
3. What might be the downside of relying on prayer for healing?

Is There Common Ground?

Can we influence the course of our own illnesses? Can emotions, stress management, and prayer prevent or cure disease? In a telephone poll of 1,004 Americans conducted by *Time*/CNN in June 1996, 82 percent indicated that they believed in the healing power of personal prayer. Three-fourths felt that praying for someone else could help cure their illness. Interestingly, fewer than two-thirds of doctors say they believe in God. Benson, who developed the "relaxation response," thinks there is a strong link between religious commitment and good health. He contends that people do not have to have a professed belief in God to reap the psychological and physical rewards of the "faith factor."

Benson defined the faith factor as the combined force of the relaxation response and the placebo effect. In "God at the Bedside" (*New England Journal of Medicine*, March 18, 2004), physician Jerome Groopman is asked by a patient to pray for her after receiving a diagnosis of cancer. Dr. Groopman, although religious, considers prayer and religion a private matter. He debated over whether or not he should sidestep the patient's request or should he cross a boundary from the purely professional to the personal and join her in prayer. The article addresses his solution to dealing with this difficult issue.

Dr. Bernard Siegel, writing in his bestseller *Love, Medicine and Miracles* (Harper & Row, 1986), argues that there are no "incurable diseases, only incurable people" and that illness is a personality flaw. In "Welcome to the Mind/Body Revolution," *Psychology Today* (July/August 1993), author Marc Barash further discusses how the mind and immune system influence each other. The journal *Social Science and Medicine* published a literature review in July 2006 entitled "Do Religious/Spiritual Coping Strategies Affect Illness Adjustment in Patients with Cancer? A Systematic Review of the Literature." The study found mixed results. Some researchers determined that religion influenced the outcome of disease while other did not. The authors also found that many of the studies showed methodological flaws, echoed by Michael Shermer. Mixed results were also found in a study that reviewed the effects of prayer on coping after open heart surgery. The authors determined that despite the growing evidence for effects of religious factors on cardiac health, findings are not always consistent, especially among older and sicker populations. See "Long Term Adjustment After Surviving Open Heart Surgery: The Effect of Using Prayer for Coping Replicated in a Prospective Design," *Gerontologist*, December 2010.

In *You Don't Have to Die: Unraveling the AIDS Myth* (Burton Goldberg Group, 1994), a chapter entitled "Mind-Body Medicine" discusses the body's innate healing capabilities and the role of self-responsibility in the healing process. A long-term AIDS survivor who traveled the country interviewing other long-term survivors found that the one thing they all shared was the belief that AIDS was survivable. They all also accepted the reality of their diagnosis but refused to see their condition as a death sentence.

Additional Resources

Güthlin, C., Anton, A., Kruse, J., & Walach, H. (2012). Subjective concepts of chronically ill patients using distant healing. *Qualitative Health Research*, *22*(3), 320–331.

Mouch, C., & Sonnega, A. (2012). Spirituality and recovery from cardiac surgery: A review. *Journal of Religion & Health*, *51*(4), 1042–1060.

Park, C., Lim, H., Newlon, M., Suresh, D., & Bliss, D. (2014). Dimensions of religiousness and spirituality as predictors of well-being in advanced chronic heart failure patients. *Journal of Religion & Health*, *53*(2), 579–590.

Poloma, M. M. (2012). Testing prayer: Science and healing. *Journal for the Scientific Study of Religion,* *51*(4), 825–827.

Stewart, M. (2014). Spiritual assessment: A patient-centered approach to oncology social work practice. *Social Work in Health Care, 53*(1), 59–73.

Internet References . . .

Ethics in Medicine: Spirituality and Medicine

http://eduserv.hscer.Washington.edu/bioethics/topics/spirit.html

MedScape: The Online Resource for Better Patient Care

www.medscape.com

WebMD

www.webmd.com/balance/features/can-prayer-heal

Unit 4

UNIT

Sexuality and Gender Issues

*F*ew issues could be of greater controversy than those concerning gender and sexuality. Recent generations of Americans have rejected "traditional" sexual roles and values, which has resulted in more opportunities and great equality for women. On the other hand, societal changes have seen a significant increase in babies born out of wedlock, babies born to increasingly older parents, the spread of sexually transmitted diseases, and a rise in legal abortions. Many of these issues such as abortion, birth control, and right to life versus pro–choice remain controversial and may never be fully resolved. This section addresses many of the concerns associated with sexuality, gender, and health.

Selected, Edited, and with Issue Framing Material by:
Eileen L. Daniel, *SUNY College at Brockport*

ISSUE

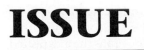

Is It Necessary for Pregnant Women to Completely Abstain from All Alcoholic Beverages?

YES: National Organization on Fetal Alcohol Syndrome, from "Is It Completely Safe and Risk-Free to Drink a Little Alcohol While Pregnant, Such as a Glass of Wine?" *nofas.org* (2013)

NO: Emily Oster, from "I Wrote That It's OK to Drink While Pregnant. Everyone Freaked Out. Here's Why I'm Right," *slate.com* (2013)

Learning Outcomes

After reading this issue, you will be able to:

- Discuss the risks associated with alcohol consumption during pregnancy.
- Discuss the characteristics of fetal alcohol syndrome.
- Assess the argument that limited amounts of alcohol during pregnancy may not be harmful to the child.

ISSUE SUMMARY

YES: The National Organization on Fetal Alcohol Syndrome provides evidence that even moderate quantities of alcohol can damage a developing fetus and cites new research indicating that even small amounts of alcoholic beverages consumed during pregnancy may be harmful.

NO: Economics professor Emily Oster argues that there are almost no studies on the effects of moderate drinking during pregnancy and that small amounts of alcohol are unlikely to have much effect.

In 1973, a paper was published in the British medical journal *The Lancet*. It described a pattern of birth defects that occurred among children born of alcoholic women and was called "fetal alcohol syndrome" or FAS ("Recognition of the Fetal Alcohol Syndrome in Early Infancy," *Lancet,* vol. 2, 1973). Since that time, thousands of studies have supported the relationship between heavy alcohol consumption during pregnancy and resulting birth defects. One controversial point related to FAS, however, is the amount of alcohol that must be consumed to cause danger to the developing baby. It seems that some threshold must exist though it's unclear what that is.

In their 1973 study, Jones and Smith correlated FAS only among children born to alcohol-abusing women. While the researchers were successful in bringing the syndrome to international attention, it also created apprehension that any amount of alcohol consumption during pregnancy could cause danger to the child. Many doctors and researchers believe that even minute levels of alcohol intake during pregnancy can cause FAS, resulting in a panic that may have exaggerated the dangers of *any* consumption.

Fortunately, FAS is relatively uncommon, though the United States has one of the highest rates in the developed world. This may be related to the pattern of alcohol consumption in this country. In many European countries, alcohol is often consumed daily, whereas in the United States alcohol intake is more confined to weekends. This results in higher blood alcohol levels on those days. In addition, there are other variables that increase the risk of FAS that cannot be linked solely to the amount of alcohol consumed. For example, women who binge drink are much more likely to bear children with the pattern of birth defects linked to FAS than women who consume the same total amount of alcohol over a period of time. In addition to binge drinking, a pregnant woman's health is another significant factor. Women who bear children with FAS often have liver disease and nutritional deficiencies including anemia, infections, and other conditions that exacerbate alcohol's effects on the fetus. Older mothers and those who have given birth to several children are also at greater risk to have children with FAS. While binge drinking, other health issues, and age are important risk factors, the two most significant conditions along with alcohol consumption are low income and cigarette smoking. Low income is related to poor diet, smoking and other drug use, and exposure to pollutants such as lead. Smoking is also a factor in FAS because it contains toxins that reduce blood flow and level of oxygen available to the fetus.

While it appears that heavy alcohol consumption, particularly binge drinking, combined with smoking, poor diet, low income, and concomitant health problems increase the risk of FAS, is there an absolutely safe level of consumption during pregnancy? Two recent studies suggest that alcohol use during pregnancy may be more dangerous for the child than previously thought. In one study, researchers found symptoms of FAS in children whose mothers drank two drinks per day at certain stages of pregnancy. The children born of these women were found to be unusually small and/or had learning or behavioral problems. The researchers also found other defects associated with FAS at a higher rate than expected ("Epidemiology of FASD in a Province in Italy: Prevalence and Characteristics of Children in a Random Sample of Schools," *Alcoholism: Clinical and Experimental Research,* September 2006). A second study confirmed that FAS is not the only concern associated with alcohol consumption during pregnancy. It's also a risk factor for alcohol abuse among the children born of these women ("In Utero Alcohol Exposure and Prediction of Alcohol Disorders in Early Adulthood: A Birth Cohort Study," *Archives of General Psychiatry,* September 2006).

It's apparent that heavy use of alcohol during pregnancy increases the risk of FAS. What is unclear is the risk associated with any amount of alcohol. A 25-year study of babies born to mother who were social drinkers found that even low intakes of alcohol had measurable effects on their babies. The study concluded that no minimum level of drinking was absolutely safe. See "When Two Drinks Are Too Many," *Psychology Today,* May/June 2004.

The following two selections address whether it is safe for pregnant women to drink during pregnancy. The National Organization on Fetal Alcohol Syndrome argues that even a small amount of alcohol can damage a developing fetus and cites new research that indicates that moderate consumption of alcoholic beverages during pregnancy may be harmful and that it's safer to avoid drinking.

Economics professor Emily Oster counters that there are almost no studies on the effects of moderate drinking during pregnancy and that small amounts of alcohol consumed during pregnancy are unlikely to have much harmful effect.

YES ↵

National Organization on Fetal Alcohol Syndrome

Is It Completely Safe and Risk-Free to Drink a Little Alcohol While Pregnant, Such as a Glass of Wine?

No. According to the CDC and the U.S. Surgeon General, "There is no known safe amount of alcohol to drink while pregnant. There is also no safe time during pregnancy to drink and no safe kind of alcohol." According to the American Academy of Pediatrics: "There is no safe amount of alcohol when a woman is pregnant. Research evidence is that even drinking small amounts of alcohol while pregnant can lead to miscarriage, stillbirth, prematurity, or sudden infant death syndrome."

When you drink alcohol, so does your developing baby. Any amount of alcohol, even in one glass of wine, passes through the placenta from the mother to the growing baby. Developing babies lack the ability to process, or metabolize, alcohol through the liver or other organs. They absorb all of the alcohol and have the same blood alcohol concentration as the mother. It makes no difference if the alcoholic drink consumed is a distilled spirit or liquor such as vodka, beer, or wine.

Alcohol is a teratogen, a toxic substance to a developing baby, and can interfere with healthy development causing brain damage and other birth defects. Most babies negatively affected by alcohol exposure have no physical birth defects. These children have subtle behavioral and learning problems that are often undiagnosed or misdiagnosed as Autism or Attention Deficit Disorder instead of one of the Fetal Alcohol Spectrum Disorders.

If you know a woman who is having difficulty abstaining from alcohol, the NOFAS mentoring network, The Circle of Hope, helps and supports women who have used alcohol or illicit drugs while pregnant.

Medical Studies

Several research studies available through the Collaborative Initiative on FASD (CIFASD):

The University of Queensland, 2013. This study finds "women who regularly drink as little as two glasses of wine per drinking session while pregnant can adversely impact their child's results at school."

Alcoholism: Clinical and Experimental Research, 2012. The study concludes, "Reduced birth length and weight, microcephaly, smooth philtrum, and thin vermillion border are associated with specific gestational timing of prenatal alcohol exposure and are dose-related without evidence of a threshold. Women should continue to be advised to abstain from alcohol consumption from conception throughout pregnancy."

International Journal of Epidemiology, 2012. This study states, "Even low amounts of alcohol consumption during early pregnancy increased the risk of spontaneous abortion substantially."

Alcohol Research & Health, 2011. This study found that drinking at low to moderate levels during pregnancy is associated with miscarriage, stillbirth, preterm delivery, and sudden infant death syndrome (SIDS).

Alcohol, Health, and Research World, 1997. This study states, "even a small amount of alcohol may affect child development."

Common Myths

Myth: My doctor said it's fine to have a glass of wine or two while pregnant.

Your doctor might not be informed about the risk of prenatal alcohol exposure or could be uncomfortable talking with you about the risks to your embryo or fetus associated with prenatal alcohol use. Unfortunately, many doctors are not properly educated about the risks associated with prenatal alcohol exposure. The American Congress of Obstetricians and Gynecologists (ACOG) advises women to not consume any alcohol while pregnant. Some doctors tell women that it's okay to drink a little wine because they are not comfortable talking with women who might not be interested in abstaining from alcohol or have difficulty doing so.

Myth: My friends or family members drank a bit and their kids are fine.

Every pregnancy is different. Not everyone who drinks while pregnant will have a child with measurable problems at birth, adolescence, or even adulthood, just like not every cigarette smoker will develop lung cancer. The fact remains that alcohol is toxic to the developing baby. Why take the risk?

Also, some children may have subtle damage from being exposed to alcohol that is not evident until school-age or later, such as problems with learning and behavior. In many of these cases, the problems are most often not linked to the prenatal alcohol exposure, inhibiting an accurate diagnoses and delaying appropriate intervention. According to Dr. Susan Astley Ph.D. and Dr. Therese Grant Ph.D., "Children exposed to and damaged by prenatal alcohol exposure look deceptively good in the preschool years. The full impact of their alcohol exposure will not be evident until their adolescent years."

Myth: There is no evidence of any effects from just one drink.

Dr. Michael Charness of Harvard Medical School gives just one example: "We've been able to show very striking effects of alcohol on the L1 cell adhesion molecule, a critical molecule for development, at concentrations of alcohol that a woman would have in her blood after just one drink."

Myth: A little bit of wine helps to reduce stress and can be healthy while pregnant.

The potential benefits of alcohol use during pregnancy to the *mother* are separate from and are outweighed by the potential risk to the mother's developing child. The scientific and medical research is very clear: No published biomedical research has found any risk-free benefit of prenatal alcohol exposure for the embryo or fetus. Hundreds of papers have conclusively demonstrated that alcohol use has the potential to cause both physical and functional damage to a growing baby.

The good news is that the vast majority of women in the U.S. stop drinking alcohol when they are pregnant. Those who continue drinking may do so because they do not understand the risks of continued drinking or because alcohol is a part of their lifestyle that they do not want to or cannot give up. Women commonly cite the need to relax as one of the reasons they drink during

pregnancy even if they understand the risks. Pregnant women should ask their doctor about the diet and exercise that is appropriate for them, and to relax they might listen to soothing music, pamper themselves, take a bath, read, eliminate guilt, try deep breathing or meditation, schedule time for themselves with no responsibilities or distractions, and don't hesitate to ask their friends and family for help if they feel overwhelmed or uncomfortable.

Myth: On a holiday or special occasion, it's perfectly fine to at least have a few celebratory sips.

The human body functions the same, whether it's a holiday or not. Alcohol does not somehow lose its toxicity in utero because it happens to be New Year's Eve, or because wine is consumed instead of whiskey, or because the drinker has an advanced academic degree and a high socioeconomic status. The risk of prenatal alcohol exposure is not a risk to the health of the expectant mother; it is a risk to the development of her offspring.

The guidance to abstain from alcohol when pregnant is not intended to interfere with a woman's lifestyle choice to consume alcohol or in any way judge a woman for choosing to enjoy her favorite alcoholic beverage; it is intended to eliminate the chance her baby will have even the slightest reduction in their intellectual and physical abilities.

Myth: One glass of wine is not enough for the developing baby to even be exposed to the alcohol.

Any alcohol consumed by a pregnant woman is passed to the developing baby, even if it's a small amount. There is no threshold of prenatal alcohol consumption below which the baby is not exposed.

Myth: Drinking wine is better than using heroin or cocaine while pregnant.

Alcohol, including wine, causes far more damage to the developing baby than any other drug. The Institute of Medicine says, "Of all the substances of abuse (including cocaine, heroin, and marijuana), alcohol produces by far the most serious neurobehavioral effects in the fetus." No type of alcohol or illicit drugs consumed during pregnancy are completely without risk.

Myth: You have to be an alcoholic to drink enough to cause real damage.

The medical research is clear: Drinking at a level *below* the threshold for alcoholism can still cause damage to the growing baby. There are many women who are not alcoholics that have children with measurable effects of alcohol exposure. Damage can be caused by a pregnant woman's lack of awareness of the risks—not only as a result of her alcoholism.

Myth: Alcohol can only cause physical deformities. If the baby looks normal, it must be fine.

The vast majority (over 85%) of children with damage from prenatal alcohol exposure have *no* physical birth defects, only cognitive and/or behavioral consequences. There is such a wide range of effects that most subtle behavioral and cognitive difficulties are rarely diagnosed as alcohol-related.

Myth: It is alarming and even condescending for a doctor or anyone else to advise a woman to abstain from alcohol during pregnancy.

In the United States 50% of pregnancies are unplanned, so it is possible that the first time a woman is told that alcohol can harm her pregnancy is after she is already pregnant and has been drinking. It is important for physicians to advise the woman of the risks of alcohol use during pregnancy, be nonjudgmental, and provide guidance for an appropriate intervention if necessary. If a woman has been drinking alcohol during her pregnancy, the earlier she stops the greater the chance that her child will not have alcohol-related birth defects.

All women should be reminded of the risk of prenatal alcohol exposure. If a woman is informed of the risk and decides to drink, that is her decision—NOFAS is opposed to any rules, regulations, or statutes that seek to punish or sanction women for drinking alcohol during pregnancy. Practitioners should always inform their patients about the risks of known exposures.

It is important for pregnant women to be reminded that proper nutrition, good general health, and early and regular prenatal doctor visits might help reduce the effects of light drinking during pregnancy. It is believed that some women have a genetic predisposition that increases the vulnerability of their embryo or fetus to alcohol exposure, and, consequently, some women have a genetic make-up that reduces their vulnerability for having an alcohol-effected birth. However, the scientific community does not know for sure whether or not these genetic and epigenetic factors (changes in how genes are expressed without altering the underlying DNA sequence) contribute to the vulnerable pregnancies for certain women.

The Simple Approach

Thousands of pieces of research have shown alcohol to be a neurotoxin in utero. That means alcohol is a *toxic substance* to the developing baby just like carbon monoxide and lead. Alcohol causes the death of developing brain cells in the embryo or fetus. Common sense advises not exposing a developing baby to *any* amount of a toxic substance.

Medical experts on light drinking during pregnancy—watch on Youtube

Official Recommendations

United States Surgeon General Advisory

The most comprehensive review of alcohol and pregnancy research to date has been conducted by the Office of the Surgeon General within the Office of the Assistant Secretary for Health in the Office of the Secretary, U.S. Department of Health and Human Services. The Surgeon General first advised women to abstain from alcohol during pregnancy in 1981, and issued a new advisory in 2005.

The advisory states in part, "Based on the current, best science available we now know the following:

- No amount of alcohol consumption can be considered safe during pregnancy;
- Alcohol can damage the embryo or fetus at any stage of pregnancy;
- Damage can occur in the earliest weeks of pregnancy, even before a woman knows she is pregnant;
- The cognitive effects and behavioral problems resulting from prenatal alcohol exposure are lifelong."

"For these reasons:

- A pregnant woman should not drink alcohol during pregnancy;
- A pregnant woman who has already consumed alcohol during pregnancy should stop in order to minimize further risk;
- A woman who is considering becoming pregnant should abstain from alcohol."

About half of all pregnancies are unplanned. As a result, many women consume alcohol without knowing that they are pregnant. The Surgeon General's advisory also suggests that women of childbearing age should consult their physician about how best to reduce the risk of prenatal alcohol exposure.

Recommendations

Centers for Disease Control and Prevention
There is no known safe amount of alcohol to drink while pregnant. There is also no safe time during pregnancy to drink and no safe kind of alcohol.

National Institute on Alcohol Abuse and Alcoholism
No amount of alcohol is safe for pregnant women to drink.

American Academy of Pediatrics
The American Academy of Pediatrics recommends women who are pregnant or planning a pregnancy avoid drinking any alcohol.

American College of Obstetricians and Gynecologists
ACOG reiterates its long-standing position that no amount of alcohol consumption can be considered safe during pregnancy.

March of Dimes
Drinking alcohol when you're pregnant can be very harmful to your baby. It can cause your baby to have a range of lifelong health conditions.

National Arc
There is no absolute safe amount of alcohol that a woman can drink during pregnancy. Risk of FASD increase as the amount of alcohol consumed increases.

Baby Center
All public health officials in the United States recommend that pregnant women, as well as women who are trying to conceive, play it safe by steering clear of alcohol entirely.

Statements from Medical Experts

Dr. Kenneth Jones—First Named "Fetal Alcohol Syndrome" in 1973

"When talking about the prenatal effects of alcohol we usually think exclusively about the dose, the strength, and the timing of alcohol exposure. However, perhaps even more important are factors involving the mother—her genetic background and nutritional status to name just two. Based on those maternal factors, what may be a completely safe amount of alcohol for one woman to drink during her pregnancy may be a serious problem for another woman's developing fetus. Without knowing those genetic and nutritional factors that are critically involved with the way a woman metabolizes alcohol, it is not possible to make any generalizations about a 'safe' amount of alcohol during pregnancy. What may be 'safe' for one woman may be 'devastating' for another woman's unborn baby."

Dr. Michael Charness—Harvard Medical School

"Moderate levels of alcohol have been shown to disrupt the activity of a number of molecules that are critical for normal brain development. One such example, the L1 cell adhesion molecule, guides the migration of brain cells and the formation of connections between brain cells. Children with mutations in the L1 gene have developmental disabilities and brain malformations, and, importantly, the function of the L1 molecule is also disrupted by concentrations of alcohol that a woman would have in her blood after a single drink. These kinds of experiments support the view that women who are pregnant or trying to conceive would be safer to abstain from alcohol than to engage in even occasional light drinking.

Absence of proof is not proof of absence. The absence of evidence for developmental abnormalities in women who drink small amounts occasionally during pregnancy does not prove that light drinking is safe. Clinical studies do not have the power to detect small effects of alcohol on brain development, and even significant effects might be missed if the wrong test is used or if testing is conducted at the wrong developmental period. More practically, it is impossible to assure a mother who drinks lightly during pregnancy that her drinking did not result in a small drop in the IQ of her child. Light drinking is not essential to the health or well being of a pregnant woman, so why take a chance?"

If You Already Drank While Pregnant

If you have just found out you are pregnant and you have been drinking alcohol, stop drinking now and talk with your doctor. Any time during pregnancy that you stop drinking you increase the chance that your baby will not be affected by alcohol.

If you are finding it difficult to stop drinking, help is available. Visit your doctor to talk about your drinking, or find a professional in your area using the Substance Abuse and Treatment Facility Locator. You can also contact NOFAS or at (800) 66-NOFAS.

Alcohol and Pregnancy Science

Alcohol, like the chemical element mercury, is a confirmed teratogen (a substance that interferes with normal prenatal development). Alcohol can cause central nervous system (brain and spinal cord) malformations with associated neurobehavioral dysfunction. By comparison, lead is a neurotoxin but not a teratogen in that it produces neurobehavioral dysfunction in the absence of brain and spinal cord malformations.

Science definitively recognizes that when a pregnant woman consumes alcohol, the alcohol crosses the placenta into the blood supply of the developing embryo or fetus. An embryo or fetus has neither the developed organ systems nor enzymes able to metabolize alcohol.

The first paper in the medical literature describing a constellation of birth defects linked to prenatal alcohol exposure was published in France in 1968 by Dr. Paul Lemoine.

The first paper in U.S. medical literature appeared in 1973 authored by Drs. David Smith and Ken Lyons Jones. As of 2012, nearly 4,000 papers have been published confirming the toxicity of alcohol to the embryo or fetus, the underlying mechanisms of alcohol-induced damage to the embryo or fetus, and the physical and functional birth defects related to prenatal alcohol exposure.

No published study has suggested that alcohol is not a teratogen or demonstrated that prenatal alcohol use has any potential benefit to human development.

The basic and biomedical research demonstrates that alcohol damages the developing brain through multiple actions at different cellular sites interfering with normal development by disrupting cell migration, cell functions, and causing cell death.

Alcohol can cause damage to multiple regions of the brain, specifically to the corpus collosum (connects brain hemispheres), cerebellum (consciousness and voluntary processes), basal ganglia (movement and cognition), hippocampus (emotional behavior and memory), hypothalamus (sensory input), among other neural regions.

Ethanol is the principal psychoactive constituent in alcoholic beverages. In utero it has been found to:

- Interfere with normal proliferation of nerve cells;
- Increase the formation of free radicals—cell damaging molecular fragments;
- Alter cells ability to regulate cell growth, division and survival;
- Impair the development and function of astocytes, cells that guide the migration of nerve cells to their proper places;
- Interfere with the normal adhesion of cells to one another;
- Alter the formation of axons, nerve cell extensions that conduct impulses away from the cell body;
- Alter the pathways of biochemical or electrical signals within cells;
- Alter the expression of genes, including genes that regulate cell development.

Human development occurs in an orderly process of biochemical and structural transition during which new constituents are being formed and spatially arranged throughout gestation. At any time in the span of development these ongoing processes can be subtly or severely disturbed or abruptly halted resulting in abnormal development or fetal death.

Therefore, at any time alcohol is present it has the potential to harm development. For example, the hallmark facial dysmorphology associated with Fetal Alcohol Syndrome will only occur if alcohol is present during the specific window of development.

Of all the substances of abuse, including marijuana, cocaine and heroin, alcohol produces by far the most serious neurobehavioral effects on the embryo or fetus.

Women at Risk

Factors known to contribute to the risk of having a child with alcohol-related birth defects include biological susceptibility, poor nutrition, poor general health, and a lack of prenatal care.

Some light and moderate drinkers have offspring with identifiable birth defects while some women who consume alcohol throughout pregnancy have offspring without any apparent or quantifiable birth defects. Research is currently exploring both the genetic and protective factors involved in the manifestation of alcohol-related birth defects.

An examination of sociodemographic factors indicated that generally more older women (~30 or 35 years old and older) drink during pregnancy, but younger women (~24 years old or younger) face higher risks of binge drinking or drinking in the few months prior to recognizing they are pregnant. With regard to race and ethnicity, White women report a higher prevalence of alcohol use than Black or Hispanic women, although Hispanic women may increase use as they become more acculturated in the United States. Differences in prevalence based on geographic location appeared potentially important, with binge drinking more prevalent in the North-central sections of the United States and less so in the Southeast. Higher education and higher income were linked specifically to higher rates of alcohol use during pregnancy in some studies.

Key Facts on Alcohol and Pregnancy

There is no safe amount or type of alcohol to consume during pregnancy. Any amount of alcohol, even if it's just one glass of wine, passes from the mother to the baby. It makes no difference if the alcohol is wine, beer, or liquor or distilled spirits (vodka, rum, tequila, etc.)

A developing baby can't process alcohol. Developing babies lack the ability to process alcohol with their liver, which is not fully formed. They absorb all of the alcohol and have the same blood alcohol concentration as the mother.

Alcohol causes more harm than heroin or cocaine during pregnancy. The Institute of Medicine says, "Of all the substances of abuse (including cocaine, heroin, and marijuana), alcohol produces by far the most serious neurobehavioral effects in the fetus." No type of alcohol or illicit drugs consumed during pregnancy are completely without risk.

Alcohol used during pregnancy can result in FASD. An estimated 40,000 newborns each year are believed to have an FASD, Fetal Alcohol Spectrum Disorders, with damage ranging from major to subtle.

1 in 100 newborns in the U.S. might have FASD, nearly the same rate as Autism. FASD is more prevalent than Down Syndrome, Cerebral Palsy, SIDS, Cystic Fibrosis, and Spina Bifida combined. Alcohol use during pregnancy is the leading preventable cause of birth defects, developmental disabilities, and learning disabilities.

NATIONAL ORGANIZATION ON FETAL ALCOHOL SYNDROME (NOFAS) is a nonprofit public health charitable organization focused on the issue of fetal alcohol syndrome and fetal alcohol spectrum disorders (FASD).

Emily Oster

➡ **NO**

I Wrote That It's OK to Drink While Pregnant. Everyone Freaked Out. Here's Why I'm Right.

When I was pregnant, I wondered, as many women do: Can I have a drink? It is well-known that drinking to excess during pregnancy is dangerous, and perhaps less well known but still true, that even one or two episodes of binge drinking can be harmful. But what about an occasional glass of wine with dinner?

Expert opinions on this differ. *What to Expect When You're Expecting* says no alcohol. *Panic-Free Pregnancy* says an occasional drink is fine. A 2010 survey asked obstetricians, "How much alcohol can a pregnant woman consume without risk of adverse pregnancy outcomes?" Sixty percent of the OBs said none, but the other 40 percent said some alcohol was fine. The American Congress of Obstetricians and Gynecologists (ACOG) says no amount of alcohol has been shown to be safe, but the U.K. equivalent (the Royal College of Obstetricians and Gynecologists) says that while not drinking is the safest option, "Small amounts of alcohol during pregnancy have not been shown to be harmful."

My obstetrician said a few drinks a week was fine. But as with everything else, amid this disagreement, I needed to go to the data myself.

I reviewed many, many studies, but I focused in on ones that compare women who drank lightly or occasionally during pregnancy to those who abstained. The best of these studies are ones that separate women into several groups—for example: no alcohol, a few drinks a week, one drink a day, more than one drink a day—and that limit the focus to women who say they never had a binge drinking episode. With these parameters, we can really hone in on the question of interest: What is the impact of having an occasional drink, assuming that you never overdo it?

I summarize two studies in detail in my book: one looking at alcohol consumption by pregnant women and behavior problems for the resulting children up to age 14 and one looking at alcohol in pregnancy and test performance at age 14. Both show no difference between the children of women who abstain and those who drink up to a drink a day. I summarize two others in less detail: one looking at IQ scores at age 8 and a more recent one looking at IQ scores at age 5. These also demonstrate no impact of light drinking on test scores.

I argue that based on this data, many women may feel comfortable with an occasional glass of wine—even up to one a day—in later trimesters. (More caution in the first trimester—no more than two drinks a week—because of some evidence of miscarriage risk.)

Although this discussion takes up only a small share of the book, it has garnered the loudest reaction, much of it outrage. NOFAS, a fetal alcohol syndrome advocacy group, issued a press release even before the book came out saying I was harmful and irresponsible. Amazon reviews of the book—at least some of them by people who explicitly said they would never read it—attacked me and anyone who had a drink during pregnancy as an alcoholic. One commented on my daughter: "Emily Oster claims that her 2-year old daughter is perfectly healthy, yet the full impact of the alcohol exposure on her child will not be evident until the adolescent years."

The president of ACOG has vehemently disagreed with me, saying in a radio interview about occasional drinking that alcohol in pregnancy is more dangerous than heroin or cocaine. Of course, there has been occasional public agreement from OBs (and much more private agreement).

Some of the arguments made in response to the book are tangential. Commenters wish that there was more in the book about the dangers of fetal alcohol syndrome, more discussion of the risks of binge drinking. I spend only a page on this, since it is not the question I believe most readers of the book are asking.

Some of them are philosophical. People ask, "Why take the risk?" since there is no benefit to the baby. But this ignores the fact that we are always making choices that could carry some risk and have no benefit to the baby. Driving in a car carries some risk to your baby, and your fetus does not benefit from that vacation you took. Or they ask, "Is it so hard to give up drinking for nine months?" The answer is, of course, no, but because you might enjoy the occasional beer, it seems worth at least asking the question about the risks.

Then there is the criticism that I cherry-picked studies to fit the story. This certainly isn't the case; the fact that the book doesn't summarize all 23,000 studies in PubMed on alcohol in pregnancy reflects the desire to identify the most reliable and largest and present those. Still, it's reasonable to ask whether there are studies that I missed that tell a different story.

One fact that has been cited to me a number of times, including by the ACOG president, is: "One in 7 children with fetal alcohol syndrome had a mother who drank one to eight drinks per week in the first trimester." The implication is that even light drinking early on (which would be much closer to one than eight drinks) is dangerous. But this claim doesn't come from a study; it comes from a statement made in a letter to the editor, and it's therefore impossible to evaluate critically. One to eight drinks a week could mean eight drinks on one night, for instance, and that is known to be dangerous.

Another study that has been mentioned prominently relates prenatal alcohol exposure to behavior problems in young adulthood. Although some have suggested that this paper identifies impacts of having one drink per day, the analysis actually relates behavior problems to a measure of average daily intake—which includes people having more than that, sometimes a lot more. It's true that some people evaluated in this study drink lightly, but others do not, and by lumping them together it is very difficult to draw conclusions about the light drinkers.

There is a much more technically complex study that I certainly would have included in the book if it had come out in time. It shows that light maternal drinking is associated with small IQ decreases for people with some particular genetic variants. Light maternal drinking is also associated with small IQ increases in people with some other genetic variants. This suggests that further studies may be useful in evaluating genetic risks, although it doesn't provide a lot of guidance at this time.

The bottom line is that the criticism fails to identify studies that have the features we would want: a population that is never binge drinking and a data analysis that looks separately at women who drink lightly and those who drink more. In the book I discuss one study like this, which does argue there are impacts on behavior at one drink per day, but the study fails to adjust for differences across groups, like whether the father lives at home or if there was prenatal cocaine use, among other things.

Like alcohol, Tylenol, caffeine, and anti-nausea drugs like Zofran are substances that—in moderation—are thought to be safe during pregnancy. But they are also substances that in excessive doses could be dangerous. Some women decide that they will therefore avoid them altogether because they cannot be sure. And many women, seeing the evidence in the book on alcohol, will still choose to avoid it.

But others will see the data, like the data on caffeine or Tylenol, and choose to have an occasional drink, as I did. The value of the data is not that it leads us all to the same choice, just that it introduces a concrete way to make that choice.

EMILY OSTER is an associate professor of economics at Brown University.

EXPLORING THE ISSUE

Is It Necessary for Pregnant Women to Completely Abstain from All Alcoholic Beverages?

Critical Thinking and Reflection

1. What are the short- and long-term effects of fetal alcohol syndrome?
2. Will consuming small amounts of alcohol necessarily cause damage to a developing fetus? Explain.
3. Why is it so difficult to determine a safe level of alcohol consumption during pregnancy?

Is There Common Ground?

Since its medical recognition in 1973, fetal alcohol syndrome (FAS) has progressed from a little known condition to a major public health issue. The condition has been characterized by exaggerated and unproved claims particularly the cause and impact of the condition. The second author discusses the fact that there is likely a safe threshold for alcohol consumption during pregnancy and that FAS typically occurs among women who consume the highest amount of alcohol and/or binge drink. Binge drinking among women of childbearing age is common in the United States, which has one of the world's highest rates of FAS. In a recent study, researchers determined that one in six women in the United States continues to drink during pregnancy and one in seven consumes more than seven drinks per week; 3 percent drinks more than 14 drinks per week. Thirteen percent of U.S. women aged 18–44 binge drink. The estimated number of childbearing-age women who engaged in binge drinking rose from 6.2 million in 2001 to 7.1 million in 2003, an increase of 0.9 million. A study involving over 4,000 randomly selected women showed that 30.3 percent of all women reported drinking alcohol at some time during pregnancy, of which 8.3 percent reported binge drinking (more than four drinks on one occasion). "Alcohol Consumption by Women Before and During Pregnancy" (*Maternal and Child Health Journal*, March 2009).

Fortunately, most women who use alcohol reduce their intake dramatically once they realize they are pregnant. A recent article, however, indicated that among 12,611 mothers from Maryland who gave birth to live infants between 2001 and 2008, nearly 8 percent of the study subjects admitted to drinking alcoholic beverages during the last 3 months of their pregnancy (*Obstetrics & Gynecology*, February, 2011). But doctors still don't know that risk or harm, if any, results from light to moderate alcohol intake during pregnancy, which is why they caution pregnant women to abstain. For ethical reasons, there have been few if any studies conducted on pregnant women to determine if small to moderate intake of alcohol is harmful. And to confuse the issue, some effects of alcohol consumption during pregnancy may not be apparent until a child starts school or even later in life. Child developmental and behavioral characteristics were examined from the 9-month data point of the Early Childhood Longitudinal Studies—Birth Cohort, a prospective nationally representative study. Several findings showed clear patterns between the amount of prenatal alcohol consumed and sensory regulation, mental, and motor development outcomes. Undesirable social engagement and child interaction were found to be statistically significant at the prenatal alcohol level of one to three drinks per week. Children exposed to four or more drinks per week showed statistically significant and clinically passive behavior on three sensory regulation variables ("Maternal Alcohol Consumption During Pregnancy and Infant Social, Mental, and Motor Development," *Journal of Early Intervention*, March 2010). Clearly, excessive alcohol consumption during pregnancy has negative effects on fetal growth and development. Less consistent relationships have been shown for the correlation between light to moderate maternal alcohol consumption during pregnancy with health outcomes in the offspring. Researchers in the study "Associations of Light and Moderate Maternal Alcohol Consumption With Fetal Growth Characteristics in Different Periods of Pregnancy: The Generation R Study" examined the associations of light to moderate maternal alcohol consumption with various fetal growth characteristics measured in different periods of pregnancy and found various levels of impairment among the children of women who consumed alcohol during their pregnancies (*International Journal of Epidemiology*, June 2010).

Although individual differences in reaction to alcohol prevents determining a "safe level" of drinking for all pregnant women, encouraging total abstinence from alcohol during pregnancy is prudent though not necessarily based on research. The changes in fetal activity associated with one or two drinks clearly indicate that the fetus reacts to low levels of alcohol. But these changes don't necessarily mean the fetus is damaged. Until relationships are considerably stronger than the evidence now indicates, the research does not support the consensus that low levels of alcohol intake pose a danger to the developing baby. Even though scientists can't prove small amounts of alcohol are harmful, they can't prove they aren't. On the other hand, setting a realistic threshold may be more effective than encouraging women to completing forgo alcohol. Setting a definite limit, two or fewer drinks per day, for example, may be more realistic to those women who continue to drink during pregnancy. Prevention efforts have not been particularly effective among women who drink at levels that pose the greatest risk to their fetus ("Motivational Interventions in Prenatal Clinics," *Alcohol Research & Health,* vol. 25, 2001). They may be able

to reduce rather than eliminate all alcohol which could result in a reduced risk for FAS.

Additional Resources

Buxton, B. (2005). *Damaged angels: An adoptive mother discovers the tragic toll of alcohol in pregnancy.* New York: Carroll & Graf.

Cannon, M., Guo, J., Denny, C., Green, P., Miracle, H., Sniezek, J., & Floyd, R. (2015). Prevalence and characteristics of women at risk for an alcohol-exposed pregnancy (AEP) in the United States: Estimates from the National Survey of Family Growth. *Maternal & Child Health Journal, 19*(4), 776–782.

Chen, J. (2012). Maternal alcohol use during pregnancy, birth weight and early behavioral outcomes. *Alcohol & Alcoholism, 47*(6), 649–656.

Powers, J., McDermott, L., Loxton, D., & Chojenta, C. (2013). A prospective study of prevalence and predictors of concurrent alcohol and tobacco use during pregnancy. *Maternal & Child Health Journal, 17*(1), 76–84.

Sullum, J. (2012). Drink up, moms! *Reason, 44*(5), 13–14.

Internet References . . .

March of Dimes Foundation

www.marchofdimes.com

National Clearinghouse for Alcohol and Drug Information

www.health.org

National Organization on Fetal Alcohol Syndrome: NOFAS

www.nofas.org

Selected, Edited, and with Issue Framing Material by:
Eileen L. Daniel, *SUNY College at Brockport*

ISSUE

Should Pro-Life Health Providers Be Allowed to Deny Prescriptions on the Basis of Conscience?

YES: **John A. Menges,** from "Public Hearing on HB4346 Before the House State Government Administration Committee," Illinois House State Government Administration Committee (2006)

NO: **R. Alta Charo,** from "The Celestial Fire of Conscience—Refusing to Deliver Medical Care," *The New England Journal of Medicine* (2005)

Learning Outcomes
After reading this issue, you will be able to: • Discuss why some pharmacists refuse to dispense certain medications. • Understand the mechanisms of the morning after pill. • Assess the legality of a pharmacist refusing to filling prescriptions.

ISSUE SUMMARY

YES: Pharmacist John A. Menges believes that it is his right to refuse to dispense any medication that is designed to end a human life.

NO: Attorney R. Alta Charo argues that health care professionals who protect themselves from the moral consequences of their actions may do so at their patients' risk.

A trend has been making news recently. The Pharmacists' Refusal Clause also known as the Conscience Clause allows pharmacists to refuse to fill certain prescriptions because of their own moral objections to the medication. These medications are mostly birth control pills and the "morning after pill," which can be used as emergency contraception. Though nearly all states offer some type of legal protection for health care providers who refuse to provide certain women's health care services, only three states—Arkansas, Mississippi, and South Dakota—specifically protect pharmacists who refuse to dispense birth control and emergency contraceptive pills. While only a limited number of states have passed refusal clause legislation specific to pharmacists, more and more states are considering adding it.

In the past several years there have been reports of pharmacists who refused to fill prescriptions for birth control and emergency contraceptive pills. In some of these instances, the pharmacists who refused service were fired, but in others, no legal action was taken. As a result, some women have left their drug stores without getting their pills and not sure where to go to have their prescriptions filled.

While doctors may refuse to perform abortions or other procedures that they morally object to, should pharmacists have the same right? They are members of the health care team and should be treated as medical professionals. Society does not demand that professionals abandon their morals as a condition of their employment. On the other hand, there are a number of reasons against a pharmacist's right to object. First and foremost is the right of a patient to receive timely medical treatment. Pharmacists may refuse to fill prescriptions for emergency contraception because they believe that drug ends a life. Although the patient may disapprove of abortion, she may not share the pharmacist's beliefs about birth control. If she becomes pregnant, she may then consider abortion, an issue she could have avoided if allowed to fill prescriptions for the morning after pill. Other concerns include the time-sensitive nature of the morning after pill, which must be taken within 72 hours of intercourse to effectively prevent pregnancy. Women who are refused the medication by one pharmacist may not be able to get the drug from another. This is especially true if she lives in an area with only one pharmacy. Also, low-income women may not have the time or resources to locate a pharmacy that would fill the prescription.

Other potential abuses could also arise. For instance, some pharmacists may object to filling drugs to treat AIDS if they believe HIV-positive individuals are engaged in behaviors they consider immoral such as IV drug use or homosexual relations. A pharmacist who does not believe in extramarital sex might refuse to fill a prescription for Viagra for an unmarried man. Could a pharmacist's objections here be considered invasive? Further, because a pharmacist does not have access to a patient's medical records or history, refusing to fill a prescription could be medically harmful.

While arguments could be made for both sides, it appears that there needs to be a compromise between the needs of a patient and the moral beliefs of a pharmacist. In the YES and NO selections, physician John Menges argues that health providers' consciences must be respected. R. Alta Charo counters that a provider's conscience can be in conflict with legitimate medical needs of a patient.

YES ←

John A. Menges

Public Hearing on HB4346 Before the House State Government Administration Committee

[I am] one of the 4 fired Walgreens pharmacists. I was fired for not signing a policy saying that I would indeed fill a prescription if presented with it. I did not see a prescription! Walgreens does not respect a pharmacist's right to choose. I was one of Walgreens' best pharmacists prior to this issue. I had no problem with telling someone when a pharmacist would be available to fill a prescription. I can not fill the prescriptions myself but I try to the best of my ability to not take a side because I want to be able to tell people that this drug can end a life if a woman does have questions. By taking the position I take I find women asking questions. I believe many women wouldn't use this drug if they knew how it can work. If a woman is going to make a real choice as the other side says then the woman needs to have access to both "pro-choice" pharmacist and pro-life pharmacist like myself, so her choice is an informed choice. I pray that by trying to take a neutral position on this issue that some women will listen and some children will live.

The one thing I could not be neutral on is the issue of dispensing. When my three supervisors fired me, I told them "It feels very good knowing that my Faith and Religion is more important to me than a paycheck."

The following is a testimony I gave on a House bill earlier this year [2006].

Testimony

I would like to thank Rep. Granberg for introducing this bill and all members of this committee for giving me the opportunity to speak to you today.

My name is JOHN A. MENGES and I am a licensed pharmacist in the state of Illinois. I am one of the four pharmacists who lost my job with Walgreens for failing to sign an Emergency Contraceptive Policy that violated my religious beliefs. To make things clear to all members of this committee during the 8 months I worked following

the Governor's mandate I was not presented with a prescription to fill. During the 3 years I worked at Walgreens I can only recall being presented with prescriptions for this medication 3 times and during that time I estimate that I filled over 71,000 prescriptions.

I am here today because I can not dispense any drug designed to end a human life. Before I enter any discussion of these drugs I would like to try to clarify some terminology. For me human life begins when fertilization occurs. Fertilization is the point at which the sperm penetrates the egg. Life for me is the issue. The redefining of the terms "pregnancy" and "conception" in 1965 by the American College of Obstetricians and Gynecologists only confuse this life issue more. Prior to 1965 "pregnancy" and "conception" began at fertilization when life begins. Now "pregnancy" and "conception" begins at implantation of the embryo in the uterus. This still doesn't negate the fact that embryologists world-wide agree unanimously that human life begins at fertilization. This does explain why the morning after pill is classified as a contraceptive by the FDA and not as an abortafacient and I hope this clarifies why many say this drug doesn't end a pregnancy. Understanding the terminology enables one to realize how confusing the words fertilization, pregnancy, and conception have become. With this very simple explanation of the terminology I want to remind you that the beginning of human life at the point of fertilization is the issue for me. I hold human life at this stage in development with the same respect I hold for any human life.

The drugs I was referring to as I tried to explain some definitions are classified as "emergency contraceptives" by the FDA. Presently "Plan B" also known as the "morning after pill" is the only drug approved to be used for emergency contraception but most oral contraceptives can be dosed to work as emergency contraception. Emergency contraceptive doses are doses that are higher than doses of regular birth control. To simplify my discussion of emergency contraceptives I will limit my discussion

Menges, John A. Illinois House State Government Administration Committee, February 15, 2006.

to "Plan B." Plan B consists of two Progestin tablets containing 0.75 mg of levonorgestrel. The first tablet is to be taken within 72 hours of intercourse and the second tablet 12 hours after the first dose. Without getting into too much detail here the problem I have is the significant post-fertilization mechanism of action by which these drugs work. The mechanisms of action stated in the manufacturers prescribing information include preventing ovulation, altering tubal transport of sperm and/or ova, or inhibiting implantation by altering the endometrium. The time during a woman's menstrual cycle plays an important role in what mechanism of action is at work. The menstrual cycle can last anywhere from 21 to 40 days. Ovulation usually occurs 14 to 15 days before the end of the cycle. If emergency contraception is given early in the cycle it is more likely to prevent ovulation. But during this time ovulation and pregnancy are less likely to occur anyway. As the time for ovulation nears the chance for emergency contraception to prevent ovulation will lessen to the effect that ovulation can occur in some instances after emergency contraception has been taken. Once ovulation has occurred and fertilization has taken place any mechanism that prevents this implantation is the ending of human life.

So what am I doing as a pharmacist if I can't dispense a drug approved by the FDA? Believe me I asked myself this question when the first emergency contraceptive was approved by the FDA in 1998. I was a pharmacy manager in a supermarket pharmacy at the time. My number one priority as pharmacy manager is the same as it is today and that is customer service to my patients. I have always made it known to my employees, supervisors, and patients that I work first for the patient. My employer was a direct beneficiary of this as I always made them look good. The day the first emergency contraceptive was approved I talked with the staff pharmacist who worked with me about his thoughts. Neither of us could dispense emergency contraceptives as it went against everything we believed in. The question I and many pharmacists had to answer was which patient do we serve? Do we serve the women requesting emergency contraceptive or the human life she could be carrying? I could not make a decision to participate in ending any human life so my decision was to refer women and answer any questions they might have if and when the situation arose.

So here I am almost 8 years after the first emergency contraceptives were approved and I can only recall 5 times that I have been faced with prescriptions. Three of those prescriptions I saw while employed with Walgreens.

Not that a person can derive any statistical conclusions from 5 prescriptions but I didn't have incident with any of those encounters. In fact I have been thanked for my willingness to talk about emergency contraceptives as many pharmacists avoid the issue. This leads me to the moral issue I read about in different editorials. My choice to step aside and not fill these prescriptions in no way is a reflection of me trying to push my morals on others. It is my upholding my moral beliefs for myself. Our government allows women to make this choice and my actions have never prevented any women from exercising her choice. I have a choice too and my choice is not to dispense any medication that will end a human life. Those are morals that I have to live up to. The people who think I try to push my morals on others need to ask themselves why I dispense medication to patients who have just had an abortion for pain and bleeding. I give these patients the same respect I give every patient. The answers are simple as I went into pharmacy to help people not hurt people. I don't ask questions as to why people need my help because morals don't play a role in my helping people. I went into pharmacy to care for people and help them improve their lives. I love the profession of pharmacy because of all the good I am able to do as a pharmacist. Pharmacy goes beyond the counseling, recommendations and referrals I give. It is much more than my filling prescriptions fast and accurately. It is the respect I give every patient. I listen to my patients and help them when I can. I will never intentionally do any harm to any patient.

On November 28th of last year I lost my job because of my conscience objective to filling a medication that ends human life. My employer fired me for not signing policy asking me to violate my conscience. During the 8 months following the Governor's mandate I was not presented with a prescription to fill. Even though I believe I am currently covered under The Health Care Right of Conscience Act, I would like to ask every member of the house to vote YES on HB 4346. I am one of a small minority of pharmacists in this state who can't fill these medications. By voting YES on HB 4346 you will protect other pharmacists from having to endure what I, my wife, and my 2 children have had to endure these past months. It is difficult to explain my feelings. It hurts.

Without saying anymore I would like to answer any questions members might have. Thank You.

JOHN A. MENGES is a licensed pharmacist.

R. Alta Charo

➡ **NO**

The Celestial Fire of Conscience—Refusing to Deliver Medical Care

Apparently heeding George Washington's call to "labor to keep alive in your breast that little spark of celestial fire called conscience," physicians, nurses, and pharmacists are increasingly claiming a right to the autonomy not only to refuse to provide services they find objectionable, but even to refuse to refer patients to another provider and, more recently, to inform them of the existence of legal options for care.

Largely as artifacts of the abortion wars, at least 45 states have "conscience clauses" on their books—laws that balance a physician's conscientious objection to performing an abortion with the profession's obligation to afford all patients nondiscriminatory access to services. In most cases, the provision of a referral satisfies one's professional obligations. But in recent years, with the abortion debate increasingly at the center of wider discussions about euthanasia, assisted suicide, reproductive technology, and embryonic stem-cell research, nurses and pharmacists have begun demanding not only the same right of refusal, but also—because even a referral, in their view, makes one complicit in the objectionable act—a much broader freedom to avoid facilitating a patient's choices.

A bill recently introduced in the Wisconsin legislature, for example, would permit health care professionals to abstain from "participating" in any number of activities, with "participating" defined broadly enough to include counseling patients about their choices. The privilege of abstaining from counseling or referring would extend to such situations as emergency contraception for rape victims, in vitro fertilization for infertile couples, patients' requests that painful and futile treatments be withheld or withdrawn, and therapies developed with the use of fetal tissue or embryonic stem cells. This last provision could mean, for example, that pediatricians—without professional penalty or threat of malpractice claims—could refuse to tell parents about the availability of varicella vaccine for their children, because it was developed with the use of tissue from aborted fetuses.

This expanded notion of complicity comports well with other public policy precedents, such as bans on federal funding for embryo research or abortion services, in which taxpayers claim a right to avoid supporting objectionable practices. In the debate on conscience clauses, some professionals are now arguing that the right to practice their religion requires that they not be made complicit in any practice to which they object on religious grounds.

Although it may be that, as Mahatma Gandhi said, "in matters of conscience, the law of majority has no place," acts of conscience are usually accompanied by a willingness to pay some price. Martin Luther King, Jr., argued, "An individual who breaks a law that conscience tells him is unjust, and who willingly accepts the penalty of imprisonment in order to arouse the conscience of the community over its injustice, is in reality expressing the highest respect for law."

What differentiates the latest round of battles about conscience clauses from those fought by Gandhi and King is the claim of entitlement to what newspaper columnist Ellen Goodman has called "conscience without consequence."

And of course, the professionals involved seek to protect only themselves from the consequences of their actions—not their patients. In Wisconsin, a pharmacist refused to fill an emergency-contraception prescription for a rape victim; as a result, she became pregnant and subsequently had to seek an abortion. In another Wisconsin case, a pharmacist who views hormonal contraception as a form of abortion refused not only to fill a prescription for birth-control pills but also to return the prescription or transfer it to another pharmacy. The patient, unable to take her pills on time, spent the next month dependent on less effective contraception. Under Wisconsin's proposed law, such behavior by a pharmacist would be entirely legal and acceptable. And this trend is not limited to pharmacists and physicians; in Illinois, an emergency medical technician refused to take a woman to an abortion clinic, claiming that her own Christian beliefs prevented her from transporting the patient for an elective abortion.

At the heart of this growing trend are several intersecting forces. One is the emerging norm of patient autonomy, which has contributed to the erosion of the professional stature of medicine. Insofar as they are reduced to mere purveyors of medical technology, doctors no longer have extraordinary privileges, and so their notions of extraordinary duty—house calls, midnight duties, and charity care—deteriorate as well. In addition, an emphasis on mutual responsibilities has been gradually supplanted by an emphasis on individual rights. With autonomy and rights as the preeminent social values comes a devaluing of relationships and a diminution of the difference between our personal lives and our professional duties.

Finally, there is the awesome scale and scope of the abortion wars. In the absence of legislative options for outright prohibition, abortion opponents search for proxy wars, using debates on research involving human embryos, the donation of organs from anencephalic neonates, and the right of persons in a persistent vegetative state to die as opportunities to rehearse arguments on the value of biologic but nonsentient human existence. Conscience clauses represent but another battle in these so-called culture wars.

Most profoundly, however, the surge in legislative activity surrounding conscience clauses represents the latest struggle with regard to religion in America. Should the public square be a place for the unfettered expression of religious beliefs, even when such expression creates an oppressive atmosphere for minority groups? Or should it be a place for religious expression only if and when that does not in any way impinge on minority beliefs and practices? This debate has been played out with respect to blue laws, school prayer, Christmas crèche scenes, and workplace dress codes.

Until recently, it was accepted that the public square in this country would be dominated by Christianity. This long-standing religious presence has made atheists, agnostics, and members of minority religions view themselves as oppressed, but recent efforts to purge the public square of religion have left conservative Christians also feeling subjugated and suppressed. In this culture war, both sides claim the mantle of victimhood—which is why health care professionals can claim the right of conscience as necessary to the nondiscriminatory practice of their religion, even as frustrated patients view conscience clauses as legalizing discrimination against them when they practice their own religion.

For health care professionals, the question becomes: What does it mean to be a professional in the United States? Does professionalism include the rather old-fashioned notion of putting others before oneself? Should professionals avoid exploiting their positions to pursue an agenda separate from that of their profession? And perhaps most crucial, to what extent do professionals have a collective duty to ensure that their profession provides nondiscriminatory access to all professional services?

Some health care providers would counter that they distinguish between medical care and nonmedical care that uses medical services. In this way, they justify their willingness to bind the wounds of the criminal before sending him back to the street or to set the bones of a battering husband that were broken when he struck his wife. Birth control, abortion, and in vitro fertilization, they say, are lifestyle choices, not treatments for diseases.

And it is here that licensing systems complicate the equation. Such a claim would be easier to make if the states did not give these professionals the exclusive right to offer such services. By granting a monopoly, they turn the profession into a kind of public utility, obligated to provide service to all who seek it. Claiming an unfettered right to personal autonomy while holding monopolistic control over a public good constitutes an abuse of the public trust—all the worse if it is not in fact a personal act of conscience but, rather, an attempt at cultural conquest.

Accepting a collective obligation does not mean that all members of the profession are forced to violate their own consciences. It does, however, necessitate ensuring that a genuine system for counseling and referring patients is in place, so that every patient can act according to his or her own conscience just as readily as the professional can. This goal is not simple to achieve, but it does represent the best effort to accommodate everyone and is the approach taken by virtually all the major medical, nursing, and pharmacy societies. It is also the approach taken by the governor of Illinois, who is imposing an obligation on pharmacies, rather than on individual pharmacists, to ensure access to services for all patients.

Conscience is a tricky business. Some interpret its personal beacon as the guide to universal truth. But the assumption that one's own conscience is the conscience of the world is fraught with dangers. As C.S. Lewis wrote, "Of all tyrannies, a tyranny sincerely exercised for the good of its victims may be the most oppressive. It would be better to live under robber barons than under omnipotent moral busybodies. The robber baron's cruelty may sometimes sleep, his cupidity may at some point be satiated; but those who torment us for our own good will torment us without end for they do so with the approval of their own conscience."

R. Alta Charo teaches law and bioethics at the University of Wisconsin Law and Medical Schools.

EXPLORING THE ISSUE

Should Pro-Life Health Providers Be Allowed to Deny Prescriptions on the Basis of Conscience?

Critical Thinking and Reflection

1. Why might refusal to dispense morning after pills lead to a "slippery slope"?
2. Should health providers ever have the right to refuse to provide medical care or dispense medications they do not support?
3. What problems might develop if pharmacists have the right to refuse to fill all prescriptions?

Is There Common Ground?

In the years since *Roe v. Wade*, state and federal legislatures have seen a growth in conscience clauses. Many pro-choice advocates perceive these clauses as another way to limit a woman's right to choose. Within weeks of the *Roe* decision in the early 1970s, Congress adopted legislation that permitted individual health care providers receiving federal funding or working for organizations receiving such funding to refuse to perform or assist in performing abortions or sterilizations if these procedures violated their moral or religious beliefs. The provision also prohibited discrimination against these providers because of the refusal to perform abortions or sterilizations. Currently, 45 states allow health care providers to refuse to be involved in abortions. Also, 12 states allow health care providers to refuse to provide sterilization, while 13 states allow providers to refuse to provide contraceptive services or information related to contraception.

Pharmacists who refuse to fill prescriptions for birth control pills or emergency contraception largely believe that these medications are actually a method of abortion. In a paper published in the *Archives of Family Medicine* (2000), physicians Walter Larimore and Joseph B. Stanford stated that birth control pills have the potential of interrupting development of the fertilized egg after fertilization. Emergency contraception or the morning after pill also has been seen as a means of abortion. It prevents pregnancy by either preventing fertilization or preventing implantation of a fertilized egg in the uterus. The morning after pill is often confused with RU-486, which is clearly a method of abortion. Unlike RU-486, emergency contraception cannot disrupt an established pregnancy and

cannot cause an abortion. Clearly, better education about the methods of action of these drugs would be valuable.

Solutions have been proposed to enable patients to receive the drugs prescribed by their physicians. As a rule, it would make sense for pharmacists who will not dispense a drug to have an obligation to meet their customers' needs by referring them to other pharmacies. Pharmacists who object to filling prescriptions for birth control pills or emergency contraception might ensure that there is a pharmacist on duty who will fill the prescription or refer their customers elsewhere.

In some countries, customers can purchase the drug without a prescription. In the United States, a prescription can only be filled by a licensed pharmacist. As a result, pharmacists are the last link in the chain of delivery. The author believes it is not acceptable to allow refusals in urban areas where pharmacies are plentiful, but forbid them in rural settings, where pharmacies are scarce. Rather, there should be strong public policy requiring that all pharmacists dispense emergency contraception to customers who request it, regardless of pharmacists' moral or religious objections. In "Claims of Conscience: Setting the Ground Rules When Rights Collide," *Humanist* (September/October 2009), the author discusses right of conscience claims, which allow pharmacists to refuse to fill morning after pill prescriptions. The author notes that these claims can be taken too far. It takes a result-oriented approach to the ethical argument so that if another pharmacist is available to fill the legal prescription, it would allow a conscience refusal but not otherwise. See also "Pharmacist Conscience Clauses and Access to Oral Contraceptives" (*Journal of Medical Ethics*, July 2008). This paper examines the pharmacists' role and their professional and moral obligations to patients in the light of recent refusals by pharmacists to dispense oral contraceptives.

This issue raises important questions about public health and individual rights. Should pharmacists have a right to reject prescriptions for birth control pills, emergency contraception, Viagra, or any other drug that may be morally objectionable to them?

Additional Resources

Davidson, L. A., Pettis, C. T., Joiner, A. J., Cook, D. M., & Klugman, C. M. (2010). Religion and conscientious objection: A survey of pharmacists' willingness to dispense medications. *Social Science & Medicine, 71*(1), 161–165.

Dubow, S. (2015). "A constitutional right rendered utterly meaningless": Religious exemptions and reproductive politics, 1973–2014. *Journal of Policy History, 27*(1), 1–35.

Kelleher, J. (2010). Emergency contraception and conscientious objection. *Journal of Applied Philosophy, 27*(3), 290–304.

Lewis, J. D., & Sullivan, D. M. (2012). Abortifacient potential of emergency contraceptives. *Ethics & Medicine: An International Journal of Bioethics, 28*(3), 113–120.

Marshall, C. (2013). The spread of conscience clause legislation. *Human Rights, 39*(2), 15–16.

Internet References . . .

American Pharmacists Association

www.aphanet.org/

National Right to Life

www.nrlc.org/

Pharmacists for Life International

www.pfli.org/

Selected, Edited, and with Issue Framing Material by:
Eileen L. Daniel, *SUNY College at Brockport*

ISSUE

Should the Cervical Cancer Vaccine for Girls Be Compulsory?

YES: Cynthia Dailard, from "Achieving Universal Vaccination Against Cervical Cancer in the United States: The Need and the Means," *Guttmacher Policy Review* (2006)

NO: Gail Javitt, Deena Berkowitz, and Lawrence O. Gostin, from "Assessing Mandatory HPV Vaccination: Who Should Call the Shots?" *Journal of Law, Medicine & Ethics* (2008)

Learning Outcomes

After reading this issue, you will be able to:

- Discuss why many parents oppose having their daughters vaccinated against cervical cancer.
- Assess the risk associated with contracting the HPV virus.
- Identify the side effects associated with the vaccine.

ISSUE SUMMARY

YES: The late Cynthia Dailard, a senior public policy associate at the Guttmacher Institute, argues that universal vaccination is needed because virtually all cases of cervical cancer are linked to the human papillomavirus. Most infected people are unaware of their infection, which is linked to nearly 10,000 cases of cervical cancer.

NO: Professors Gail Javitt, Deena Berkowitz, and Lawrence O. Gostin believe that mandating the cervical cancer vaccine raises significant legal, ethical, and social concerns. They are also concerned about the long-term safety and effectiveness of the vaccine.

A number of infectious diseases are almost completely preventable through childhood immunization. These include diphtheria, meningitis, pertussis (whooping cough), tetanus, polio, measles, mumps, and rubella (German measles). Largely as a result of widespread vaccination, these once-common diseases have become relatively rare. Before the introduction of the polio vaccine in 1955, polio epidemics occurred each year. In 1952, a record 20,000 cases were diagnosed, as compared to the last outbreak in 1979, when only 10 cases were identified.

While vaccination is a life saver, it may also be controversial. In June 2006, the Food and Drug Administration approved a new immunization called Gardisil, used to prevent diseases caused by the sexually transmitted human papillomavirus (HPV). The virus causes genital warts and cervical cancer. The Centers for Disease Control and Prevention has determined that up to 50 percent of all sexually active men and women in the United States will be infected with HPV at some time in their life. The infection is especially common among women aged 20–24. About 20 states are considering making the vaccination a requirement, while Texas has already done so. Many parents and lawmakers are opposed to the mandatory vaccination for a variety of reasons: the vaccine doesn't target all types of HPV, it doesn't prevent diseases caused by these other types, and while HPV affects both sexes, it's usually recommended for girls. Other reasons for the opposition include the relatively high cost of the vaccine, the fact that many people don't understand that HPV causes cervical cancer, and questions about its long-term safety.

The Centers for Disease Control and Prevention supports getting as many girls vaccinated as early and as fast as possible. They believe this vaccination will reduce the incidence and prevalence of cervical cancer among older women and lessen the spread of this highly infectious disease. The American Cancer Society also supports early and widespread vaccination of young girls.

In the United States it is believed that a valid way to lower the expense of the HPV vaccine and to educate the public on the advantages of vaccination is to make it compulsory for girls entering school. Vaccinations for mumps, measles, rubella, and hepatitis B (which is also sexually transmitted) are currently required. While there is value in preventing cervical cancer, which is estimated to be the most common sexually transmitted infection in the United States, many parents have concerns over manda-

tory vaccination to prevent a sexually transmitted disease. Some parents believe that young girls should be encouraged to abstain from sexual relations rather than being forced to receive the vaccination.

In the YES and NO selections, the late Cynthia Dailard, a senior public policy associate at the Guttmacher Institute, argued that universal vaccination was needed because virtually all cases of cervical cancer are linked to the human papillomavirus. Most infected people are unaware of their infection, which is linked to nearly 10,000 cases of cervical cancer. Professors Gail Javitt, Deena Berkowitz, and Lawrence Gostin believe that mandating the cervical cancer vaccine raises significant legal, ethical, and social concerns. They are also concerned over the long-term safety and effectiveness of the relatively new vaccine.

YES ↵

Cynthia Dailard

Achieving Universal Vaccination Against Cervical Cancer in the United States: The Need and the Means

The advent of a vaccine against the types of human papillomavirus (HPV) linked to most cases of cervical cancer is widely considered one of the greatest health care advances for women in recent years. Experts believe that vaccination against HPV has the potential to dramatically reduce cervical cancer incidence and mortality particularly in resource-poor developing countries where cervical cancer is most common and deadly. In the United States, the vaccine's potential is likely to be felt most acutely within low-income communities and communities of color, which disproportionately bear the burden of cervical cancer.

Because HPV is easily transmitted through sexual contact, the vaccine's full promise may only be realized through near-universal vaccination of girls and young women prior to sexual activity—a notion reflected in recently proposed federal guidelines. And history, as supported by a large body of scientific evidence, suggests that the most effective way to achieve universal vaccination is by requiring children to be inoculated prior to attending school. Yet the link between HPV and sexual activity—and the notion that HPV is different than other infectious diseases targeted by vaccine school entry requirements—tests the prevailing justification for such efforts. Meanwhile, any serious effort to achieve universal vaccination among young people with this relatively expensive vaccine will expose holes in the public health safety net that, if left unaddressed, have the potential to exacerbate longstanding disparities in cervical cancer rates among American women.

The Case for Universal Vaccination

Virtually all cases of cervical cancer are linked to HPV, an extremely common sexually transmitted infection (STI) that is typically asymptomatic and harmless; most people never know they are infected, and most cases resolve on their own. It is estimated that approximately three in four Americans contract HPV at some point in their lives, with most cases acquired relatively soon after individuals have sex for the first time. Of the approximately 30 known types of HPV that are sexually transmitted, more than 13 are associated with cervical cancer. Yet despite the prevalence of HPV, cervical cancer is relatively rare in the United States; it generally occurs only in the small proportion of cases where a persistent HPV infection goes undetected over many years. This is largely due to the widespread availability of Pap tests, which can detect precancerous changes of the cervix that can be treated before cancer sets in, as well as cervical cancer in its earliest stage, when it is easily treatable.

Still, the American Cancer Society estimates that in 2006, almost 10,000 cases of invasive cervical cancer will occur to American women, resulting in 3,700 deaths. Significantly, more than half of all U.S. women diagnosed with cervical cancer have not had a Pap test in the last three years. These women are disproportionately low income and women of color who lack access to affordable and culturally competent health services. As a result, the incidence of cervical cancer is approximately 1.5 times higher among African American and Latina women than among white women; women of color are considerably more likely than whites to die of the disease as well. Two new HPV vaccines—Gardasil, manufactured by Merck & Company, and Cervarix, manufactured by GlaxoSmithKline—promise to transform this landscape. Both are virtually 100% effective in preventing the two types of HPV responsible for 70% of all cases of cervical cancer; Gardasil also protects against two other HPV types associated with 90% of all cases of genital warts. Gardasil was approved by the federal Food and Drug Administration (FDA) in June; GlaxoSmithKline is expected to apply for FDA approval of Cervarix by year's end.

Following FDA approval, Gardasil was endorsed by the Centers for Disease Control and Prevention's Advisory

Dailard, Cynthia. From *Guttmacher Policy Review*, vol. 9, no. 4, Fall 2006, pp. 12–16. Copyright © 2006 by Guttmacher Institute. Reprinted by permission.

Committee on Immunization Practices (ACIP), which is responsible for maintaining the nation's schedule of recommended vaccines. ACIP recommended that the vaccine be routinely administered to all girls ages 11–12, and as early as age nine at a doctor's discretion. Also, it recommended vaccination of all adolescents and young women ages 13–26 as part of a national "catch-up" campaign for those who have not already been vaccinated.

The ACIP recommendations, which are closely followed by health care professionals, reflect the notion that to eradicate cervical cancer, it will be necessary to achieve near-universal vaccination of girls and young women prior to sexual activity, when the vaccine is most effective. Experts believe that such an approach has the potential to significantly reduce cervical cancer deaths in this country and around the world. Also, high vaccination rates will significantly reduce the approximately 3.5 million abnormal Pap results experienced by American women each year, many of which are caused by transient or persistent HPV infections. These abnormal Pap results require millions of women to seek follow-up care, ranging from additional Pap tests to more invasive procedures such as colposcopies and biopsies. This additional care exacts a substantial emotional and even physical toll on women, and costs an estimated $6 billion in annual health care expenditures. Finally, widespread vaccination fosters "herd immunity," which is achieved when a sufficiently high proportion of individuals within a population are vaccinated that those who go unvaccinated—because the vaccine is contraindicated for them or because they are medically underserved, for example—are essentially protected.

The Role of School Entry Requirements

Achieving high vaccination levels among adolescents, however, can be a difficult proposition. Unlike infants and toddlers, who have frequent contact with health care providers in the context of well-child visits, adolescents often go for long stretches without contact with a health care professional. In addition, the HPV vaccine is likely to pose particular challenges, given that it must be administered three times over a six-month period to achieve maximum effectiveness.

A large body of evidence suggests that the most effective means to ensure rapid and widespread use of childhood or adolescent vaccines is through state laws or policies that require children to be vaccinated prior to enrollment in day care or school. These school-based immunization requirements, which exist in some form in all 50 states, are widely credited for the success of immunization programs

in the United States. They have also played a key role in helping to close racial, ethnic and socioeconomic gaps in immunization rates, and have proven to be far more effective than guidelines recommending the vaccine for certain age-groups or high-risk populations. Although each state decides for itself whether a particular vaccine will be required for children to enroll in school, they typically rely on ACIP recommendations in making their decision.

In recent months, some commentators have noted that as a sexually transmitted infection, HPV is "different" from other infectious diseases such as measles, mumps or whooping cough, which are easily transmitted in a school setting or threaten school attendance when an outbreak occurs. Some socially conservative advocacy groups accordingly argue that the HPV vaccine does not meet the historical criteria necessary for it to be required for children attending school; many of them also contend that abstinence outside of marriage is the real answer to HPV. They welcome the advent of the vaccine, they say, but will oppose strenuously any effort to require it for school enrollment.

This position reflects only a limited understanding of school-based vaccination requirements. These requirements do not exist solely to prevent the transmission of disease in school or during childhood. Instead, they further society's strong interest in ensuring that people are protected from disease throughout their lives and are a highly efficient means of eradicating disease in the larger community. For example, states routinely require school-age children to be vaccinated against rubella (commonly known as German measles), a typically mild illness in children, to protect pregnant women in the community from the devastating effects the disease can have on a developing fetus. Similarly, states currently require vaccination against certain diseases, such as tetanus, that are not "contagious" at all, but have very serious consequences for those affected. And almost all states require vaccination against Hepatitis B, a blood borne disease which can be sexually transmitted.

Moreover, according to the National Conference of State Legislatures (NCSL), all 50 states allow parents to refuse to vaccinate their children on medical grounds, such as when a vaccine is contraindicated for a particular child due to allergy, compromised immunity or significant illness. All states except Mississippi and West Virginia allow parents to refuse to vaccinate their children on religious grounds. Additionally, 20 states go so far as to allow parents to refuse to vaccinate their children because of a personal, moral or other belief. Unlike a medical exemption, which requires a parent to provide documentation from a physician, the process for obtaining nonmedical exemptions can vary widely by state.

NCSL notes that, in recent years, almost a dozen states considered expanding their exemption policy. Even absent any significant policy change, the rate of parents seeking exemptions for nonmedical reasons is on the rise. This concerns public health experts. Research shows that in states where exemptions are easier to obtain, a higher proportion of parents refuse to vaccinate their children; research further shows that these states, in turn, are more likely to experience outbreaks of vaccine-preventable diseases, such as measles and whooping cough. Some vaccine program administrators fear that because of the social sensitivities surrounding the HPV vaccine, any effort to require the vaccine for school entry may prompt legislators to amend their laws to create nonmedical exemptions where they do not currently exist or to make existing exemptions easier to obtain. This has the potential not only to thwart the effort to stem the tide of cervical cancer, but to foster the spread of other vaccine-preventable diseases as well.

Financing Challenges Laid Bare

Another barrier to achieving universal vaccination of girls and young women will be the high price of the vaccine. Gardasil is expensive by vaccine standards, costing approximately $360 for the three-part series of injections. Despite this high cost, ACIP's endorsement means that Gardasil will be covered by most private insurers; in fact, a number of large insurers have already announced they will cover the vaccine for girls and young women within the ACIP-recommended age range. Still, the Institute of Medicine estimates that approximately 11% of all American children have private insurance that does not cover immunization, and even those with insurance coverage may have to pay deductibles and copayments that create a barrier to care.

Those who do not have private insurance or who cannot afford the out-of-pocket costs associated with Gardasil will need to rely on a patchwork system of programs that exist to support the delivery of subsidized vaccines to low-income and uninsured individuals. In June, ACIP voted to include Gardasil in the federal Vaccines for Children program (VFC), which provides free vaccines largely to children and teenagers through age 18 who are uninsured or receive Medicaid. The program's reach is significant: In 2003, 43% of all childhood vaccine doses were distributed by the VFC program.

The HPV vaccine, however, is not just recommended for children and teenagers; it is also recommended for young

THE POTENTIAL ROLE OF FAMILY PLANNING CLINICS IN AN HPV VACCINE "CATCH-UP" CAMPAIGN

Family planning clinics, including those funded under Title X of the Public Health Service Act, have an important role to play in a national "catch-up" campaign to vaccinate young women against HPV. This is particularly true for women ages 19–26, who are too old to receive free vaccines through the federal Vaccines for Children program but still fall within the ACIP-recommended age range for the HPV vaccine.

Almost 4,600 Title X–funded family planning clinics provide subsidized family planning and related preventive health care to just over five million women nationwide. In theory, Title X clinics are well poised to offer the HPV vaccine, because they already are a major provider of STI services and cervical cancer screening, providing approximately six million STI (including HIV) tests and 2.7 million Pap tests in 2004 alone. Because Title X clients are disproportionately low income and women of color, they are at particular risk of developing cervical cancer later in life. Moreover, most Title X clients fall within the ACIP age recommendations of 26 and under for the HPV vaccine (59% are age 24 or younger, and 18% are ages 25–29); many of these women are uninsured and may not have an alternative source of health care.

Title X funds may be used to pay for vaccines linked to improved reproductive health outcomes, and some Title X clinics offer the Hepatitis B vaccine (which can be sexually transmitted). Although many family planning providers are expressing interest in incorporating the HPV vaccine into their package of services, its high cost—even at a discounted government purchase price—is likely to stand in the way. Clinics that receive Title X funds are required by law to charge women based on their ability to pay, with women under 100% of the federal poverty level (representing 68% of Title X clients) receiving services completely free of charge and those with incomes between 100–250% of poverty charged on a sliding scale. While Merck has expressed an interest in extending its patient assistance program to publicly funded family planning clinics, it makes no promises. In fact, a statement on the company's Web site says that "Due to the complexities associated with vaccine funding and distribution in the public sector, as well as the resource constraints that typically exist in public health settings, Merck is currently evaluating whether and how a vaccine assistance program could be implemented in the public sector."

adult women up through age 26. Vaccines are considered an "optional" benefit for adults under Medicaid, meaning that it is up to each individual state to decide whether or not to cover a given vaccine. Also, states can use their own funds and federal grants to support the delivery of subsidized vaccines to low-income or uninsured adults. Many states, however, have opted instead to channel these funds toward childhood-vaccination efforts, particularly as vaccine prices have grown in recent years. As a result, adult vaccination rates remain low and disparities exist across racial, ethnic and socioeconomic groups—mirroring the disparities that exist for cervical cancer.

In response to all this, Merck in May announced it would create a new "patient assistance program," designed to provide all its vaccines free to adults who are uninsured, unable to afford the vaccines and have an annual household income below 200% of the federal poverty level ($19,600 for individuals and $26,400 for couples). To receive free vaccines, patients will need to complete and fax forms from participating doctors' offices for processing by Merck during the patients' visits. Many young uninsured women, however, do not seek their care in private doctors' offices, but instead rely on publicly funded family planning clinics for their care, suggesting the impact of this program may be limited (see box).

Thinking Ahead

Solutions to the various challenges presented by the HPV vaccine are likely to have relevance far beyond cervical cancer. In the coming years, scientific breakthroughs in the areas of immunology, molecular biology and genetics will eventually permit vaccination against a broader range of acute illnesses as well as chronic diseases. Currently, vaccines for other STIs such as chlamydia, herpes and HIV are in various stages of development. Also under study are vaccines for Alzheimer's disease, diabetes and a range of cancers. Vaccines for use among adolescents will also be increasingly common. A key question is, in the future, will individuals across the economic spectrum have access to these breakthrough medical advances or will disadvantaged individuals be left behind?

When viewed in this broader context, the debate over whether the HPV vaccine should be required for school enrollment may prove to be a healthy one. If the HPV vaccine is indeed "the first of its kind," as some have characterized it, it has the potential to prompt communities across the nation to reconsider and perhaps reconceive the philosophical justification for school entry requirements. Because the U.S. health care system is fragmented, people have no guarantee of health insurance coverage or access to affordable care. School entry requirements might therefore provide an important opportunity to deliver public health interventions that, like the HPV vaccine, offer protections to individuals who have the potential to become disconnected from health care services later in life. Similar to the HPV vaccine's promise of cervical cancer prevention, these benefits may not be felt for many years, but nonetheless may be compelling from a societal standpoint. And bearing in mind that school dropout rates begin to climb as early as age 13, middle school might be appropriately viewed as the last public health gate that an entire age-group of individuals pass through together—regardless of race, ethnicity or socioeconomic status.

Meanwhile, the cost and affordability issues raised by the HPV vaccine may help draw attention to the need to reform the vaccine-financing system in this country. In 2003, the Institute of Medicine proposed a series of reforms designed to improve the way vaccines are financed and distributed. They included a national insurance benefit mandate that would apply to all public and private health care plans and vouchers for uninsured children and adults to receive immunizations through the provider of their choice. Legislation introduced by Rep. Henry Waxman (D-CA) and Sen. Edward Kennedy (D-MA), called the Vaccine Access and Supply Act, adopts a different approach. The bill would expand the Vaccines for Children program, create a comparable Vaccines for Adults program, strengthen the vaccine grant program to the states and prohibit Medicaid cost-sharing requirements for ACIP-recommended vaccines for adults.

Whether the HPV vaccine will in fact hasten reforms of any kind remains to be seen. But one thing is clear: If the benefits of this groundbreaking vaccine cannot be enjoyed by girls and women who are disadvantaged by poverty or insurance status, then it will only serve to perpetuate the disparities in cervical cancer rates that have persisted in this country for far too long.

Cynthia Dailard was a senior public policy associate at the Guttmacher Institute and a NEPRHA board member.

Gail Javitt, Deena Berkowitz,
and Lawrence O. Gostin

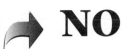 **NO**

Assessing Mandatory HPV Vaccination: Who Should Call the Shots?

I. Introduction

The human papillomavirus (HPV) is the most common sexually transmitted infection worldwide. In the United States, more than six million people are infected each year. Although most HPV infections are benign, two strains of HPV cause 70 percent of cervical cancer cases.[1] Two other strains of HPV are associated with 90 percent of genital warts cases.[2]

In June 2006, the Food and Drug Administration (FDA) approved the first vaccine against HPV. Sold as Gardasil, the quadrivalent vaccine is intended to prevent four strains of HPV associated with cervical cancer, precancerous genital lesions, and genital warts.[3] Following FDA approval, the national Advisory Committee on Immunization Practices (ACIP) recommended routine vaccination for girls ages 11–12 with three doses of quadrivalent HPV vaccine.[4] Thereafter, state legislatures around the country engaged in an intense effort to pass laws mandating vaccination of young girls against HPV. This activity was spurred in part by an intense lobbying campaign by Merck, the manufacturer of the vaccine.[5]

The United States has a robust state-based infrastructure for mandatory vaccination that has its roots in the 19th century. Mandating vaccination as a condition for school entry began in the early 1800s and is currently required by all 50 states for several common childhood infectious diseases.[6] Some suggest that mandatory HPV vaccination for minor females fits squarely within this tradition.

Nonetheless, state efforts to mandate HPV vaccination in minors have raised a variety of concerns on legal, ethical, and social grounds. Unlike other diseases for which state legislatures have mandated vaccination for children, HPV is neither transmissible through casual contact nor potentially fatal during childhood. It also would be the first vaccine to be mandated for use exclusively in one gender. As such, HPV vaccine presents a new context for considering vaccine mandates.

In this paper, we review the scientific evidence supporting Gardasil's approval and the legislative actions in the states that followed. We then argue that mandatory HPV vaccination at this time is both unwarranted and unwise. While the emergence of an HPV vaccine refects a potentially significant public health advance, the vaccine raises several concerns. First, the long-term safety and effectiveness of the vaccine are unclear, and serious adverse events reported shortly after the vaccine's approval raise questions about its short-term safety as well. In light of unanswered safety questions, the vaccine should be rolled out slowly, with risks carefully balanced against benefits in individual cases. Second, the legal and ethical justifications that have historically supported state-mandated vaccination do not support mandating HPV vaccine. Specifically, HPV does not threaten an imminent and significant risk to the health of others. Mandating HPV would therefore constitute an expansion of the state's authority to interfere with individual and parental autonomy. Engaging in such expansion in the absence of robust public discussion runs the risk of creating a public backlash that may undermine the goal of widespread HPV vaccine coverage and lead to public distrust of established childhood vaccine programs for other diseases. Third, the current sex-based HPV vaccination mandates present constitutional concerns because they require only girls to be vaccinated. Such concerns could lead to costly and protracted legal challenges. Finally, vaccination mandates will place economic burdens on federal and state governments and individual practitioners that may have a negative impact on the provision of other health services. In light of these potentially adverse public health, economic, and societal consequences, we believe that it is premature for states to add HPV to the list of state-mandated vaccines.

II. Background

Before discussing in detail the basis for our opposition to mandated HPV vaccination, it is necessary to review the public health impact of HPV and the data based on which the FDA approved the vaccine. Additionally, to understand the potentially widespread uptake of HPV vaccine mandates, we review the state legislative activities that have occurred since the vaccine's approval.

A. HPV Epidemiology

In the United States, an estimated 20 million people, or 15 percent of the population, are currently infected with HPV.[7] Modeling studies suggest that up to 80 percent of sexually active women will have become infected with the virus at some point in their lives by the time they reach age 50.[8] Prevalence of HPV is highest among sexually active females ages 14–19.[9]

Human papillomavirus comprises more than 100 different strains of virus, of which more than 30 infect the genital area.[10] The majority of HPV infections are transient, asymptomatic, and cause no clinical problems. However, persistent infection with high risk types of HPV is the most important risk factor for cervical cancer precursors and invasive cervical cancer. Two strains in particular, 16 and 18, have been classified as carcinogenic to humans by the World Health Organization's international agency for research on cancer.[11] These strains account for 70 percent of cervical cancer cases[12] and are responsible for a large proportion of anal, vulvar, vaginal, penile, and urethral cancers.[13]

More than 200,000 women die of cervical cancer each year.[14] The majority of these deaths take place in developing countries, which lack the screening programs and infrastructure for diagnosis, treatment, and prevention that exist in the United States. In the U.S., it is estimated that there were about 9,700 cases of invasive cervical cancer and about 3,700 deaths from cervical cancer in 2006, as compared with 500,000 cases and 288,000 deaths worldwide.[15]

Two other HPV types, 6 and 11, are associated with approximately 90 percent of anogenital warts. They are also associated with low grade cervical disease and recurrent respiratory papillomatosis (RRP), a disease consisting of recurrent warty growths in the larynx and respiratory tract. Juvenile onset RRP (JORRP), a rare disorder caused by exposure to HPV during the peripartum period, can cause significant airway obstruction or lead to squamous cell carcinoma with poor prognosis.[16]

Although HPV types 6, 11, 16, and 18 are associated with significant morbidity and mortality, they have a fairly low prevalence in the U.S. population. One study of sexually active women ages 18 to 25 found HPV 16 and 18 prevalence to be 7.8 percent.[17] Another study found overall prevalence of types 6, 11, 16, and 18 to be 1.3 percent, 0.1 percent, 1.5 percent, and 0.8 percent, respectively.[18]

B. Gardasil Safety and Effectiveness

Gardasil was approved based on four randomized, double blind, placebo-controlled studies in 21,000 women ages 16 to 26. Girls as young as nine were included in the safety and immunogenicity studies but not the efficacy studies. The results demonstrated that in women without prior HPV infection, Gardasil was nearly 100 percent effective in preventing precancerous cervical lesions, precancerous vaginal and vulvar lesions, and genital warts caused by vaccine-type HPV. Although the study period was not long enough for cervical cancer to develop, the prevention of these cervical precancerous lesions was considered a valid surrogate marker for cancer prevention. The studies also show that the vaccine is only effective when given prior to infection with high-risk strains.[19]

Gardasil is the second virus-like particle (VLP) vaccine to be approved by the FDA; the first was the Hepatitis B vaccine. VLPs consist of viral protein particles derived from the structural proteins of a virus. These particles are nearly identical to the virus from which they were derived but lack the virus's genetic material required for replication, so they are noninfectious and nononcogenic. VLPs offer advantages over more traditional peptide vaccines as the human body is more highly attuned to particulate antigens, which leads to a stronger immune response since VLP vaccines cannot revert to an infectious form, such as attenuated particles or incompletely killed particles.

No serious Gardasil-related adverse events were observed during clinical trials. The most common adverse events reported were injection site reactions, including pain, redness, and swelling.[20] The most common systemic adverse reactions experienced at the same rate by both vaccine and placebo recipients were headache, fever, and nausea. Five vaccine recipients reported adverse vaccine-related experiences: bronchospasm, gastroenteritis, headache with hypertension, joint movement impairment near injection site, and vaginal hemorrhage. Women with positive pregnancy tests were excluded from the studies, as were some women who became pregnant following receipt of either vaccine or placebo. The incidence of spontaneous pregnancy loss and congenital anomalies were similar in both groups.[21] Gardasil was assigned pregnancy risk category B by the FDA on the basis that animal reproduction studies failed to demonstrate a risk to the fetus.[22]

As of June 2007, the most recent date for which CDC has made data available, there were 1,763 reports of potential side effects following HPV vaccination made to the CDC's Vaccine Adverse Event Reporting System (VAERS). Ninety-four of these were defined as serious, including 13 unconfirmed reports of Guillain-Barre syndrome (GBS), a neurological illness resulting in muscle weakness and sometimes in paralysis. The CDC is investigating these cases. Seven deaths were also reported among females who received the vaccine, but the CDC stated that none of these deaths appeared to be caused by vaccination.[23]

Although the FDA approved the vaccine for females ages 9–26, based on the data collected in those age groups, the ACIP recommendation for vaccination is limited to females ages 11–12. This recommendation was based on several considerations, including age of sexual debut in the United States and the high probability of HPV acquisition within several years of sexual debut, cost-effectiveness evaluations, and the established young adolescent health care visit at ages 11–12 when other vaccines are also recommended.

C. State Legislative Actvivities

Since the approval of Gardasil, legislators in 41 states and the District of Columbia have introduced legislation addressing the HPV vaccine.[24] Legislative responses to Gardasil have focused on the following recommendations: (1) mandating HPV vaccination of minor girls as a condition for school entrance; (2) mandating insurance coverage for HPV vaccination or providing state funding to defray or eliminate cost of vaccination; (3) educating the public about the HPV vaccine; and/or (4) establishing committees to make recommendations about the vaccine.

In 2007, 24 states and the District of Columbia introduced legislation specifically to mandate the HPV vaccine as a condition for school entry.[25] Of these, only Virginia and Washington, D.C. passed laws requiring HPV vaccination. The Virginia law requires females to receive three properly spaced doses of HPV vaccine, with the first dose to be administered before the child enters sixth grade. A parent or guardian may refuse vaccination for his child after reviewing "materials describing the link between the human papillomavirus and cervical cancer approved for such use by the Board of Health."[26] The law will take effect October 1, 2008.

Additionally, the D.C. City Council passed the HPV Vaccination and Reporting Act of 2007, which directs the mayor to establish an HPV vaccination program "consistent with the standards set forth by the Centers for Disease Control for all females under the age of 13 who are residents of the District of Columbia."[27] The program includes a "requirement that the parent or legal guardian of a female child enrolling in grade 6 for the first time submit certification that the child has received the HPV vaccine" and a provision that "allows a parent or guardian to opt out of the HPV vaccination requirement." It also directs the mayor to develop reporting requirements "for the collection and

analyzation [sic] of HPV vaccination data within the District of Columbia Department of Health," including "annual reporting to the Department of Health as to the immunization status of each female child entering grade 6." The law requires Congressional approval in order to take effect.

In contrast, an Executive Order issued by the Texas governor was thwarted by that state's legislature. Executive Order 4, signed by Governor Rick Perry on February 4, 2007, would have directed the state's health department to adopt rules mandating the "age appropriate vaccination of all female children for HPV prior to admission to the sixth grade."[28] It would have allowed parents to "submit a request for a conscientious objection affidavit form via the Internet." However, H.B. 1098, enacted by the Texas state legislature on April 26, 2007, states that HPV immunization is "not required for a person's admission to any elementary or secondary school," and "preempts any contrary order issued by the governor."[29] The bill was filed without the governor's signature and became effective on May 8, 2007.

Of the 22 other states in which legislation mandating HPV vaccination was introduced in 2007, all would have required girls to be vaccinated somewhere between ages 11 and 13 or before entry into sixth grade. Most would have provided for some sort of parental or guardian exemption, whether for religious, moral, medical, cost, or other reasons. However, vaccine mandate bills in California and Maryland were withdrawn.

Bills requiring insurance companies to cover HPV vaccination or allocating state funds for this purpose were enacted in eight states.[30] Eight states also enacted laws aimed at promoting awareness of the HPV vaccine using various mechanisms, such as school-based distribution of educational materials to parents of early adolescent children.[31] Finally, three states established expert bodies to engage in further study of HPV vaccination either instead of or as an adjunct to other educational efforts.[32]

In total, 41 states and D.C. introduced legislation addressing HPV vaccination in some manner during the 2007 legislative session, and 17 of these states enacted laws relating to HPV vaccination.

III. Why Mandating HPV Is Premature

The approval of a vaccine against cancer-causing HPV strains is a significant public health advance. Particularly in developing countries, which lack the health care resources for routine cervical cancer screening, preventing HPV infection has the potential to save millions of lives. In the face of such a dramatic advance, opposing government-mandated HPV vaccination may seem foolhardy, if not heretical. Yet strong legal, ethical, and policy arguments underlie our position that state-mandated HPV vaccination of minor females is premature.

A. Long-Term Safety and Effectiveness of the Vaccine Is Unknown

Although the aim of clinical trials is to generate safety and effectiveness data that can be extrapolated to the general population, it is widely understood that such trials cannot reveal all possible adverse events related to a product. For this reason, post-market adverse event reporting is required for all manufacturers of FDA-approved products, and post-market surveillance (also called "phase IV studies") may be required in certain circumstances. There have been numerous examples in recent years in which unforeseen adverse reactions following product approval led manufacturers to withdraw their product from the market. For example, in August 1998, the FDA approved Rotashield, the first vaccine for the prevention of rotavirus gastroenteritis in infants. About 7,000 children received the vaccine before the FDA granted the manufacturer a license to market the vaccine. Though a few cases of intussusception, or bowel obstruction, were noted during clinical trials, there was no statistical difference between the overall occurrence of intussusception in vaccine compared with placebo recipients. After administration of approximately 1.5 million doses of vaccine, however, 15 cases of intussusception were reported, and were found to be causally related to the vaccine. The manufacturer subsequently withdrew the vaccine from the market in October 1999.[33]

In the case of HPV vaccine, short-term clinical trials in thousands of young women did not reveal serious adverse effects. However, the adverse events reported since the vaccine's approval are, at the very least, a sobering reminder that rare adverse events may surface as the vaccine is administered to millions of girls and young women. Concerns have also been raised that other carcinogenic HPV types not contained in the vaccines will replace HPV types 16 and 18 in the pathological niche.

The duration of HPV vaccine-induced immunity is unclear. The average follow-up period for Gardasil during clinical trials was 15 months after the third dose of the vaccine. Determining long-term efficacy is complicated by the fact that even during naturally occurring HPV infection, HPV antibodies are not detected in many women. Thus, long-term, follow-up post-licensure studies cannot rely solely upon serologic measurement of HPV-induced antibody titers. One study indicates that protection against persistent HPV 16 infection remained

at 94 percent 3.5 years after vaccination with HPV 16.[34] A second study showed similar protection for types 16 and 18 after 4.5 years.[35]

The current ACIP recommendation is based on assumptions about duration of immunity and age of sexual debut, among other factors. As the vaccine is used for a longer time period, it may turn out that a different vaccine schedule is more effective. In addition, the effect on co-administration of other vaccines with regard to safety is unknown, as is the vaccines' efficacy with varying dose intervals. Some have also raised concerns about a negative impact of vaccination on cervical cancer screening programs, which are highly effective at reducing cervical cancer mortality. These unknowns must be studied as the vaccine is introduced in the broader population.

At present, therefore, questions remain about the vaccine's safety and the duration of its immunity, which call into question the wisdom of mandated vaccination. Girls receiving the vaccine face some risk of potential adverse events as well as risk that the vaccine will not be completely protective. These risks must be weighed against the state's interest in protecting the public from the harms associated with HPV. As discussed in the next section, the state's interest in protecting the public health does not support mandating HPV vaccination.

B. Historical Justifications for Mandated Vaccination Are Not Met

HPV is different in several respects from the vaccines that first led to state-mandated vaccination. Compulsory vaccination laws originated in the early 1800s and were driven by fears of the centuries-old scourge of smallpox and the advent of the vaccine developed by Edward Jenner in 1796. By the 1900s, the vast majority of states had enacted compulsory smallpox vaccination laws.[36] While such laws were not initially tied to school attendance, the coincidental rise of smallpox outbreaks, growth in the number of public schools, and compulsory school attendance laws provided a rationale for compulsory vaccination to prevent the spread of smallpox among school children as well as a means to enforce the requirement by barring unvaccinated children from school.[37] In 1827, Boston became the first city to require all children entering public school to provide evidence of vaccination.[38] Similar laws were enacted by several states during the latter half of the 19th century.[39]

The theory of herd immunity, in which the protective effect of vaccines extends beyond the vaccinated individual to others in the population, is the driving force behind mass immunization programs. Herd immunity theory proposes that, in diseases passed from person to person, it is difficult to maintain a chain of infection when large numbers of a population are immune. With the increase in number of immune individuals present in a population, the lower the likelihood that a susceptible person will come into contact with an infected individual. There is no threshold value above which herd immunity exists, but as vaccination rates increase, indirect protection also increases until the infection is eliminated.

Courts were soon called on to adjudicate the constitutionality of mandatory vaccination programs. In 1905, the Supreme Court decided the seminal case, *Jacobson v. Massachusetts*,[40] in which it upheld a population-wide smallpox vaccination ordinance challenged by an adult male who refused the vaccine and was fined five dollars. He argued that a compulsory vaccination law was "hostile to the inherent right of every freeman to care for his own body and health in such way as to him seems best." The Court disagreed, adopting a narrower view of individual liberty and emphasizing the duties that citizens have towards each other and to society as a whole. According to the Court, the "liberty secured by the Constitution of the United States . . . does not import an absolute right in each person to be, at all times and in all circumstances, wholly freed from restraint. There are manifold restraints to which every person is necessarily subject for the common good." With respect to compulsory vaccination, the Court stated that "[u]pon the principle of self-defense, of paramount necessity, a community has the right to protect itself against an epidemic of disease which threatens the safety of its members." In the Court's opinion, compulsory vaccination was consistent with a state's traditional police powers, i.e., its power to regulate matters affecting the health, safety, and general welfare of the public.

In reaching its decision, the Court was influenced both by the significant harm posed by smallpox—using the words "epidemic" and "danger" repeatedly—as well as the available scientific evidence demonstrating the efficacy of the vaccine. However, the Court also emphasized that its ruling was applicable only to the case before it, and articulated principles that must be adhered to for such an exercise of police powers to be constitutional. First, there must be a public health necessity. Second, there must be a reasonable relationship between the intervention and public health objective. Third, the intervention may not be arbitrary or oppressive. Finally, the intervention should not pose a health risk to its subject. Thus, while *Jacobson* "stands firmly for the proposition that police powers authorize states to compel vaccination for the public good," it also indicates that "government power must be exercised reasonably to pass constitutional scrutiny."[41] In the 1922 case *Zucht v. King*,[42] the Court reaffirmed its ruling in *Jacobson* in the context of a school-based smallpox vaccination mandate.

The smallpox laws of the 19th century, which were almost without exception upheld by the courts, helped lay the foundation for modern immunization statutes. Many modern-era laws were enacted in response to the transmission of measles in schools in the 1960s and 1970s. In 1977, the federal government launched the Childhood Immunization Initiative, which stressed the importance of strict enforcement of school immunization laws.[43] Currently, all states mandate vaccination as a condition for school entry, and in deciding whether to mandate vaccines, are guided by ACIP recommendations. At present, ACIP recommends vaccination for diphtheria, tetanus, and acellular pertussis (DTaP), Hepatitis B, polio, measles, mumps, and rubella (MMR), varicella (chicken pox), influenza, rotavirus, haemophilus Influenza B (HiB), pneumococcus, Hepatitis A, meningococcus, and, most recently HPV. State mandates differ; for example, whereas all states require DTaP, polio, and measles in order to enter kindergarten, most do not require Hepatitis A.[44]

HPV is different from the vaccines that have previously been mandated by the states. With the exception of tetanus, all of these vaccines fit comfortably within the "public health necessity" principle articulated in *Jacobson* in that the diseases they prevent are highly contagious and are associated with significant morbidity and mortality occurring shortly after exposure. And, while tetanus is not contagious, exposure to *Clostridium tetani* is both virtually unavoidable (particularly by children, given their propensity to both play in the dirt and get scratches), life threatening, and fully preventable only through vaccination. Thus, the public health necessity argument plausibly extends to tetanus, albeit for different reasons.

Jacobson's "reasonable relationship" principle is also clearly met by vaccine mandates for the other ACIP recommended vaccines. School-aged children are most at risk while in school because they are more likely to be in close proximity to each other in that setting. All children who attend school are equally at risk of both transmitting and contracting the diseases. Thus, a clear relationship exists between conditioning school attendance on vaccination and the avoidance of the spread of infectious disease within the school environment. Tetanus, a noncontagious disease, is somewhat different, but school-based vaccination can nevertheless be justified in that children will foreseeably be exposed within the school environment (e.g., on the playground) and, if exposed, face a high risk of mortality.

HPV vaccination, in contrast, does not satisfy these two principles. HPV infection presents no public health necessity, as that term was used in the context of *Jacobson*. While non-sexual transmission routes are theoretically possible, they have not been demonstrated. Like other sexually transmitted diseases which primarily affect adults, it is not immediately life threatening; as such, cervical cancer, if developed, will not manifest for years if not decades. Many women will never be exposed to the cancer-causing strains of HPV; indeed the prevalence of these strains in the U.S. is quite low. Furthermore, many who are exposed will not go on to develop cervical cancer. Thus, conditioning school attendance on HPV vaccination serves only to coerce compliance in the absence of a public health emergency.[45]

The relationship between the government's objective of preventing cervical cancer in women and the means used to achieve it—that is, vaccination of all girls as a condition of school attendance—lacks sufficient rationality. First, given that HPV is transmitted through sexual activity, exposure to HPV is not directly related to school attendance.[46] Second, not all children who attend school are at equal risk of exposure to or transmission of the virus. Those who abstain from sexual conduct are not at risk for transmitting or contracting HPV. Moreover, because HPV screening tests are available, the risk to those who choose to engage in sexual activity is significantly minimized. Because it is questionable how many school-aged children are actually at risk—and for those who are at risk, the risk is not linked to school attendance—there is not a sufficiently rational reason to tie mandatory vaccination to school attendance.

To be sure, the public health objective that proponents of mandatory HPV vaccination seek to achieve is compelling. Vaccinating girls before sexual debut provides an opportunity to provide protection against an adult onset disease. This opportunity is lost once sexual activity begins and exposure to HPV occurs. However, that HPV vaccination may be both medically justified and a prudent public health measure is an insufficient basis for the state to compel children to receive the vaccine as a condition of school attendance.

C. In the Absence of Historical Justification, the Government Risks Public Backlash by Mandating HPV Vaccination

Childhood vaccination rates in the United States are very high; more than half of the states report meeting the Department of Health and Human Services (HHS) Healthy People 2010 initiative's goal of 95 percent vaccination coverage for childhood vaccination.[47] However, from its inception, state mandated vaccination has been accompanied by a small but vocal anti-vaccination movement. Opposition has historically been "fueled by general distrust of government, a rugged sense of individualism, and concerns about the efficacy and safety of vaccines."[48] In recent years, vaccination programs also have been a "victim of their tremendous success,"[49] as dreaded diseases such as measles and polio have largely disappeared in the United States, taking with them the fear that motivated past generations. Some have noted with alarm the rise in the number of parents opting out of vaccination and of resurgence in anti-vaccination rhetoric making scientifically unsupported allegations that vaccination causes adverse events such as autism.[50]

The rash of state legislation to mandate HPV has led to significant public concern that the government is overreaching its police powers authority. As one conservative columnist has written, "[F]or the government to mandate the expensive vaccine for children would be for Big Brother to reach past the parents and into the home."[51] While some dismiss sentiments such as this one as simply motivated by right wing moral politics, trivializing these concerns is both inappropriate and unwise as a policy matter. Because sexual behavior is involved in transmission, not all children are equally at risk. Thus, it is a reasonable exercise of a parent's judgment to consider his or her child's specific risk and weigh that against the risk of vaccination.

To remove parental autonomy in this case is not warranted and also risks parental rejection of the vaccine because it is perceived as coercive. In contrast, educating the public about the value of the vaccine may be highly effective without risking public backlash. According to one poll, 61 percent of parents with daughters under 18 prefer vaccination, 72 percent would support the inclusion of information about the vaccine in school health classes, and just 45 percent agreed that the vaccine should be included as part of the vaccination routine for all children and adolescents.[52]

Additionally, Merck's aggressive role in lobbying for the passage of state laws mandating HPV has led to some skepticism about whether profit rather than public health has driven the push for state mandates.[53] Even one proponent of state-mandated HPV vaccination acknowledges that Merck "overplayed its hand" by pushing hard for legislation mandating the vaccine.[54] In the face of such criticisms, the company thus ceased its lobbying efforts but indicated it would continue to educate health officials and legislators about the vaccine.[55]

Some argue that liberal opt-out provisions will take care of the coercion and distrust issues. Whether this is true will depend in part on the reasons for which a parent may opt out and the ease of opting out. For example, a parent may not have a religious objection to vaccination in general, but nevertheless may not feel her 11-year-old daughter is at sufficient risk for HPV to warrant vaccination. This sentiment may or may not be captured in a "religious or philosophical" opt-out provision.

Even if opt-out provisions do reduce public distrust issues for HPV, however, liberal opt outs for one vaccine may have a negative impact on other vaccine programs. Currently, with the exception of those who opt out of all vaccines on religious or philosophical grounds, parents must accept all mandated vaccines because no vaccine-by-vaccine selection process exists, which leads to a high rate of vaccine coverage. Switching to an "a la carte" approach, in which parents can consider the risks and benefits of vaccines on a vaccine-by-vaccine basis, would set a dangerous precedent and may lead them to opt out of other vaccines, causing a rise in the transmission of these diseases. In contrast, an "opt in" approach to HPV vaccine would not require a change in the existing paradigm and would still likely lead to a high coverage rate.

D. Mandating HPV for Girls and Not Boys May Violate Constitutional Principles of Equality and Due Process

1. VACCINATION OF MALES MAY PROTECT THEM FROM HPV-RELATED MORBIDITY

The HPV vaccine is the first to be mandated for only one gender. This is likely because the vaccine was approved for girls and not boys. Data demonstrating the safety and immunogenicity of the vaccine are available for males aged 9–15 years. Three phase 1 studies demonstrated that safety, tolerance, and immunogenicity of the HPV vaccine were similar to men and women. The first two studies focused on HPV 16 and 11, respectively, while the third study demonstrated high levels of immunogenicity to prophylactic HPV 6/11/16/18 vaccine in 10–15-year-old males.[56] Phase III clinical trials examining the vaccine's efficacy in men and adolescent boys are currently underway, with results available in the next couple of years.[57]

HPV infection is common among men.[58] One percent of the male population aged 15–49 years has genital warts, with peak incidence in the 20–24-year-old age group.[59] A recent cohort study found the 24-month cumulative incidence of HPV infection among 240 men aged 18–20 years to be 62.4 percent, nearly double the incidence of their female counterparts.[60] This result may have been due to the increased sensitivity of the new HPV-PCR-based testing procedure used in the study. Nonetheless, the results

reaffirm that HPV is common and multifocal in males. Males with genital warts have also been shown to carry the genital type specific HPV virus on their fingertips.[61] While HPV on fingertips may be due to autoinoculation, it may also represent another means of transmission.[62] Men are also at risk for HPV-related anogenital cancers. Up to 76 percent of penile cancers are HPV DNA positive.[63] Fifty-eight percent of anal cancers in heterosexual men and 100 percent among homosexual men are positive for HPV DNA.[64] Therefore, assuming vaccine efficacy is confirmed in males, they also could be protected through HPV vaccination.

2. INCLUDING MALES IN HPV VACCINATION MAY BETTER PROTECT THE PUBLIC THAN FEMALE VACCINATION ALONE

As no clinical trial data on vaccine efficacy in men has been published to date, mathematical models have been used to explore the potential benefits and cost effectiveness of vaccinating boys in addition to girls under various clinical scenarios. Even under the most generous assumption about vaccine efficacy in males and females, cost-effective analyses have found contradictory results. Several studies suggest that if vaccine coverage of women reaches 70–90 percent of the population, then vaccinating males would be of limited value and high cost.[65] Ruanne Barnabas and Geoffrey Garnett found that a multivalent HPV vaccine with 100 percent efficacy targeting males and females 15 years of age with vaccine coverage of at least 66 percent was needed to decrease cervical cancer by 80 percent. They concluded that vaccinating men in addition to women had little incremental benefit in reducing cervical cancer,[66] that vaccine acceptability in males is unknown, and that in a setting with limited resources, the first priority in reducing cervical cancer mortality should be to vaccinate females.

Yet several models argue in favor of vaccinating males. Vaccination not only directly protects through vaccine-derived immunity, but also indirectly through herd immunity, meaning a level of population immunity that is sufficient to protect unvaccinated individuals. If naturally acquired immunity is low and coverage of women is low, then vaccinating men will be of significant benefit. James Hughes et al. found that a female-only monovalent vaccine would be only 60–75 percent as efficient as a strategy that targets both genders.[67] Elamin Elbasha and Erik Dasbach found that while vaccinating 70 percent of females before the age of 12 would reduce genital warts by 83 percent and cervical cancer by 78 percent due to HPV 6/11/16/18, including men and boys in the program would further reduce the incidence of genital warts, CIN, and cervical cancer by 97 percent, 91 percent, and 91 percent, respectively.[68] In all mathematical models, lower female coverage made vaccination of men and adolescent boys more cost effective, as did a shortened duration of natural immunity.

All the models include parameters that are highly inferential and lacking in evidence, such as duration of vaccine protection, reactivation of infections, transmission of infection, and health utilities. The scope of the models is limited to cervical cancer, cancer-in-situ, and genital warts. None of the models accounts for HPV-related anal, head, and neck cancers, or recurrent respiratory papillomatosis. As more data become available, the scope of the models will be broadened and might strengthen the argument in favor of vaccinating males. Given that male vaccination may better protect the public than female vaccination alone, female-specific mandates may be constitutionally suspect, as discussed below.

3. THE GOVERNMENT MUST ADEQUATELY JUSTIFY ITS DECISION TO MANDATE VACCINATION IN FEMALES ONLY

While courts have generally been deferential to state mandate laws, this deference has its limits. In 1900, a federal court struck a San Francisco Board of Health resolution requiring all Chinese residents to be vaccinated with a serum against bubonic plague about which there was little evidence of efficacy. Chinese residents were prohibited from leaving the area unless they were vaccinated. The court struck down the resolution as an unconstitutional violation of the Equal Protection and Due Process clauses. The court found that there was not a defensible scientific rationale for the board's approach and that it was discriminatory in targeting "the Asiatic or Mongolian race as a class." Thus, it was "not within the legitimate police power" of the government.[69]

A sex-based mandate for HPV vaccination could be challenged on two grounds: first, under the Equal Protection Clause because it distinguishes based on gender and second, under the Due Process Clause, because it violates a protected interest in refusing medical treatment. In regard to the Equal Protection concerns, courts review laws that make sex-based distinctions with heightened scrutiny: the government must show that the challenged classification serves an important state interest and that the classification is at least substantially related to serving that interest. To be sure, courts would likely view the goal of preventing cervical cancer as an important public health objective. However, courts would also likely demand that the state justify its decision to burden females with the risks of vaccination, and not males, even though males also contribute to HPV transmission,

will benefit from an aggressive vaccination program of females, and also may reduce their own risk of disease through vaccination.

With respect to the Due Process Clause, the Supreme Court has, in the context of right-to-die cases, recognized that individuals have a constitutionally protected liberty interest in refusing unwanted medical treatment.[70] This liberty interest must, however, be balanced against several state interests, including its interest in preserving life. Mandated HPV laws interfere with the right of girls to refuse medical treatment, and therefore could be challenged under the Due Process Clause. Whether the government could demonstrate interests strong enough to outweigh a girl's liberty interest in refusing vaccination would depend on the strength of the government's argument that such vaccination is life-saving and the extent to which opt outs are available and easily exercised in practice.

Even if courts upheld government mandates as consistent with the Due Process and Equal Protection clauses, such mandates remain troubling in light of inequalities imposed by sex-based mandates and the liberty interests that would be compromised by HPV mandates, therefore placing deeply cherished national values at risk.

E. Unresolved Economic Concerns

Mandated HPV vaccination may have negative unintended economic consequences for both state health departments and private physicians, and these consequences should be thoroughly considered before HPV vaccination is mandated. In recent years, state health departments have found themselves increasingly strapped by the rising number of mandated vaccines. Some states that once provided free vaccines to all children have abandoned the practice due to rising costs. Adding HPV could drive more states to abandon funding for other vaccinations and could divert funding from other important public health measures. At the federal level, spending by the federal Vaccines for Children program, which pays for immunizations for Medicaid children and some others, has grown to $2.5 billion, up from $500 million in 2000.[71] Such rapid increases in budgetary expenses affect the program's ability to assist future patients. Thus, before HPV vaccination is mandated, a thorough consideration of its economic consequences for existing vaccine programs and other non-vaccine programs should be undertaken.

The increasing number of vaccines has also has placed a burden on physicians in private practice. Currently, about 85 percent of the nation's children get all or at least some of their inoculations from private physicians' offices.[72] These offices must purchase vaccines and then wait for reimbursement from either government or private insurers. Some physicians have argued that the rising costs of vaccines and the rising number of new mandatory vaccines make it increasingly difficult for them to purchase vaccinations initially and that they net a loss due to insufficient reimbursement from insurers. Adding HPV to the list of mandated vaccines would place further stress on these practices, and could lead them to reduce the amount of vaccines they purchase or require up-front payment for these vaccines. Either of these steps could reduce access not only to HPV but to all childhood vaccines.

Access to HPV is one reason that some proponents favor state mandates. They argue that in the absence of a state mandate, parents will not know to request the vaccine, or will not be able to afford it because it will not be covered by insurance companies or by federal or state programs that pay for vaccines for the uninsured and underinsured. However, mandates are not the only way to increase parental awareness or achieve insurance coverage. In light of the potentially significant economic consequences of state mandates, policymakers should consider other methods of increasing parental awareness and insurance coverage that do not also threaten to reduce access to those who want vaccination.

IV. Conclusion

Based on the current scientific evidence, vaccinating girls against HPV before they are sexually active appears to provide significant protection against cervical cancer. The vaccine thus represents a significant public health advance. Nevertheless, mandating HPV vaccination at the present time would be premature and ill-advised. The vaccine is relatively new, and long-term safety and effectiveness in the general population is unknown. Vaccination outcomes of those voluntarily vaccinated should be followed for several years before mandates are imposed. Additionally, the HPV vaccine does not represent a public health necessity of the type that has justified previous vaccine mandates. State mandates could therefore lead to a public backlash that will undermine both HPV vaccination efforts and existing vaccination programs. Finally, the economic consequences of mandating HPV are significant and could have a negative impact on financial support for other vaccines as well as other public health programs. These consequences should be considered before HPV is mandated.

The success of childhood vaccination programs makes them a tempting target for the addition of new vaccines that, while beneficial to public health, exceed the original justifications for the development of such programs and impose new financial burdens on both the government, private physicians, and, ultimately, the public. HPV will not be the last disease that state legislatures will attempt to prevent through mandatory vaccination. Thus, legislatures and public health advocates should consider carefully the consequences of altering the current paradigm for mandatory childhood vaccination and should not mandate HPV vaccination in the absence of a new paradigm to justify such an expansion.

Note

The views expressed in this article are those of the authors and do not reflect those of the Genetics and Public Policy Center or its staff.

References

1. D. Saslow et al., "American Cancer Society Guideline for Human Papillomavirus (HPV) Vaccine Use to Prevent Cervical Cancer and Its Precursors," *CA: A Cancer Journal for Clinicians* 57, no. 1 (2007): 7–28.
2. Editorial, "Should HPV Vaccination Be Mandatory for All Adolescents?" *The Lancet* 368, no. 9543 (2006): 1212.
3. U.S. Food and Drug Administration, *FDA Licenses New Vaccine for Prevention of Cervical Cancer and Other Diseases in Females Caused by Human Papillomavirus: Rapid Approval Marks Major Advancement in Public Health, Press Release,* June 8, 2006, *available at* . . . (last visited March 5, 2008).
4. Centers for Disease Control and Prevention, *CDC's Advisory Committee Recommends Human Papillomavirus Virus Vaccination,* Press Release, June 29, 2006, *available at* . . . (last visited March 5, 2008).
5. A. Pollack and S. Saul, "Lobbying for Vaccine to Be Halted," *New York Times,* February 21, 2007, *available at* . . . (last visited March 14, 2008).
6. Centers for Disease Control and Prevention, *Childcare and School Immunization Requirements, 2005–2006, August 2006, available at* . . . (last visited March 5, 2008).
7. Centers for Disease Control and Prevention, "A Closer Look at Human Papillomavirus (HPV)," 2000, *available at* . . . (last visited March 5, 2008); Centers for Disease Control and Prevention, "Genital HPV Infection—CDC Fact Sheet," May 2004, *available at* . . . (last visited March 5, 2008).
8. See Saslow et al., *supra* note 1.
9. S. D. Datta et al., "Sentinel Surveillance for Human Papillomavirus among Women in the United States,

2003–2004," in Program and Abstracts of the 16th Biennial Meeting of the International Society for Sexually Transmitted Diseases Research, Amsterdam, The Netherlands, July 10–13, 2005.

10. Centers for Disease Control and Prevention, "Human Papillomavirus (HPV) Infection," July 2, 2007, *available at* . . . (last visited March 5, 2008).

11. J. R. Nichols, "Human Papillomavirus Infection: The Role of Vaccination in Pediatric Patients," *Clinical Pharmacology and Therapeutics* 81, no. 4 (2007) 607–610.

12. See Saslow et al., *supra* note 1.

13. J. M. Walboomers et al., "Human Papillomavirus Is a Necessary Cause of Invasive Cervical Cancer Worldwide," *Journal of Pathology* 189, no. 1 (1999) 12–19.

14. J. K. Chan and J. S. Berek, "Impact of the Human Papilloma Vaccine on Cervical Cancer," *Journal of Clinical Oncology* 25, no. 20 (2007): 2975–2982.

15. See Saslow et al., *supra* note 1.

16. B. Simma et al., "Squamous-Cell Carcinoma Arising in a Non-Irradiated Child with Recurrent Respiratory Papillomatosis," *European Journal of Pediatrics* 152, no. 9 (1993): 776–778.

17. E. F. Dunne et al., "Prevalence of HPV Infection among Females in the United States," *JAMA* 297, no. 8 (2007): 813–819.

18. L. E. Markowitz et al., "Quadrivalent Human Papillomavirus Vaccine: Recommendations of the Advisory Committee on Immunization Practices (ACIP)," *Morbidity and Mortality Weekly Report* 55, no. RR-2 (2007): 1–24.

19. L. A. Koutsky et al., "A Controlled Trial of a Human Papillomavirus Type 16 Vaccine," *New England Journal of Medicine* 347, no. 21 (2002): 1645–1651; D. R. Brown et al., "Early Assessment of the Efficacy of a Human Papillomavirus Type 16L1 Virus-Like Particle Vaccine," *Vaccine* 22, nos. 21–22 (2004): 2936–2942; C. M. Wheeler, "Advances in Primary and Secondary Interventions for Cervical Cancer: Human Papillomavirus Prophylactic Vaccines and Testing," *Nature Clinical Practice Oncology* 4, no. 4 (2007): 224–235; L. L. Villa et al., "Prophylactic Quadrivalent Human Papillomavirus (Types 6, 11, 16, and 18) L1 Virus-Like Particle Vaccine in Young Women: A Randomized Double-Blind Placebo-Controlled Multicentre Phase II Efficacy Trial," *The Lancet Oncology* 6, no. 5 (2005): 271–278; see Saslow, *supra* note 1.

20. *Id.* (Villa).

21. See Wheeler, *supra* note 19.

22. N. B. Miller, *Clinical Review of Biologics License Application for Human Papillomavirus 6, 11, 16, 18 L1 Virus Like Particle Vaccine (S. cerevisiae) (STN 125126*

GARDASIL), Manufactured by Merck, Inc.," Food and Drug Administration, June 8, 2006, *available at* . . . (last visited March 5, 2008).

23. Centers for Disease Control and Prevention, *HPV Vaccine—Questions and Answers for the Public,* June 28, 2007, *available at* . . . (last visited April 2, 2008).

24. National Conference of State Legislatures, "HPV Vaccine," July 11, 2007, *available at* . . . (last visited March 5, 2008).

25. *Id.*

26. S.B. 1230, 2006 Session, Virginia (2007); H.B. 2035, 2006 Session, Virginia (2007).

27. *HPV Vaccination and Reporting Act of 2007,* B.17–0030, 18th Council, District of Columbia (2007).

28. Governor of the State of Texas, Executive Order RP65, February 2, 2007, *available at* . . . (last visited March 5, 2008).

29. S.B. 438, 80th Legislature, Texas (2007); H.B. 1098, 80th Legislature, Texas (2007).

30. The states are Colorado, Maine, Nevada, New Mexico, New York, North Dakota, Rhode Island, and South Carolina. See National Conference of State Legislatures, *supra* note 24.

31. The states are Colorado, Indiana, Iowa, North Carolina, North Dakota, Texas, Utah, and Washington. *Id.* (National Conference of State Legislatures).

32. The states are Maryland, Minnesota, and New Mexico. *Id.* (National Conference of State Legislatures).

33. Centers for Disease Control and Prevention, *RotaShield (Rotavirus) Vaccine and Intussusception,* 2004, *available at* . . . (last visited March 14, 2008); M. B. Rennels, "The Rotavirus Vaccine Story: A Clinical Investigator's View," *Pediatrics* 106, no. 1 (2000): 123–125.

34. C. Mao et al., "Efficacy of Human Papilomavirus-16 Vaccine to Prevent Cervical Intraepithelial Neoplasia: A Randomized Controlled Trial," *Obstetrics and Gynecology* 107, no. 1 (2006): 18–27.

35. L. L. Villa et al., "Immunologic Responses Following Administration of a Vaccine Targeting Human Papillomavirus Types 6, 11, 16 and 18," *Vaccine* 24, no. 27–28 (2006): 5571–5583; D. M. Harper et al., "Sustained Efficacy Up to 4.5 Years of a Bivalent L1 Virus-Like Particle Vaccine against Human Papillomavirus Types 16 and 18: Follow Up from a Randomized Controlled Trial," *The Lancet* 367, no. 9518 (2006): 1247–1255.

36. J. G. Hodge and L. O. Gostin, "School Vaccination Requirements: Historical, Social, and Legal Perspectives," *Kentucky Law Journal* 90, no. 4 (2001-2002): 831–890.

37. J. Duffy, "School Vaccination: The Precursor to School Medical Inspection," *Journal of the History of Medicine and Allied Sciences* 33, no. 3 (1978): 344–355.

38. See Hodge and Gostin, *supra* note 36.

39. *Id.*

40. *Jacobson v. Commonwealth of Massachusetts,* 197 U.S. 11 (1905).

41. L. O. Gostin and J. G. Hodge, "The Public Health Improvement Process in Alaska: Toward a Model Public Health Law," *Alaska Law Review* 17, no. 1 (2000): 77–125.

42. *Zucht v. King,* 260 U.S. 174 (1922).

43. A. R. Hinman et al., "Childhood Immunization: Laws That Work," *Journal of Law, Medicine & Ethics* 30, no. 3 (2002): 122–127; K. M. Malone and A. R. Hinman, "Vaccination Mandates: The Public Health Imperative and Individual Rights," in R. A. Goodman et al., *Law in Public Health Practice* (New York: Oxford University Press, 2006).

44. See Centers for Disease Control and Prevention, *supra* note 6.

45. B. Lo, "HPV Vaccine and Adolescents' Sexual Activity: It Would Be a Shame if Unresolved Ethical Dilemmas Hampered This Breakthrough," *BMJ* 332, no. 7550 (2006): 1106–1107.

46. R. K. Zimmerman, "Ethical Analysis of HPV Vaccine Policy Options," *Vaccine* 24, no. 22 (2006): 4812–4820.

47. C. Stanwyck et al., "Vaccination Coverage among Children Entering School—United States, 2005–06 School Year," *JAMA* 296, no. 21 (2006): 2544–2547.

48. See Hodge and Gostin, *supra* note 36.

49. S. P. Calandrillo, "Vanishing Vaccinations: Why Are So Many Americans Opting Out of Vaccinating Their Children?" *University of Michigan Journal of Legal Reform* 37 (2004): 353–440.

50. *Id.*

51. B. Hart, "My Daughter Won't Get HPV Vaccine," *Chicago Sun Times, February* 25, 2007, at B6.

52. J. Cummings, "Seventy Percent of U.S. Adults Support Use of the Human Papillomavirus (HPV) Vaccine: Majority of Parents of Girls under 18 Would Want Daughters to Receive It," *Wall Street Journal Online* 5, no. 13 (2006), *available at . . .* (last visited March 5, 2008).

53. J. Marbella, "Sense of Rush Infects Plan to Require HPV Shots," *Baltimore Sun,* January 30, 2007, *available at . . .* (last visited March 14, 2008).

54. S. Reimer, "Readers Worry about HPV Vaccine: Doctors Say It's Safe," *Baltimore Sun,* April 3, 2007.

55. A. Pollack and S. Saul, "Lobbying for Vaccine to Be Halted," *New York Times,* February 21, 2007, *available at . . .* (last visited March 14, 2008).

56. J. Partridge and L. Koutsky, "Genital Human Papillomavirus in Men," *The Lancet Infectious Diseases* 6, no. 1 (2006): 21–31.

57. See Markowitz et al., *supra* note 18.

58. *Id.*

59. See Partridge and Koutsky, *supra* note 56.

60. J. Partridge, "Genital Human Papillomavirus Infection in Men: Incidence and Risk Factors in a Cohort of University Students," *Journal of Infectious Diseases* 196, no. 15 (2007): 1128–1136. It should be noted that the higher incidence might be due to the increased sensitivity of the HPV-PCR-based testing procedure used in this recent study.

61. *Id.*

62. J. Kim, "Vaccine Policy Analysis Can Benefit from Natural History Studies of Human Papillomavirus in Men," *Journal of Infectious Diseases* 196, no. 8 (2007): 1117–1119.

63. See Partridge and Koutsky, *supra* note 56.

64. *Id.*

65. R. V. Barnabas, P. Laukkanen, and P. Koskela, "Epidemiology of HPV 16 and Cervical Cancer in Finland and the Potential Impact of Vaccination: Mathematical Modeling Analysis," *PLoS Medicine* 3, no. 5 (2006): 624–632.

66. *Id.*

67. J. P. Hughess, G. P. Garnett, and L. Koutsky, "The Theoretical Population Level Impace of a Prophylactic Human Papillomavirus Vaccine," *Epidemiology* 13, no. 6 (2002): 631–639.

68. D. Elbasha, "Model for Assessing Human Papillomavirus Vaccination Strategies," *Emerging Infectious Diseases* 13, no. 1 (January 2007): 28–41. Please note that these researchers are employed by Merck, the producer of Gardasil vaccine.

69. *Wong Wai v. Williamson,* 103 F. 1 (N.D. Cal. 1900).

70. *Vacco v. Quill,* 521 U.S. 793 (1997); *Washington v. Glucksberg,* 521 U.S. 702 (1997).

71. A. Pollack, "Rising Costs Make Doctors Balk at Giving Vaccines," *New York Times,* March 24, 2007.

72. *Id.*

GAIL JAVITT is the law and policy director at the Genetics and Public Policy Center in Washington, D.C. She is also a research scientist in the Berman Institute of Bioethics at Johns Hopkins University in Baltimore, Maryland.

DEENA BERKOWITZ is an assistant professor of pediatrics at George Washington University School of Medicine and Health Sciences in Washington, D.C.

LAWRENCE O. GOSTIN is an associate dean, the Linda D. and Timothy J. O'Neil Professor of Global Health Law, the faculty director of the O'Neil Institute for National and Global Health Law, and the director of the Center for Law and the Public's Health at Georgetown University Law Center in Washington, D.C.

EXPLORING THE ISSUE

Should the Cervical Cancer Vaccine for Girls Be Compulsory?

Critical Thinking and Reflection

1. Discuss why the vaccine is controversial.
2. What are the laws governing vaccinations for school children in the United States?
3. Why is it important to try to prevent and treat cervical cancer, especially among women?

Is There Common Ground?

Currently, all 50 states require children to be vaccinated for a variety of illnesses before enrolling in school. Exemptions apply for children whose parents' religious beliefs prohibit vaccinations. Some children are exempt for medical reasons, which must be certified by their doctors. However, almost all children are vaccinated by the time they enter school. The recent development of Gardasil could add another shot to what many children receive by age 5. Should all states make it mandatory for school attendance?

There is considerable opposition to the HPV vaccination due partly to the increasing trend among some parents to refuse to have their children vaccinated. These parents believe, erroneously, that many vaccines are more dangerous than the diseases they prevent. The HPV vaccine adds the additional element of parents' beliefs that their children will remain abstinent until marriage. Abstinence provides effective and absolute protection against this sexually transmitted infection. Unfortunately, by age 19, nearly 70 percent of American girls are sexually active. Another concern among parents is that the vaccine will actually increase sexual activity among teens by removing the threat of HPV infection.

Some additional arguments against the HPV vaccine maintain that cervical cancer is different from measles or polio, diseases that are spread through casual contact. While cervical cancer kills approximately 3,700 women each year in the United States, and nearly 10,000 cases are diagnosed, the disease has a high survival rate though treatment can leave women infertile. In addition, cervical cancer deaths have dropped 75 percent from 1955 to 1992 and the numbers continue to decrease due to the widespread use of the Pap smear. Most women diagnosed with cervical cancer today either have never had a Pap smear or did not have one on a regular basis. Would it make more sense to use public funds to ensure all women have access to Pap smears? Also, not all viral strains are prevented through the use of the vaccine and women would still need to have routine Pap smears. Also, what if the vaccine causes health issues later in life? To determine the safety of Gardasil, researchers conducted a systematic review and meta-analysis to determine the effectiveness and safety of vaccines against cervical cancer. They concluded that the HPV vaccines are safe, well tolerated, and highly effective in preventing infections and cervical diseases among young females. The authors determined, however, that long-term efficacy and safety need to be addressed in future trials. See "Efficacy and Safety of Prophylactic Vaccines Against Cervical HPV Infection and Diseases among Women: A Systematic Review & Meta-Analysis," *BMC Infectious Diseases* (2011).

The American Cancer Society continues to endorse mandatory vaccination for HPV for all girls before entering school. They contend that since not all women get regular Pap smears, the vaccine would be a way to effectively prevent cervical cancer among American women. Attorney R. Alta Charo supports mandatory vaccination with Gardasil and is concerned that "cancer prevention has fallen victim to the culture wars."

Additional Resources

Clayton, J. (2012). Clinical approval: Trials of an anticancer jab. *Nature, 488*(7413), S4–S6.

Dooren, J. (2012, October 2). Study finds HPV vaccine Gardasil safe. *Wall Street Journal—Eastern Edition*, p. D2.

Jenson, H. B. (2012). Community (herd) immunity follows HPV vaccination. (Cover story). *Infectious Disease Alert, 31*(12), 133–134.

Mahoney, D. J., Stojdl, D. F., & Laird, G. (2014). Virus therapy for cancer. *Scientific American, 311*(5), 54–59.

Tomljenovic, L., & Shaw, C. A. (2012). Too fast or not too fast: The FDA's approval of Merck's HPV vaccine Gardasil. *Journal of Law, Medicine & Ethics, 40*(3), 673–681.

Internet References . . .

American Cancer Society

www.cancer.org

HPV—Centers for Disease Control and Prevention

www.cdc.gov/vaccines/pubs/vis/downloads/vis-hpv-gardasil.pdf

U.S. National Institutes of Health (NIH)

www.nih.gov

U.S. National Library of Medicine

www.nlm.nih.gov

World Health Organization

www.who.int/en

Selected, Edited, and with Issue Framing Material by:
Eileen L. Daniel, *SUNY College at Brockport*

ISSUE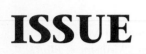

Is There a Valid Reason for Routine Infant Male Circumcision?

YES: Hanna Rosin, from "The Case Against the Case Against Circumcision; Why One Mother Heard All of the Opposing Arguments, Then Circumcised Her Sons Anyway," *New York Magazine* (2009)

NO: Michael Idov, from "Would You Circumcise This Baby? Why a Growing Number of Parents, Especially in New York and Other Cities, Are Saying No to the Procedure" *New York Magazine* (2009)

Learning Outcomes

After reading this issue, you will be able to:

• Discuss the health risks associated with infant male circumcision.
• Distinguish the difference between routine circumcision and religious rituals.
• Understand the health benefits associated with male circumcision.

ISSUE SUMMARY

YES: Writer Hanna Rosin argues that male circumcision decreases the risk of disease transmission and that people who oppose the operation are filled with anger that transcends the actual outcome.

NO: Michael Idov, author and contributing editor of *New York Magazine*, counters that newborns feel pain and that there is no valid medical reason to perform the surgery.

Male circumcision is the removal of the foreskin (prepuce) from the penis, and in the United States it is typically performed shortly after birth. In the Jewish religion, male circumcision is considered a commandment from God. It is also a common practice among Muslims. Worldwide, about 30 percent of males are circumcised and of those, about two-thirds are Muslim. About 55–65 percent of all newborn boys are circumcised in the United States each year, although this rate varies by region (western states have the lowest rates and the north central region has the highest). Up to 20 percent of men who are not circumcised during the newborn periods will be circumcised sometime later in life. Circumcision is much more common in the United States, Canada, and the Middle East than in other parts of the world. Currently, the United States is the only country in the developed world where the majority of male infants are circumcised for nonreligious reasons.

Circumcision is an elective procedure that has both pros and cons. As a benefit, circumcised infants are less likely to develop urinary tract infections (UTIs), especially in the first year of life. UTIs are about 10 times more common in uncircumcised infants compared with circumcised ones. However, even with this increased risk of UTIs, only 1 percent or less of uncircumcised baby boys are typically affected. Circumcised men may also be at lower risk for penile cancer, although the disease is uncommon in both circumcised and uncircumcised males. Some studies indicate that circumcision might also help protect against sexually transmitted diseases including AIDS/HIV. Irritation, inflammation, infection, and other problems of the penis occur more frequently among uncircumcised males since it is easier to keep a circumcised penis clean. There are also claims that circumcision affects the sensitivity of the tip of the penis, decreasing or increasing sexual pleasure later in life.

While circumcision appears to offer some medical benefits, it also carries potential risks since it is a surgical procedure. Complications of newborn circumcision are rare, occurring in between 0.2 and 3 percent of cases. Of these, the most frequent are treatable minor bleeding and local infection. Anesthesia is used more frequently now than in the past to prevent the newborn from feeling pain.

There are also negative outcomes of a psychological nature that have been anecdotally reported. These include sexual dysfunction of various forms and degrees, including impotence; awareness of a loss of normal protective, sensory, and mechanical functioning; anger; resentment; feelings of parental betrayal; feeling (awareness) of being mutilated; feelings of one's right to a normal intact body having been violated and removed; feelings of not being whole and natural; addictions or dependencies; sense of anatomical and sexual inferiority to genitally intact (non-circumcised) men; foreskin (or intact penis) envy. The quality and quantity of long-term psychologically negative effects of infant circumcision on men, however, have never been scientifically investigated.

Medical practice has long respected an adult's right to self-determination in health care decision making through the practice of informed consent. This process requires the physician to explain any procedure or treatment and to address the risks, benefits, and alternatives for the patient to make an informed choice. Since infants or small children lack the ability to decide for themselves, parents must make these choices. However, it is often uncertain as to what is in the best interest of any individual patient. In cases such as the decision to perform a circumcision shortly after birth when there are potential benefits and risks and the procedure is not essential to the child's current well-being, it is the parents who determine what is in the best interest of the child. In the United States, it is valid for the parents to take into account cultural, religious, and ethnic traditions, in addition to medical factors, when making this choice.

Overall, infant male circumcision is neither essential nor harmful to a boy's health. The American Academy of Pediatrics (AAP) and the American Academy of Family Physicians (AAFP) do not endorse the procedure as a way to prevent any of the medical conditions mentioned previously. The AAP also does not find sufficient evidence to medically recommend circumcision or argue against it.

In the YES and NO selections, Hanna Rosin argues that male circumcision decreases the risk of disease transmission and that people who oppose the operation are filled with anger that transcends the actual outcome. Author and contributing editor of *New York Magazine* Michael Idov counters that newborns feel pain and that there is no valid medical reason to perform the surgery.

YES ↵

Hanna Rosin

The Case Against the Case Against Circumcision; Why One Mother Heard All of the Opposing Arguments, Then Circumcised Her Sons Anyway

Anyone with a heart would agree that the Jewish bris is a barbaric event. Grown-ups sit chatting politely, wiping the cream cheese off their lips, while some religious guy with minimal medical training prepares to slice up a newborn's penis. The helpless thing wakes up from a womb-slumber howling with pain. I felt near hysterical at both of my sons' brisses. Pumped up with new-mother hormones, I dug my nails into my palms to keep from clawing the rabbi. For a few days afterward, I cursed my God and everyone else for creating the bloody mess in the diaper. But then the penis healed and assumed its familiar heart shape and I promptly forgot about the whole trauma. Apparently some people never do.

I am Jewish enough that I never considered not circumcising my sons. I did not search the web or call a panel of doctors to fact-check the health benefits, as a growing number of wary Americans now do. Despite my momentary panic, the words "genital mutilation" did not enter my head. But now that I have done my homework, I'm sure I would do it again—even if I were not Jewish, didn't believe in ritual, and judged only by cold, secular science.

Every year, it seems, a new study confirms that the foreskin is pretty much like the appendix or the wisdom tooth—it is an evolutionary footnote that serves no purpose other than to incubate infections. There's no single overwhelming health reason to remove it, but there are a lot of smaller health reasons that add up. It's not critical that any individual boy get circumcised. For the growing number of people who feel hysterical at the thought, just don't do it. But don't ruin it for the rest of us. It's perfectly clear that on a grand public-health level, the more boys who get circumcised, the better it is for everyone.

Twenty years ago, this would have been a boring, obvious thing to say, like feed your baby rice cereal before bananas, or don't smoke while pregnant. These days, in certain newly enlightened circles on the East and West Coasts, it puts you in league with Josef Mengele. Late this summer, when *The New York Times* reported that the U.S. Centers for Disease Control might consider promoting routine circumcision as a tool in the fight against AIDS, the vicious comments that ensued included references to mass genocide.

There's no use arguing with the anti-circ activists, who only got through the headline of this story before hunting down my e-mail and offering to pay for me to be genitally mutilated. But for those in the nervous middle, here is my best case for why you should do it. Biologists think the foreskin plays a critical role in the womb, protecting the penis as it is growing during the third month of gestation. Outside the womb, the best guess is that it once kept the penis safe from, say, low-hanging thorny branches. Nowadays, we have pants for that.

Circumcision dates back some 6,000 years and was mostly associated with religious rituals, especially for Jews and Muslims. In the nineteenth century, moralists concocted some unfortunate theories about the connection between the foreskin and masturbation and other such degenerate impulses. The genuinely useful medical rationales came later. During the World War II campaign in North Africa, tens of thousands of American GIs fell short on their hygiene routines. Many of them came down with a host of painful and annoying infections, such as phimosis, where the foreskin gets too tight to retract over the glans. Doctors already knew about the connection to sexually transmitted diseases and began recommending routine circumcision.

In the late eighties, researchers began to suspect a relationship between circumcision and transmission of HIV, the virus that causes AIDS. One researcher wondered why certain Kenyan men who see prostitutes get infected and others don't. The answer, it turned out, was that the ones who don't were circumcised. Three separate trials in Uganda, Kenya, and South Africa involving over

10,000 men turned up the same finding again and again. Circumcision, it turns out, could reduce the risk of HIV transmission by at least 60 percent, which, in Africa, adds up to 3 million lives saved over the next twenty years. The governments of Uganda and Kenya recently started mass-circumcision campaigns.

These studies are not entirely relevant to the U.S. They apply only to female-to-male transmission, which is relatively rare here. But the results are so dramatic that people who work in AIDS prevention can't ignore them. Daniel Halperin, an AIDS expert at the Harvard School of Public Health, has compared various countries, and the patterns are obvious. In a study of 28 nations, he found that low circumcision rates (fewer than 20 percent) match up with high HIV rates, and vice versa. Similar patterns are turning up in the U.S. as well. A team of researchers from the CDC and Johns Hopkins analyzed records of over 26,000 heterosexual African-American men who showed up at a Baltimore clinic for HIV testing and denied any drug use or homosexual contact. Among those with known HIV exposure, the ones who did turn out to be HIV-positive were twice as likely to be uncircumcised. There's no causal relationship here; foreskin does not cause HIV transmission. But researchers guess that foreskins are more susceptible to sores, and also have a high concentration of certain immune cells that are the main portals for HIV infection.

Then there are a host of other diseases that range from rare and deadly to ruin your life to annoying. Australian physicians give a decent summary: "STIs such as carcinogenic types of human papillomavirus (HPV), genital herpes, HIV, syphilis and chancroid, thrush, cancer of the penis, and most likely cancer of the prostate, phimosis, paraphimosis, inflammatory skin conditions such as balanoposthitis, inferior hygiene, sexual problems, especially with age and diabetes, and, in the female partners, HPV, cervical cancer, HSV-2, and chlamydia, which is an important cause of infertility." The percentages vary in each case, but it's clear that the foreskin is a public-health menace.

Edgar Schoen, now a professor emeritus of pediatrics at the University of California San Francisco, has been pushing the pro-circumcision case since 1989, when he chaired an American Academy of Pediatrics Task Force on the practice. The committee later found insufficient evidence to recommend routine circumcision, but to Schoen, this is the "narrow thinking of neonatologists" who sit on the panels. All they see is a screaming baby, not a lifetime of complications. In the meantime, sixteen states have eliminated Medicaid coverage for circumcision, causing the rates among Hispanics, for one, to plummet. For Schoen and Halperin and others, this issue has become primarily a question of "health-care parity for the poor."

The people whom circumcision could help the most are now the least likely to get it.

This mundane march of health statistics has a hard time competing with the opposite side, which is fighting for something they see as fundamental: a right not to be messed with, a freedom from control, and a general sense of wholeness. For many circumcision opponents, preventive surgery is a bizarre, dystopian disruption. I can only say that in public health, preventive surgery is pretty common—appendix and wisdom teeth, for example. "If we could remove the appendix in a three- or four-minute operation without cutting into the abdomen, we would," says Schoen. Anesthesia is routine now, so the infants don't suffer the way they used to. My babies didn't seem to howl more than they did in their early vaccines, particularly the one where they "milk" the heel for blood.

Sexual pleasure comes up a lot. Opponents of circumcision often mention studies of "penile sensitivity regions," showing the foreskin to be the most sensitive. But erotic experience is a rich and complicated affair, and surely can't be summed up by nerve endings or friction or "sensitivity regions." More-nuanced studies have shown that men who were circumcised as adults report a decrease in sexual satisfaction when they were forced into it, because of an illness, and an increase when they did it of their own will. In a study of Kenyan men who volunteered for circumcision, 64 percent reported their penis to be "much more sensitive" and their ease of reaching orgasm much greater two years after the operation. In a similar study, Ugandan women reported a 40 percent increase in sexual satisfaction after their partners were circumcised. Go figure. Surely this is more psychology than science.

People who oppose circumcision are animated by a kind of rage and longing that seems larger than the thing itself. Websites are filled with testimonies from men who believe their lives were ruined by the operation they had as an infant. I can only conclude that it wasn't the cutting alone that did the ruining. An East Bay doctor who came out for circumcision recently wrote about having visions of tiny foreskins rising up in revenge at him, clogging the freeways. I see what he means. The foreskin is the new fetus—the object that has been imbued with magical powers to halt a merciless, violent world—a world that is particularly callous to children. The notion resonates in a moment when parents are especially overprotective, and fantasy death panels loom. It's all very visual and compelling—like the sight of your own newborn son with the scalpel looming over him. But it isn't the whole truth.

Hanna Rosin is a senior editor for *The Atlantic* magazine.

Michael Idov
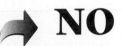 **NO**

Would You Circumcise This Baby? Why a Growing Number of Parents, Especially in New York and Other Cities, Are Saying No to the Procedure

To cut or not to cut. The choice loomed the moment New Yorkers Rob and Deanna Morea found out, three months into Deanna's pregnancy, that their first child was going to be a boy. Both had grown up with the view of circumcision as something automatic, like severing the umbilical cord. To Rob—white, Catholic, and circumcised—an intact foreskin seemed vaguely un-American. Deanna, African-American and also Catholic, dismissed the parents who don't circumcise their children as a "granola-eating, Birkenstock-wearing type of crowd." But that was before they knew they were having a son.

Circumcision is still, as it has been for decades, one of the most routinely performed surgical procedures in the United States—a million of the operations are performed every year. Yet more Americans are beginning to ask themselves the same question the Moreas did: Why, exactly, are we doing this? Having peaked at a staggering 85 percent in the sixties and seventies, the U.S. newborn-circumcision rate dropped to 65 percent in 1999 and to 56 percent in 2006. Give or take a hiccup here and there, the trend is remarkably clear: Over the past 30 years, the circumcision rate has fallen 30 percent. All evidence suggests that we are nearing the moment (2014?) when the year's crop of circumcised newborns will be in the minority.

Opposition to circumcision isn't new, of course. What is new are the opponents. What was once mostly a fringe movement has been flowing steadily into the mainstream. Today's anti-circumcision crowd are people like the Moreas—people whose religious and ideological passions don't run high either way and who arrive at their decision through a kind of personal cost-benefit analysis involving health concerns, pain, and other factors. At the same time, new evidence that circumcision can help prevent the spread of AIDS, coupled with centuries-old sentiments supporting the practice, are touching off a backlash to the backlash. Lately, arguments pro and con have grown fierce, flaring with the contentious intensity of our time.

The idea of separating the prepuce from the penis is older than the Old Testament. The first depiction of the procedure exists on the walls of an Egyptian tomb built in 2400 B.C.—a relief complete with hieroglyphics that read, "Hold him and do not allow him to faint." The notion appears to have occurred to several disparate cultures, for reasons unknown. "It is far easier to imagine the impulse behind Neolithic cave painting than to guess what inspired the ancients to cut their genitals," writes David L. Gollaher in his definitive tome *Circumcision: A History of the World's Most Controversial Surgery*. One theory suggests that the ritual's original goal was to simply draw blood from the sexual organ—to serve as the male equivalent of menstruation, in other words, and thus a rite of passage into adulthood. The Jews took their enslavers' practice and turned it into a sign of their own covenant with God; 2,000 years later, Muslims followed suit.

Medical concerns didn't enter the picture until the late-nineteenth century, when science began competing with religious belief. America took its first step toward universal secular circumcision, writes Gollaher, on "the rainy morning of February 9, 1870." Lewis Sayre, a leading Manhattan surgeon, was treating an anemic 5-year-old boy with partially paralyzed leg muscles when he noticed that the boy's penis was encased in an unusually tight foreskin, causing chronic pain. Going on intuition, Sayre drove the boy to Bellevue and circumcised him, improvising on the spot with scissors and his fingernails. The boy felt better almost immediately and fully recovered the use of his legs within weeks. Sayre began to perform circumcisions to treat paralysis—and, in at least five cases, his strange inspiration worked. When Sayre published the results in the *Transactions of the American Medical Association*, the floodgates swung open. Before long, surgeons were using circumcision to treat all manner of ailments.

There was another, half-hidden appeal to the procedure. Ever since the twelfth-century Jewish scholar and physician Maimonides, doctors realized that circumcision dulls the sensation in the glans, supposedly discouraging promiscuity. The idea was especially attractive to the Victorians, famously obsessed with the perils of masturbation. From therapeutic circumcision as a cure for insomnia there was only a short step toward circumcision as a way to dull the "out of control" libido.

In the thirties, another argument for routine circumcision presented itself. Research suggested a link between circumcision and reduced risk of penile and cervical cancer. In addition to the obvious health implications, the finding strengthened the idea of the foreskin as unclean. On par with deodorant and a daily shower, circumcision became a means of assimilating the immigrant and urbanizing the country bumpkin—a civilizing cut. And so at the century's midpoint, just as the rest of the English-speaking world began souring on the practice (the British National Health Service stopped covering it in 1949), the U.S. settled into its status as the planet's one bastion of routine neonatal circumcision—second only to Israel.

That belief held sway for decades. Men had it done to their sons because it was done to them. Generations of women came to think of the uncircumcised penis as odd. To leave your son uncircumcised was to expose him to ostracism in the locker room and the bedroom. No amount of debunking seemed to alter that. As far back as 1971, the American Academy of Pediatrics declared that there were "no valid medical indications for circumcision in the neonatal period." The following year, some 80 percent of Americans circumcised their newborns.

What changed? The shift away from circumcision is driven by a mass of converging trends. For one, we live in an age of child-centric parenting. New research suggests that the babies feel and process more than previously thought, including physical pain (see "How Much Does It Hurt?"). In a survey conducted for this story, every respondent who decided against circumcision cited "unwillingness to inflict pain on the baby" as the main reason. The movement toward healthier living is another factor. Just as people have grown increasingly wary of the impact of artificial foods in their diets and chemical products in the environment, so too have they become more suspicious of the routine use of preventive medical procedures. We've already rejected tonsillectomy and appendectomy as bad ideas. The new holistically minded

consensus seems to be that if something is there, it's there for a reason: Leave it alone. Globalization plays a part too. As more U.S. women have sex with foreign-born men, the American perception of the uncut penis as exotic has begun to fade. The decline in the number of practicing Jews contributes as well. Perhaps as a reflection of all of these typically urban-minded ideas, circumcision rates are dropping in big coastal cities at a faster rate than in the heartland. In 2006, for example, a minority of male New York City newborns were circumcised—43.4 percent. In Minnesota, the rate was 70 percent. Circumcision, you could say, is becoming a blue-state-red-state issue.

The Moreas considered all of this and more, having imbibed more information about both the pros and cons of circumcision during the last four months of Deanna's pregnancy than they care to recall. They still hadn't decided what to do until the day after their son, Anderson, was born. Then, when a nurse came to take the boy to be circumcised, the decision came clear to them. "We didn't want to put him through that—we didn't want to cut him," says Deanna. "It's mutilation. They do it to girls in Africa. No matter how accepted it is, it's mutilation."

And yet, the pendulum is already swinging back. Earlier this year, *The New York Times* published a front-page story noting that the Centers for Disease Control was considering recommending routine circumcision to help stop the spread of AIDS. The idea was based largely on studies done in Africa indicating that circumcised heterosexual men were at least 60 percent less susceptible to HIV than uncircumcised ones. The story promptly touched off a firestorm, with pro- and anti-circumcision commenters exchanging angry barbs. The CDC will now say only that it's in the process of determining a recommendation.

Caught at the crossroads of religion and science, circumcision has proved to be a free-floating symbol, attaching itself to whatever orthodoxy captures a society's imagination. Its history is driven by wildly shifting rationales: from tribal rite of passage to covenant with God to chastity guarantor to paralysis cure to cancer guard to unnecessary, painful surgery to a Hail Mary pass in the struggle with the AIDS pandemic. There's no reason to think a new rationale won't come down the pike when we least expect it. Our millennia-long quest to justify one of civilization's most curious habits continues.

Michael Idov is a contributing editor at *New York Magazine* and the author of the novel *Ground Up*.

EXPLORING THE ISSUE

Is There a Valid Reason for Routine Infant Male Circumcision?

Critical Thinking and Reflection

1. What are the medical benefits of male circumcision?
2. What role does the procedure have in religious rites? Which religions promote circumcision?
3. Describe why some individuals believe that circumcision violates a boy's body.

Is There Common Ground?

In southern Africa, the small country of Swaziland is experiencing one of the highest rates of HIV in the world. Slightly less than 20 percent of Swaziland's 1 million people are HIV positive, an epidemic linked to poverty, a lack of medical resources, and a culture in which having multiple sex partners is common. Nearly half of women ages 25–29 and men 35–39 are infected. During recent times, the average life expectancy has dropped from about 61 years to 47 due to the AIDS epidemic. To help fight the disease and prevent new cases, Swaziland has been preparing its male citizens for mass circumcision since 2006. This is in response to a 2005 study conducted in South Africa, which determined that circumcised men are as much as 60 percent less likely to contract HIV through heterosexual sex. Researchers do not fully understand why the disease rate was so much lower, but the study was so convincing that it was halted after 18 months, because preventing the uncircumcised control group from getting the procedure would not have been ethical. According to a recent article in the *Atlantic Monthly* ("The Kindest Cut," January/February 2011), there was a nationwide campaign in Swaziland to circumcise 160,000 HIV-negative males by the end of 2011. While Swaziland is in the process of circumcising thousands of men, not all researchers are convinced of the benefits of the procedure as a means to combat AIDS. In "Circumcision" (*Journal of Pediatrics & Child Health*, January/February 2011) author David Isaacs argues that there is insufficient proof of the health benefits of the procedure. However, the article "Role of the Foreskin in Male Circumcision: An Evidence-Based Review" (*Journal of Reproductive Immunology*, March 2011) presents evidence that shows HIV transmission is reduced

when a man is circumcised. Similar results were found in the study published in *Preventive Medicine* in March 2011 ("Male Circumcision as an HIV Prevention Intervention in the US: Influence of Health Care Providers and Potential for Risk Compensation"), which also found male circumcision was an HIV-prevention intervention and reduced the potential for disease transmission. While it's clear that researchers don't always agree, many studies argue that circumcision may help prevent diseases among males. Overall, the procedure remains controversial and many experts disagree on the risks and benefits.

Additional Resources

Carbery, B., Zhu, J., Gust, D. A., Chen, R. T., Kretsinger, K., & Kilmarx, P. H. (2012). Need for physician education on the benefits and risks of male circumcision in the United States. *AIDS Education & Prevention, 24*(4), 377–387.

Earp, B. D. (2012). Can religious beliefs justify circumcision? *Attorneys for the Rights of the Child Newsletter, 9*(3), 1–13.

Jacobs, A. J., & Arora, K. S. (2015). Ritual male infant circumcision and human rights. *American Journal of Bioethics, 15*(2), 30–39.

Morris, B. J., Bailey, R. C., Klausner, J. D., et al. (2012). Review: A critical evaluation of arguments opposing male circumcision for HIV prevention in developed countries. *AIDS Care, 24*(12), 1565–1575.

Starzyk, E. J., Kelley, M. A., Caskey, R. N., Schwartz, A., Kennelly, J. F., & Bailey, R. C. (2015). Infant male circumcision: Healthcare provider knowledge and associated factors. *Plos One, 10*(1), 1–14.

Internet References . . .

Cleveland Clinic Fact Sheet—Circumcision

http://my.clevelandclinic.org/services/circumcision
/hic_circumcision.aspx

Mayo Clinic Circumcision Fact Sheet

www.mayoclinic.com/health/circumcision/MY01023

Medline Plus: National Institutes of Health

www.nlm.nih.gov/medlineplus/circumcision.html

National Circumcision Resource Center

www.circumcision.org

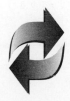

Unit 5

UNIT

Public Health Issues

*T*here are many health issues that concern the public and are affected by public policy and public health laws. The focus of public health intervention is to improve the health and quality of life of populations. This is accomplished through the prevention and treatment of disease and other physical and mental health conditions, surveillance of disease cases, enactment of public health laws (i.e., smoking bans in public, ban on "supersized" soft drinks), and the promotion of healthy behaviors. An important component of public health policy is the balance between protecting public health and the maintenance of individual freedoms.

Selected, Edited, and with Issue Framing Material by:
Eileen L. Daniel, *SUNY College at Brockport*

ISSUE

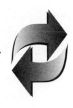

Is There a Link Between Vaccination and Autism?

YES: Alex Newman and Rebecca Terrell, from "Vaccine vs. Virus: Which Is the Bigger Threat?" *The New American* (2015)

NO: Matthew Normand and Jesse Dallery, from "Mercury Rising: Exposing the Vaccine-Autism Myth," *Skeptic* (2007)

Learning Outcomes

After reading this issue, you will be able to:

- Discuss the risk factors associated with the development of autism.
- Distinguish the various conditions associated with the autism spectrum.
- Understand the reasons for the increase in children being diagnosed with autism.
- Assess the relationship between autism and vaccination.

ISSUE SUMMARY

YES: Journalist Alex Newman and nurse Rebecca Terrell claim that while the mainstream press scoffs at any association of vaccination to autism, the rates of autism have climbed precipitously since the dawn of the MMR vaccine.

NO: Psychology professors Matthew Normand and Jesse Dallery contend that studies have failed to uncover any specific link between autism and mercury-containing thimerosal vaccines.

The brain development disorder known as autism is characterized by impaired communication and interpersonal interactions and restricted and repetitive behavior. These symptoms tend to begin before a child is 3 years old. The autism spectrum disorders (ASD) also include related conditions such as Asperger syndrome that have milder signs and symptoms.

Overall, males are affected more often than females by about 4:1. It appears that between 4 and 10 individuals per 10,000 children are affected, though recent surveys have shown a much higher prevalence of 40–60 cases per 10,000 people. While there has been much publicity over the increased numbers of autism cases identified over the past 20–30 years, there is limited evidence that the actual number of new cases has risen over this timeframe. Changes in the way autism is diagnosed have been

suggested as a reason for the increased rates. Researchers studied population groups in California and documented a rise in the number of children diagnosed with autism and a decrease in the number diagnosed with mental retardation. This may suggest that a change in diagnosis from mental retardation to autism may be responsible for the increase in the incidence of autism. It is clear that further research is needed to determine if the actual numbers of cases of autism is truly increasing.

Scientists aren't clear about what causes autism, but it's likely that both genetics and environment play a role. Researchers have identified a number of genes associated with the disorder. Research involving individuals with autism has found abnormalities in multiple regions of the brain. Other studies indicate that people with autism have unusual levels of serotonin or other neurotransmitters in the brain. These irregularities imply that autism may develop from the disruption of normal brain growth early in fetal development. These irregularities are caused by defects in genes that control brain growth and that regulate how neurons communicate with each other. While these findings are interesting, they are preliminary and require additional research.

Vaccination against infectious diseases such as measles, polio, and mumps has been a very successful preventive agent. However, because of this success, many people have forgotten how dreadful these diseases were and can be. Most of the concerns about the role of vaccines in autism have focused on the measles, mumps, and rubella (MMR) and on thimerosal, the mercury-based preservative used in some vaccines before 2001. In 1998, researcher Andrew Wakefield published a paper in the British medical journal, *Lancet*. It reported on 12 children who had autism spectrum disorder as well as bowel symptoms. In eight of these children, the parents or the child's doctor linked the MMR vaccination with the onset of the behavioral

symptoms. The paper was seized upon by the media and parents groups creating a furor that led to a significant drop in the number of British children who were vaccinated, leading to a return of mumps and measles cases in England. Interestingly, in February 2009 a special federal court ruled that there was no proven link between certain early childhood vaccines such as MMR and autism that developed in three children.

Though a special federal court ruled that there was no proven link between the MMR vaccine and autism, many parents and their doctors believe otherwise. In the following selections, Alex Newman and Rebecca Terrell argue that the MMR vaccination is linked to autism despite the denials by the mainstream press. Psychology professors Matthew Normand and Jesse Dallery disagree and contend that studies have failed to uncover any specific link between autism and mercury-containing thimerosal vaccines.

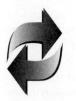

YES ↵

Alex Newman and Rebecca Terrell

Vaccine vs. Virus: Which Is the Bigger Threat?

The deaths of more than 100 children have been officially linked to receiving a measles vaccine during the past decade, according to the federal government's Vaccine Adverse Event Reporting System (VAERS). Yet the childhood measles mortality count over the same period remains at zero, according to data from the U.S. Centers for Disease Control and Prevention (CDC). Put another way, in the last 10 years an American child would have been highly more likely to die after receiving a measles shot than from contracting the disease itself. Thousands more have suffered from adverse reactions to the measles inoculation and other vaccines. The explosive numbers have massive implications for public health efforts, analysts say.

Of course, the establishment media has entirely ignored these figures in the wake of the recent Disneyland measles outbreak. As of mid-February, the number of confirmed measles cases had climbed to 113, prompting vicious attacks from mainstream media against "anti-vaxxers." In the cross hairs are parents who choose not to vaccinate their children, even though CDC officials say the epidemic was likely introduced at the Disneyland theme park by a person infected with measles overseas. *USA Today* even published a screed encouraging the jailing of parents who refuse to vaccinate their children, though it was not clear whether the Amish and other religious communities would be included in the proposed mass roundups.

Now, elements of the "mainstream" media are engaged in a damage-control effort. Media reports repeatedly and erroneously maintain that measles could not spread in a fully vaccinated society, while assuring readers of the safety and effectiveness of vaccines. In some cases, as with the *New York Times*, even the media's sources have lambasted reporters for deceiving readers with propaganda. "It seems clear to me that your reporters or writers knew exactly how they wanted to frame this story before they even conducted the interview with me, and when what I actually said didn't fit well into that story, they had to dissect and then re-combine my words in order to make them fit the intended picture that they either expected or wanted to convey," said Kelly McMenimen, the mother of an unvaccinated child whose interview was distorted, in an open letter to the *Times* editor.

However, since data revealing the truth about vaccines is publicly available online through the federal government, the facts are going viral through the alternative press. It appears the first outlet to put the information together in one report was Health Impact News, sparking a cascade of follow-up stories from various sources. HealthImpactNews.com editor Brian Shilhavy recounted that there have been no child measles deaths since 2003 in the United States, highlighting data from a CDC report issued in April of last year in response to a nationwide upsurge in measles cases.

He also used the HealthSentinel.com graph . . . , which charts a variety of official U.S. statistics illustrating measles mortality rates since 1900. Until the 1920s, more than 10 measles cases per 100,000, or 0.01 percent, resulted in death. However, by 1955, with advances in medicine and huge progress in sanitation, nutrition, and living standards, those rates steadily declined from 1900 levels to 0.03 deaths per 100,000, a mere 0.00003 percent! By the time the measles vaccine was introduced in 1963, the disease had already lost its death-grip on the developed world.

It is significant to note that, despite its reassuring jargon, the federal government's vaccination-promoting website, Vaccines.gov, chooses to ignore most pre-1963 numbers. Instead, it displays a graph illustrating the decline in overall U.S. measles cases—with no distinction of measles deaths—since the inoculation was introduced, a decidedly deceptive omission of earlier years' data.

However, the VAERS database reveals a markedly different history of the measles vaccine. After a painstaking search through this federal database of adverse effects, Shilhavy reported, "The search result contained 108 deaths over this period [i.e., 2004 to 2015—ed.], resulting from four different measles vaccines sold in the United States during the past 10 years." He continued, "This database reflects only deaths that were reported during the time frame, and therefore probably reflects a much lower number than actual deaths, since most doctors and health authorities believe vaccines are safe, and would not normally attribute a death to a vaccine and actually report it."

Indeed, results of a 2006 meta-analysis in the health journal *Drug Safety* reveal that adverse drug reactions go unreported at an alarming rate of 94 percent for prescription medications in general. And while the VAERS cautions that its reports of adverse effects do not necessarily establish a cause-and-effect relationship, and at least some of the reported deaths were probably not directly linked to the shot, the high rate of under-reporting reveals that the system almost certainly underestimates rather than overestimates the true death count. Unsuspecting parents and doctors—convinced that vaccines are entirely safe—would be unlikely to link them with sudden death, even though vaccine package inserts clearly warn of possible death or serious injury as a potential side effect. At least 77 claims have been filed with the federal National Vaccine Injury Compensation Program for deaths caused by the measles inoculation, along with over 1,000 for serious injuries, with almost 40 percent being compensated by taxpayers and 7.4 percent of cases still unresolved. Over 15,000 claims have been filed against vaccines more generally, so some of those harmed by a cocktail of vaccines that included the measles shot would likely not be included in those figures.

But now that the facts have gone viral, the largely discredited Snopes.com website is trying to discredit the facts. In its effort, the radically pro-government website has mostly attacked straw men while relying on data from Third World countries with widespread malnutrition and a dearth of basic healthcare services. It also contests the official death toll from measles cited by the CDC since 2004. Snopes chose to rely on "preliminary data" for 2009 and a 2010 CDC report claiming four people in the last decade have died from measles, though Dr. Anne Schuchat, the director of CDC's National Center for Immunization and Respiratory Diseases, told the Associated Press last year that there were zero reported deaths from measles. Separately, the CDC Division of Viral Diseases said in an e-mail that the "last documented deaths in the U.S. directly attributable to acute measles occurred in 2003." No matter which numbers are used regarding vaccine deaths and measles deaths, though, the death toll from the shots is higher in the United States over the last decade.

Meanwhile, financially strapped *Newsweek*, a Big Pharma-supported magazine still attempting to recover

after it was sold for one dollar in 2010, also piled on. In an error-riddled propaganda piece, the online outlet made the unsubstantiated statement that "it's true some people may have died as a result of the measles vaccine" but "many more would have died without them." The article cited only United Nations statistics of Third World countries, but no data from the United States, even that which is publically available.

Unsurprisingly, the CDC claims its vaccination program "eliminated" measles in 2000. "The United States was able to eliminate measles because it has a highly effective measles vaccine, a strong vaccination program that achieves high vaccine coverage in children and a strong public health system for detecting and responding to measles cases and outbreaks," the CDC argued. However, the disease still crops up annually because travelers, immigrants, and illegal aliens bring it to our shores from foreign soil.

However, as the HealthSentinel.com graph clearly shows, measles was on a downward spiral in the United States years before 1963 when the vaccine was introduced. In fact, fully vaccinated people continue to get and spread measles, as has been concluded by numerous official studies and in peer-reviewed literature. For example, as of January, CDC reported 12 percent of the California measles cases associated with Disneyland involved fully-vaccinated individuals. Interestingly, a fully-vaccinated 22-year-old woman sparked the 2011 measles outbreak in New York. Some people even get the measles from the measles vaccine, as revealed in official records.

The National Vaccine Information Center, a nonprofit educational organization and patient advocacy group that opposes government mandates on the issue, also points out on its website that the vaccine does not necessarily protect a person from measles, contrary to a false narrative pushed by misleading establishment press articles and bureaucrats. "Evidence has been published in the medical literature that vaccinated persons can get measles because either the measles vaccine fails to provide temporary vaccine-acquired immunity or the vaccine's effectiveness wanes over time," it reported. Especially problematic: Vaccines may provide temporary protection but wear off, leaving adults vulnerable to measles at a later stage in life, when the disease can be far more harmful.

Though most Americans might not know it, countless medical professionals have spoken out about the issue for decades. "After frightening you with the unlikely possibility of measles encephalitis, your doctor can rarely be counted on to tell you of the dangers associated with the vaccine he uses to prevent it," explained the late

Dr. Robert Mendelsohn in his health newsletter. "The measles vaccine is associated with encephalopathy and with a series of other complications such as SSPE (subacute sclerosing panencephalitis), which causes hardening of the brain and is invariably fatal."

"Other neurologic and sometimes fatal conditions associated with the measles vaccine include ataxia (inability to coordinate muscle movements), mental retardation, aseptic meningitis, seizure disorders, and hemiparesis (paralysis affecting one side of the body)," Dr. Mendelsohn continued after explaining that, in the developed world especially, measles is hardly a deadly plague requiring national paranoia and vaccination at gunpoint. "Secondary complications associated with the vaccine may be even more frightening. They include encephalitis, juvenile-onset diabetes, Reye's syndrome, and multiple sclerosis." In fact, still today, the package insert in the measles vaccine specifically warns of the potential for many of those problems and numerous others. "I would consider the risks associated with measles vaccination unacceptable even if there were convincing evidence that the vaccine works," the late, prominent medical doctor concluded. "There isn't." More recently, numerous high-profile doctors and experts have made similar statements, despite the overwhelming pressure and threats from government and Big Pharma to remain silent on the risks.

Manufacturer Immunity

Indeed, unlike virtually any other product or industry in the United States, the federal government protects vaccine manufacturers from liability when their products kill or injure patients. This forces victims of vaccine-related injuries—or the families of those whose deaths are linked to vaccines—to rely on the taxpayer-funded U.S. Vaccine Injury Compensation Program (VICP), rather than suing the companies that produced and sold the potentially dangerous product. With many vaccines worldwide now manufactured under World Health Organization approval in Communist China, infamous for producing dangerous and deadly products, the seriousness is even greater.

"Why does our federal government protect vaccine manufacturers from product liability lawsuits?" MaryJo Perry, co-director of Mississippi Parents for Vaccine Rights, asked in an online *USA Today* post on January 27. She noted that taxpayers have been funding the U.S. Health and Human Services Administration's VICP since 1989 to the tune of $3 billion paid to victims

of these reputedly "safe" medical products. "When citizens can't hold corporations accountable in court for the safety and effectiveness of vaccines, it is very important to protect our legal right to vaccine exemptions," Perry states.

Barbara Loe Fisher of the National Vaccine Information Center agrees. "From now on—unless we stand up and draw the line on vaccine mandates—the government can legally use police powers to force every American to get hundreds of vaccinations or be punished," she writes, "while those who are hurt by vaccination can be more easily swept under the rug and left to fend for themselves."

The National Vaccine Information Center highlights a number of vaccine injury statistics that again have been glossed over by the press. "As of January 5, 2015, there had been 946 claims filed in the federal Vaccine Injury Compensation Program for injuries and deaths following MMR vaccination, including 57 deaths and 889 serious injuries," the center reported. When other measles vaccines aside from the MMR are included, the numbers are even higher.

"Using the MedAlerts search engine, as of December 14, 2014 there had been 6,962 serious adverse events reported to the Vaccine Adverse Events Reporting System (VAERS) in connection with measles-containing vaccines since 1990," the Vaccine Information Center continued. "Over half of those serious measles vaccine-related adverse events occurred in children three years old and under. Of these measles-vaccine related adverse event reports to VAERS, 329 were deaths, with over half of the deaths occurring in children under three years of age."

Government Mandates

What motivates groups such as the Mississippi Parents for Vaccine Rights and National Vaccine Information Center is the threat of government-mandated vaccines, a troubling factor considering our current regulatory environment. Numerous state and federal measures are already in place to strip personal liberties in the name of protecting public health. Roughly 80 percent of states across the nation have, since 2002, implemented in varying degrees the Model State Emergency Health Powers Act, developed by a collaboration of government entities including the U.S. CDC and the UN World Health Organization. The act grants tremendous powers to states at the expense of personal privacy and individual freedom, allowing forced involuntary quarantines and government-mandated vaccinations during officially declared "emergencies."

On the federal level, the Public Health Service Act (PHSA), along with executive orders signed by Presidents George W. Bush and Barack Obama, established broad federal quarantine authority. In the event of public resistance to such draconian measures, Obama is prepared to deploy the military to enforce these unconstitutional policies. His Department of Defense (DoD) *Implementation Plan for Pandemic Influenza* includes "the provision of DoD assistance to civilian authorities both foreign and domestic."

In other words, a bureaucrat could deprive a U.S. citizen of his unalienable rights—for as long as said bureaucrat considers necessary—on the mere suspicion that the person being detained has been in contact with some disease. Contrast the purported federal authorities under the Public Health Service Act with the plain language in the U.S. Constitution's Fifth Amendment, which outright prohibits the deprivation of liberty without due process of law—a timeless and essential principle enshrined in the Magna Carta almost 800 years ago. State constitutions across America recognize those fundamental rights as well.

But desperate times call for desperate measures, right? Shouldn't we be willing to part with personal liberties in the interest of public health? Aren't diseases such as measles far worse than the prospect of forfeiting the Fifth Amendment?

We will deal with the legality issue shortly, but first let's consider a few points about vaccinations in general and measles in particular. First, measles is very rarely fatal, and most people recover completely. As noted earlier, between 1920 and 1955, the rate of deaths among U.S. measles cases dropped from 0.01 percent to 0.00003 percent without any help from vaccinations. Even today the global mortality rate from measles is very low at 0.00328 percent. These numbers are not meant to downplay the tragedy of individual deaths but to illustrate that we are not talking about a killer such as smallpox, so lethal that it has been used as a biological weapon of war since ancient times.

One of the main reasons for the steep early 20th-century decline in both measles cases and measles deaths was that doctors discovered the efficacy of cod-liver oil, which is rich in vitamin A. The *New England Journal of Medicine* confirmed in 1990 that vitamin A is essential in measles treatment and declared that "all children with severe measles should be given vitamin A supplements, whether or not they are thought to have a nutritional deficiency." And while vitamin A proves itself an effective therapy and protection against contracting the disease, the measles vaccine cannot promise the same.

Effective vs. Protective

Which brings us to the question of vaccine safety and effectiveness in general. Researchers may call a vaccine "effective" simply because it causes the injected person to develop antibodies. However, "it is important to understand that *effective* and *protective* in vaccine research are not synonyms," explains Dr. Sherri Tenpenny, a medical doctor and outspoken critic of vaccines. (Emphasis in original.) She cites the package insert of the HiBTiter® flu vaccine, which states that "the contribution [antibodies make] to clinical protection is unknown," and CDC literature about the pertussis vaccine, which admits, "The findings of efficacy studies have not demonstrated a direct correlation between antibody response and protection against pertussis disease." This effective-vs.-protective distinction explains how outbreaks can occur in fully immunized populations, such as the 1985 measles epidemic in a school in Corpus Christi, Texas. And as noted earlier, a number of cases in the current California outbreak involve previously immunized patients.

Long before that, the trends were similar. In 1967, for example, the UN World Health Organization declared that Ghana was measles-free after 96 percent of the population was vaccinated. But just five years later, the country suffered its most deadly outbreak of the disease. More recently, a 1990 article about measles in the *Journal of the American Medical Association* pointed out: "Although more than 95% of school-aged children in the US are vaccinated against measles, large measles outbreaks continue to occur in schools and most cases in this setting occur among previously vaccinated children."

Dr. Tenpenny recalls that she was drawn into the debate years ago when she realized that "tens of thousands have been injured and have died as a result of vaccinations." Among health problems that many parents and healthcare professionals fear could be associated with vaccines are autism, sudden infant death syndrome, allergies, juvenile diabetes, and childhood arthritis.

Yet Vaccines.gov claims, "Vaccines are some of the safest medical products available." It follows that the anti-vaccination movement is made up of parents who are inexcusably gullible and criminally irresponsible—guilty of both child abuse and endangering society with their foolhardy negligence. So goes the party line. After all, say the pro-vaccine media, measles could find no susceptible host in a fully immunized population but can only gain foothold in, and be spread by, unvaccinated people.

Why Some Parents Say No

Reputable sources, and even the CDC, expose the fallacy of such yellow journalism. Moreover, parents who reject vaccines do so out of love for their children and have morally and scientifically valid arguments. Jane Orient, M.D., executive director of the Association of American Physicians and Surgeons (AAPS), explains that many people object to vaccines that are manufactured using cells from aborted babies. Such is the case with Merck's ubiquitous MMR (measles-mumps-rubella) product, as Orient pointed out in a February 9 statement on the AAPS website.

Parents also worry about chronic adverse health conditions associated with vaccines, in particular, autism. While the mainstream press scoffs at any association, Orient notes that the rates of autism in children have climbed precipitously since the dawn of the MMR vaccine: from 1 in 10,000 children to 1 in 85. "Many factors may well contribute, but it is not unreasonable to suspect that MMR is one of them," she argues. "Measles itself can cause encephalitis (brain inflammation)—its most dreaded complication. MMR is a live-virus vaccine. And the combination could be riskier than the separate elements."

These concerns underscore the importance of preserving patients' rights to refuse medical treatment, and the reality that all medical interventions carry both benefits and risks. Regardless of whether an individual opts for or against a particular vaccine, the critical point is this: *Government has no right or authority to mandate vaccines.*

Informed Consent

AAPS clarifies the importance of the distinction. "Mandatory vaccines violate the medical ethic of informed consent," states the organization's *Fact Sheet*, which also explains that the group is not opposed to vaccines and has never taken an anti-vaccine position. It is, however, firmly opposed to government policies that violate parental informed consent. "A case could also be made that mandates for vaccines by school districts and legislatures is the de facto practice of medicine without a license."

Government-required vaccines amount to a gross violation of privacy rights and personal freedom, as well as abuse of the doctor-patient relationship. In a 1999 statement to the U.S. House Government Reform Committee, Orient explained, "The relationship of patient and physician is shattered; in administering the vaccine, the physician is serving as the agent of the state." In that role, a doctor is forced to violate the time-honored Hippocratic Oath whereby he swears to act in the best interests of his individual patient, a principle reflected in the AAPS motto: *Omnia pro aegroto*

("All for the patient"). "Instead, he is applying the new population-based ethic in which the interests of the individual patient may be sacrificed to the 'needs of society.'"

Orient stated that government-mandated vaccines mark a shocking reversal of traditional public health policy. In the past, authorities restricted individual liberty "only in case of a clear and present danger," such as a quarantine of individuals infected with a dangerous communicable disease. "Today, a child may be deprived of his liberty to associate with others, or even of his supposed right to a public education, simply because of being unimmunized," said Orient. It does not matter that he is uninfected or that he poses no "clear and present danger." He is guilty until proven innocent—or in this case, until immunized.

AAPS is not alone in its defense of informed consent to medical treatment. The National Vaccine Information Center explains that the principle of informed consent "has become a central ethical principle in the practice of modern medicine and is applied to medical interventions which involve the risk of injury or death." NVIC's members believe no exception should be made for vaccines, since the group is composed of parents whose children have been injured or have died from reactions to them.

Though there is as yet no federal vaccination mandate, each state sets its own requirements for childhood immunization as a condition for public education. The NVIC website provides detailed information about current requirements, as well as measures under way in the various state legislatures to add or remove new mandates and exemptions.

Repercussions

Despite establishment media efforts to manufacture unwarranted hysteria and demands for "medicine at gunpoint," studies and experts suggest that the approach may backfire in a major way. For one, more parents will become aware of the controversy though they may never have realized that medical professionals and studies have found vaccines to be far less than totally safe and effective.

Plus, with trust in government at historic lows, any PR efforts by politicians, lobbyists, and bureaucrats are almost assured to generate a backlash and fresh suspicions. That is unquestionably a positive development—especially when it comes to vaccines. Parents and patients should have *all* available information prior to giving consent and making important medical decisions in consultation with their doctors.

ALEX NEWMAN is a journalist and educator.
REBECCA TERRELL is a nurse and an author.

Matthew Normand and Jesse Dallery

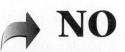 **NO**

Mercury Rising: Exposing the Vaccine-Autism Myth

On June 11, 2007, nearly 5,000 parents of autistic children filed a lawsuit against the federal government, claiming that childhood vaccines (specifically the mercury-containing thimerosal in the vaccines) caused their children's autism. The previous year the *New York Times* ran a column that was skeptical of the alleged link between autism and vaccines. It generated the following comment on an Internet message board, typical of the anecdotal analyses that perpetuate the claim:

> You say, "There is no proven link" between mercury and autism. There also is "no proven link" between going outside in the rain and cold without a hat or coat and getting the sniffles. Look at the data: the epidemic of autism mirrors the administration of vaccines with mercury. Now that they are off the shelves (more or less), the cases are going down.

Here we see how the writer dismisses scientific evidence that fails to support a link between cold and illness and vaccines and autism in favor of her personal experiences. And the vaccine-autism controversy is not constrained to a small fringe group of parents or advocates. Increasingly, people of position and power are leaping into the fray, spurred on by vocal groups demanding action. For example, an article by Robert F. Kennedy, Jr. appeared in a June 2005 issue of *Rolling Stone* magazine[1] that alleged thimerosal-containing vaccines were at the heart of the autism epidemic and, moreover, that the government was aware of this and actively engaged in a cover-up.

This article makes five points concerning the relation between thimerosal-containing vaccines and autism: (1) the dangers of mercury are well established, but this does not lead inexorably to a relationship between vaccines containing thimerosal and autism; (2) a number of well controlled studies have failed to uncover any correlation between the delivery of the vaccines and the onset of autism; (3) even if some correlation existed there are a number of alternative explanations for the correlation that do not assume any causal relationship between the vaccine and autism; (4) much attention has been given to a possible government cover up, which is certainly of concern if true but is otherwise independent of the problems with claims of a link between thimerosal and autism; and (5) the type of public hysteria manifested in the current controversy is not new and we would be well served to learn from similar controversies of recent times.

Mercury, Thimerosal, and the Potential for Harm

Science has told us unequivocally that mercury is bad for our bodies. In sufficient doses, mercury kills cells that it contacts, causes neurological damage in humans and other animals, and generally wreaks havoc on living things. Yet since the 1930s, thimerosal has been used as a preservative in vaccines.[2] One of the breakdown products of thimerosal is ethylmercury, which is an organic compound of mercury. Public concern about thimerosal is certainly understandable, but does this mean that concern about a link between vaccines and autism is justified as well? In a word, no. Mercury might do a number of nasty things to the human body, and concern about it is therefore justified, but that does not mean it causes autism.

Ethylmercury is not the same thing as its cousin, methylmercury. Cumulative and high doses of methylmercury can produce renal and neurologic damage. It can build up in the brain and stay in the body for a long time. Ethylmercury is more, well, mercurial. It is expelled rapidly from the body and it does not accumulate. Nevertheless, guidelines for the ingestion of ethylmercury were based on those for methylmercury. Around the same time these guidelines were formalized, children were receiving more vaccines that contained thimerosal. For example, in the early 1990s the Haemophilus influenzae b and hepatitis B became staple features of the vaccine schedule

Normand, Matthew; Dallery, Jesse. From *Skeptic*, vol. 13, no. 3, 2007, pp. 32–36. Copyright © 2007 by Skeptic Magazine. Reprinted by permission of Millennium Press.

for infants, which already included another thimerosal-containing vaccine (diphtheria tetanus and variants). Based on the very conservative guidelines established by the Environmental Protection Agency (EPA), it was concluded that by age two some children might be receiving excessive levels of ethylmercury when considered in the context of known risks of methylmercury exposure.[3]

Against this backdrop enter skyrocketing rates of autism diagnoses. In California, the Department of Developmental Services reported a 273% increase from 1987 to 1998 in the number of individuals served under the category of autism.[4] Surely this increase in rates was caused by an environmental source, right? In 2001, the Institute of Medicine (IOM) Immunization Safety Review Committee held a public meeting to address the link between one environmental source—thimerosal—and autism. At the meeting, Mark Blaxill, a board member of a nonprofit organization dedicated to investigating the risks of mercury exposure, presented a graph showing the *estimated* cumulative dose of thimerosal to the *estimated* prevalence of autism in California.[5] The increasing trend lines during the early 1990s were right on top of each other, about as close as you can get to perfect correlation in ecological data. Such orderly correlations are all that it takes to convince the uncritical eye.

Even before the IOM meeting, thimerosal was removed as a preservative in vaccines in the U.S., based on a request from the Food and Drug Administration (FDA) (it remains in some influenza vaccines and in some vaccines outside of the U.S.). The request was made as a precautionary measure, and not because there was evidence to accept or reject a causal relationship between thimerosal and autism. (Thimerosal is still used during manufacture of some vaccines to ensure sterility, but the trace amounts remaining are 50 times lower than when thimerosal is used as a preservative.) Since the FDA decision, a number of research reports published in some of the most esteemed peer-reviewed journals in the world have failed to find any relation between thimerosal and autism. Despite these negative findings and the removal of thimerosal from vaccines, parents, politicians and health professionals remain alarmed that children are at risk.

Much is at stake in this debate. Based on the assumption that metals such as mercury are causing autism, some parents are avoiding vaccinations altogether. Others have sought treatments like chelation therapy, which uses special chemicals to rid the body of heavy metals following acute poisoning. However, chelation is not a risk-free procedure and should not be undertaken lightly. In August of 2005, a Pittsburgh, PA area newspaper reported that a 5-year old boy with autism died following chelation therapy.

Finally, there are ongoing class action lawsuits against the manufacturers of vaccines. These lawsuits could potentially endanger the production and distribution of effective vaccines according to well-established protocols, putting scores of young children at risk.

Evidence of Harm

Let's begin with the hypothesis that thimerosal is one of the causes of autism and that it is the main culprit in the increased incidence of autism during the 1990s. This is a plausible hypothesis, but as Karl Popper taught us, a good scientific hypothesis must be falsifiable. That is, it must be possible to conceive of evidence that would prove it wrong. What evidence might suggest that the thimerosal hypothesis is false? For obvious ethical reasons, we can't perform the kind of gold-standard experiment—a randomized double-blind study—which would most convincingly indicate the lack of a causal relation. We must rely on natural experiments. One such experiment was occasioned by the removal of thimerosal in Denmark in 1992. If the thimerosal hypothesis were false, we would not expect to see changes in the rates of autism following the removal of thimerosal. In fact, the results were more robust: despite the removal of thimerosal, the rates of autism continued to climb. And not only in Denmark but in Sweden, too, where thimerosal was removed at about the same time.[6]

Another way the thimerosal hypothesis could be falsified is if it could be shown that there is no link between the amount of thimerosal exposure and the likelihood of autism. That is, we would ask if there is a dose-response relation between thimerosal exposure and developmental problems. Several studies have confirmed that there is no convincing evidence of a dose-response relation.[7] In fact, one study suggested a beneficial effect of thimerosal! For example, exposure at three months was inversely related to problems of hyperactivity, conduct, and motor development months or years later.[8] Now, these results do not imply causation, nor do they pertain to autism *per se*, but they do question the general validity of the thimerosal hypothesis.

So what of the data favoring the thimerosal hypothesis? Indeed, we must consider all sources of evidence in evaluating the truth of a claim—we must be comprehensive. Recently, some researchers have suggested that the incidence rate of autism has been on the decline since thimerosal was officially removed from vaccines in the US. If true, this would be evidence of a possible causal relationship between thimerosal and autism, and such data has been reported by one team of researchers, Mark and David Geier. Unfortunately, the study that proposed such a relationship used the Vaccine Adverse Event Reporting System (VAERS) database to make the claim.[9] The VAERS is a passive reporting system that is subject to reporting biases and errors. A health-care professional, parent, or even someone trying to prove a point[10] can enter data into the VAERS. There is no way to verify diagnoses, identify mistakes in filing, or substantiate causal hypotheses.

The irreparably flawed studies by the Geiers prompted a strong rebuke from the Centers for Disease Control (CDC) and by the American Academy of Pediatrics.[11] Simply put, the VAERS data may be useful to raise some potential questions about a phenomenon, but it certainly cannot be used to prove a hypothesis. Studies that use methods consistent with well-established scientific standards have failed to find any association between thimerosal and autism. In 2004, the Institute of Medicine concluded, "Given the lack of direct evidence for a biological mechanism and the fact that all well-designed epidemiological studies provide evidence of no association between thimerosal and autism, the committee recommends that cost-benefit assessments regarding the use of thimerosal-containing versus thimerosal-free vaccines and other biological or pharmaceutical products, whether in the United States or other countries, should not include autism as a potential risk."[12]

But what if it were determined that a strong correlation existed between the administration of thimerosal-containing vaccines and the onset of autism? Much would still be left unanswered. Consider that the average age for many vaccinations is between 12 and 18 months. Now consider that many of the "symptoms" of autism—such as social withdrawal and delayed language—aren't readily detectable until this same age or just a bit later. It could very well be that any relationship between vaccination and diagnosis is purely coincidental. If these vaccinations were not commonly given until age four, perhaps no correlation would be observed. Not to mention that the vast majority of children receive these vaccinations without incident.[13]

The bottom line is that *correlation is not causation.*

Autism Epidemic or Statistical Artifact?

Another problem for the purported vaccine-autism link is that there is good reason to be suspicious of claims of an autism epidemic. A number of factors can account for the dramatic increase in numbers, including the expansion of diagnostic criteria in 1994, and changes in criteria for inclusion in child-count data for children with autism.

Remember that 273% increase over a decade in autism spectrum disorders in California? Consider, as did the authors of a recent paper published in *Current Directions in Psychological Science,*[14] that this increase could be due to an expanded diagnostic definition of autism. The authors found that a similar expansion in the definition of "tall"—from 74.5 inches to 72 inches—generated a 273% increase if these two criteria were applied a decade apart in one county in Texas.

More important, autism is not even a "thing" that can be clearly correlated with any other thing. Unlike cancer or a broken bone, there are no discrete physical, biological, or genetic markers on which to base a diagnosis. Instead, autism is a diagnostic label based on the presence of a number of behavioral excesses and deficits. The diagnosis is subjective and subject to great variability. When you consider that many resources are made available only to those children with some formal diagnosis, it is easy to see why some diagnoses might be made with scant supporting evidence. The physician or psychologist notices some obvious learning delays and behavior problems in a patient and recognizes the need for intensive services, but the only way the family can obtain those services is if the child fits a certain diagnostic category.

Correlations are tenuous things under the best conditions. Degrade one of the variables, and you are in serious trouble. Such is the case with the autism-vaccine correlation.

A Vast Government Conspiracy?

So what do vaccine opponents make of the evidence against the vaccine-autism hypothesis? Mostly, they assert a vast conspiracy propagated by government and industry. It is proposed that government agencies such as the Centers for Disease Control and Prevention, in conjunction with scientists with varying ties to the pharmaceutical industry, have gone to great lengths to suppress evidence supporting a link between vaccines and autism. Indeed, this was the main point of Robert Kennedy Jr.'s *Rolling Stone* article. He and others claim that a conspiracy does exist and was formally discussed at a top-secret meeting in Simpsonwood, GA in 2000.

One hotly discussed result of this meeting is the purported doctoring of data by Thomas Verstraeten who, according to the vaccine opponents, presented data supporting the autism-vaccine link but later altered the data to support the opposite conclusion because he was, by then, employed by a large pharmaceutical company. Verstraeten has denied such manipulation and the data he reports support the conclusions reached by a number of other independent researchers.[15] The problem is that the only evidence of doctored data sets, dubious activity at the Simpsonwood meeting, and assorted cover-ups seems to come from a small number of zealous vaccine opponents who can offer no corroborating evidence to support the hearsay.

Now let us return to the research team purporting to have data supporting the autism-vaccine hypothesis. In addition to the flawed methods on which their conclusions are based, there are conflicts of interest that should cause one to question their motives. As it turns out, David Geier is the president of MedCon, Inc., a legal firm that seeks compensation for people claiming to have been harmed by vaccines. He also has filed, with his father Mark Geier, two patents related to a treatment for autism involving a combination of drugs and chelation. Chelation therapy is, of course, predicated on the assumption of excessive amounts of heavy metals in the blood stream of children with autism. The Geiers are clearly in a position to benefit if claims concerning a vaccine-autism link are accepted by the public.

History Repeating

A revealing aspect of this controversy is how closely it resembles past controversies, pitting science against vaccine-induced autism claims, spurred on by desperate parents, media support, and various servants of the public interest. Not so long ago, science was up against a similar set of public crusaders pushing a different cause: carcinogenic power lines. In 1979, a small, poorly controlled and poorly conducted sampling of leukemia patients in Denver, CO supposedly revealed a correlation between the patients and the proximity of their homes to high-power lines.[16] The published report of these suspect findings was largely ignored by the scientific community because of the many fatal flaws evident in the methodology. Enter Paul Brodeur, a journalist with a track record of sensationalism (in the 1960s he wrote *The Zapping of America*, a book "exposing the dangers" of microwave ovens), now warned the world of the dangers posed by power lines in his book *Currents of Death*.

No amount of scientific evidence to the contrary could persuade the journalists, advocacy groups, and legal teams demanding accountability. Of course, the million-dollar question was, "Accountability for what?" Ultimately, after numerous well-controlled studies failed to find any correlation between power-lines and cancer, the story grew cold and the public outrage slowly faded away. But not before tens of millions of dollars in research funding, decreased property values, and lawsuits were lost

because the matter was pursued long after science had delivered a verdict. Are we doomed to repeat this history with the vaccine controversy?

Clarifying Claims

Claims of a causal link between the administration of thimerosal-containing vaccines and the onset of autism are unfounded. The controversy has been driven more by public fervor than it has by science. This is not to suggest that the advocates and parents fueling the fire are malicious or intentionally misleading the public. The reality is that too many families face the unimaginable hardship of learning that their child has been diagnosed with autism and must encounter the subsequent trials and tribulations of providing the best possible care and education for their child. These parents are in desperate need of both assistance and answers. Compounding the difficulty is that many must navigate the waters of emerging science without having received the necessary training to do so. Clarifying misguided claims of causative factors can help redirect necessary resources to more promising treatments, and perhaps reveal a better understanding of the real factors that cause autism.

References

1. Kennedy, R. F., Jr. 2005. "Deadly Immunity." *Rolling Stone, 977/978*, June–July, 57–61.
2. U.S. Food and Drug Administration. n.d. *Thimerosal in Vaccines*. Accessed on March 23, 2007 from . . .
3. U.S. Food and Drug Administration. n.d.
4. Gernsbacher, M. A., Dawson, M., Goldsmith, H. H. 2005. "Three Reasons Not to Believe in an Autism Epidemic." *Current Directions in Psychological Science, 14*, 55–58.
5. Blaxill, M. 2001. "The Rising Incidence of Autism: Associations with Thimerosal." Accessed on March 23, 2007 from . . .
6. Stehr-Green P., Tull P., Stellfeld M., Mortenson P. B., Simpson D. 2003. Autism and Thimerosal Containing Vaccines: Lack of Consistent Evidence for an Association. *American Journal of Preventive Medicine, 25*, 101–106.
7. Hvild A., Stellfeld M., Wohlfahrt J., Melbye M. 2003. "Association Between Thimerosal-Containing Vaccines and Autism." *Journal of the American Medical Association, 290*, 1763–1766.
8. Heron J., Golding J.; ALSPAC Study Team. "Thimerosal Exposure in Infants and Developmental Disorders: A Prospective Cohort Study in the

United Kingdom Does Not Support a Causal Association." *Pediatrics, 114,* 577–583.

9. Geier, M. R., Geier, D. A., 2003. "Thimerosal in Childhood Vaccines, Neurodevelopment Disorders and Heart Disease in the United States." *Journal of American Physicians and Surgeons, 8,* 6–11.

10. Such a system cannot be used to prove a hypothesis. Consider that Dr. James Laidler allegedly reported that the influenza virus turned him into the Incredible Hulk, and the VAERS system accepted his report! Dr. Laidler reports that a representative of the CDC did contact him after noticing the report and, ultimately, it was deleted from the VAERS system, but only because Dr. Laidler granted permission. According to Laidler, had his permission not been granted, the report would have remained in the VAERS system. Others have reported submitting spurious reports to the VAERS system—for example that a vaccine turned someone into Wonder Woman—with similar success.

11. American Academy of Pediatrics. n.d. "Study Fails to Show a Connection Between Thimerosal and Autism." Accessed on March 23, 2007 from . . .

12. Institute of Medicine. Accessed on March 28, 2007 from . . .

13. Of course, this does not exclude the possibility that thimerosal might differentially affect an especially sensitive subset of children. Recently, researchers have reported that the neurotoxic effects of thimerosal exposure are related to autoimmune disease-sensitivity in mice. It is unclear whether these results will hold true for humans and whether such neurotoxicity has any relationship to autism, but it is an important area for further research. Unfortunately, because the "differential sensitivity" hypothesis is not yet well researched, there is no way to identify and protect those that might be at risk if it proves true. However, we know without question the dangers of disease and risks of avoiding vaccination. No matter the suspicions, the most prudent course of action is to go the vaccine route until there is real evidence to do otherwise. Also, we should note that existing evidence already casts doubt on the differential sensitivity hypothesis. If the rates of sensitivity to thimerosal remained constant before and after thimerosal was removed from vaccines, we would still expect a decrease in rates of autism. As reviewed above, this was not the case.

14. Gernsbacher, M. A., Dawson, M., Goldsmith, H. H. 2005. "Three Reasons Not to Believe in an Autism Epidemic." *Current Directions in Psychological Science, 14,* 55–58.

15. Stehr-Green et al., 2003.

16. Park, R. 2000. *Voodoo Science: The Road from Foolishness to Fraud.* Oxford: University Press.

MATTHEW NORMAND is an assistant professor of psychology at the University of the Pacific.

JESSE DALLERY is an associate professor in the behavior analysis program, Department of Psychology, the University of Florida, Gainesville.

EXPLORING THE ISSUE

Is There a Link Between Vaccination and Autism?

Critical Thinking and Reflection

1. Do parents have the right to withhold certain vaccinations from their children? On what grounds?
2. Is the government doing enough to make sure that vaccinations are safe? Explain your answer.
3. To what do you attribute the rise in diagnoses for autism? When can you say that autism started to "appear on the scene"?

Is There Common Ground?

Nine-year-old Hannah Poling had an uneventful birth and appeared to be developing normally. And then, right after receiving several routine vaccines, she became ill. Hannah recovered from her acute illness but lost her speech and eye contact and, in a matter of months, began displaying the repetitive behaviors and social withdrawal that indicate autism. Her parents reported that after her vaccinations, she just deteriorated and never came back.

Parents of children with autism have been blaming vaccines—and, especially, the mercury-based vaccine preservative thimerosal—as a cause of autism for over a decade, but researchers have repeatedly failed to identify a connection.

What is unusual about Hannah's case is that for the first time federal authorities agreed there was a connection between her autistic symptoms and the vaccines she received, though the relationship is by no means clear. A panel of medical evaluators at the Department of Health and Human Services determined that Hannah had been injured by vaccines and recommended that her family be compensated for the injuries. The panel said that Hannah had an underlying cellular disorder that was aggravated by the vaccines, causing brain damage with features of autism spectrum disorder.

The Poling case is also causing concern among public health officials, who are anxious to reassure parents that immunizations are safe and valuable. In a recent public statement, Dr. Julie Gerberding, director of the Centers for Disease Control and Prevention (CDC), insisted that "the government has made absolutely no statement about indicating that vaccines are the cause of autism, as this would be a complete mischaracterization of any of the science

that we have at our disposal today." Dr. Gerberding and other health authorities point out that the benefits of vaccines far exceed their risks. They also note that thimerosal was eliminated from routinely administered childhood vaccines manufactured after 2001, and yet autism rates have not dropped. The current CDC estimate is that 1 of 150 American children has an autism spectrum disorder.

But there are circumstances that take Hannah's case out of the ordinary. For one thing, she received an unusually large number of vaccines in 2000 (when thimerosal was still in use). Because of a series of ear infections, Hannah had lagged behind in the vaccine schedule, so in one day she was given five immunizations to prevent a total of nine diseases: measles, mumps, rubella, polio, varicella, diphtheria, pertussis, tetanus, and *Haemophilus influenzae*. A second issue in Hannah's situation is that she suffers from a mitochondrial disorder, a dysfunction in basic cell metabolism. In Hannah's case, the vaccine court determined that the underlying dysfunction of her mitochondria put her at an increased risk of injury from vaccines.

Experts on autism spectrum disorders believe that most cases are caused by a combination of genetic vulnerabilities and environmental factors. There may be hundreds of routes to autism, involving multiple combinations of genes and external variables. While it is possible thimerosal or some other aspect of vaccines is one of these factors, it has not been definitively proven and further research is needed. It's challenging to draw any clear conclusions from the case of Hannah Poling, other than the need for more research. One plausible conclusion is that pediatricians should avoid giving small children a large number of vaccines at once, even if they are thimerosal-free.

Dr. Andrew Wakefield's research, which linked autism to vaccination, has generally been discredited.

In "How the Case Against the MMR Vaccine Was Fixed" (*British Medical Journal*, August 1, 2011), the authors offer a look at the controversies raised by the paper written by Andrew Wakefield and colleagues linking autism with measles, mumps, and rubella (MMR) vaccine. The authors address details of how the discrepancies and fraudulent data in the paper were discovered. "Study Linking Vaccine to Autism Is Called Fraud" (*New York Times*, June 1, 2011) reported on the fraudulent first study to link a vaccination to autism. The research was based on doctored information about the children involved, according to a new report on the widely discredited research. The conclusions of the 1998 paper by Dr. Andrew Wakefield and his colleagues were renounced by 10 of its 13 authors and later retracted by the medical journal *The Lancet*, where it was originally published. Still, the suggestion that the combined measles, mumps, and rubella vaccine was connected to autism scared parents worldwide and vaccination rates for the MMR shot plummeted. Despite overwhelming evidence to the contrary, approximately 20 percent of Americans still believe that vaccines cause autism, a disturbing fact that will probably continue to hold true even after the early 2011 publication of a *British Medical Journal* report thoroughly debunking the 1998 paper that began the vaccine–autism scare.

Additional Resources

Buck, G., & Gatehouse, J. (2015). The real vaccine scandal. *Maclean's, 128*(7), 28–35.

DeLong, G. (2011). A positive association found between autism prevalence and childhood vaccination uptake across the U.S. population. *Journal of Toxicology & Environmental Health: Part A, 74*(14), 903–916.

Holton, A., Weberling, B., Clarke, C. E., & Smith, M. J. (2012). The blame frame: Media attribution of culpability about the MMR–autism vaccination scare. *Health Communication, 27*(7), 690–701.

Knopf, A. (2015). MMR vs. autism: A false choice. *Brown University Child & Adolescent Behavior Letter, 31*, 1–2.

Offit, P. A. (2008, May 15). Vaccines and autism revisited—The Hannah Poling case. *New England Journal of Medicine, 359*(6), 2089–2091.

Internet References . . .

Autism Society

www.autism-society.org

Centers for Disease Control: Vaccines & Immunizations

www.cdc.gov/vaccines/

Environmental Protection Agency

www.epa.gov

National Institutes of Health/Autism

www.ncbi.nlm.nih.gov

Selected, Edited, and with Issue Framing Material by:
Eileen L. Daniel, *SUNY College at Brockport*

ISSUE

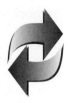

Do Cell Phones Cause Cancer?

YES: Ronald B. Herberman, from "Tumors and Cell Phone Use: What the Science Says," U.S. House of Representatives (2008)

NO: Bernard Leikind, from "Do Cell Phones Cause Cancer?" *Skeptic* (2010)

Learning Outcomes
After reading this issue, you will be able to:
• Discuss the possible mechanisms in which cell phones may trigger cancers.
• Assess other health risks associated with cell phone usage including traffic safety.
• Discuss why the long-term health implications of cell phones are unclear.
• Discuss why some countries, including France, have warned about the use of cell phones.

ISSUE SUMMARY

YES: Physician and director of the Pittsburgh Cancer Institute Ronald B. Herberman maintains that radio frequency radiation associated with cell phones is a potential health risk factor for users, especially children.

NO: Physicist Bernard Leikind argues that there is no plausible mechanism by which cell phone radiation can cause cancer.

A cell phone is a device used to make mobile telephone calls across a wide geographic area. It can make and receive telephone calls to and from the public telephone network, which includes other mobile and landline phones throughout the world. Cell phones work by connecting to a mobile network managed by a cellular phone company. In addition to operating as a telephone, mobile phones usually offer additional services including text messaging, e-mail, and Internet access along with a variety of business and gaming applications, and photography. They are extremely popular both in the United States and throughout the world. Currently, there are nearly 4.5 billion cell phones used globally.

Although cell phones have many communication advantages and are extensively used, they are also associated with health and safety risks. Cell phone use while driving is widespread, but controversial. Distractions like texting or talking on a cell phone while driving a car or other motor vehicle have been shown to increase the risk of accidents. Because of this, many areas prohibit the use of cell phones while driving and several states ban handheld cell phone use only, while allowing hands-free calling. Texting while driving is also illegal in some states.

In addition to the links between cell phone use and motor vehicle accidents, there may be a relationship between mobile phones and long-term health risks including certain cancers. Some countries, including France, have warned against the use of cell phones, especially by minors, due to health risk uncertainties. Groups of scientists claim that because mobile phone use is employing relatively new technology, long-term conclusive evidence has been impossible to determine and that the use should be restricted, or monitored closely, to be on the safe side.

Cell phones use radiation in the microwave range, which some scientists believe may be harmful to human health. In epidemiological and animal and human research, the majority show no definite causal relationship between cell phone exposure and harmful biological effects in humans. Overall, most evidence shows no harm to humans is caused by cell phones, although a significant number of individual studies do suggest such a relationship, or are inconclusive. Based upon the majority view of scientific and medical communities, the World Health Organization (WHO) has asserted that cancer is unlikely to be caused by cellular phones or their base stations and that studies have found no convincing evidence for other health problems. Some national radiation scientists have recommended measures to minimize exposure only as a precautionary approach.

While most research investigations have found no relationship between cell phones and tumor growth, at least some recent studies have found an association between cell phone use and certain kinds of brain and salivary gland cancers. A major meta analysis of 11 studies from peer-reviewed journals concluded that cell phone usage for at least 10 years may double the risk of being diagnosed with a brain tumor on the same side of the head that is most often used for cell phone conversations.

Clearly, there is no definitive answer on the potential safety issues associated with cell phone use. In the YES selection, Ronald B. Herberman, a physician and director of the Pittsburgh Cancer Institute, maintains that radio frequency radiation associated with cell phones is a potential health risk factor for users, especially children. In the NO selection, physicist Bernard Leikind argues that there is no plausible mechanism by which cell phone radiation can cause cancer.

YES ↵

Ronald B. Herberman

Tumors and Cell Phone Use: What the Science Says

Thank you for inviting me to speak with you today about the important matter of cell phones and our health. I have served as the Founding Director of the University of Pittsburgh Cancer Institute (UPCI) since 1985, and as the Founding Director of University of Pittsburgh Medical Center (UPMC) Cancer Centers since 2001. The organizations that I lead employ more than 660 oncologists, other cancer experts and research faculty and more than 2,000 other staff members. In addition to the cutting edge cancer research performed at UPCI, our cancer centers, located throughout western Pennsylvania and adjacent states, annually treat more than 27,000 new cancer patients each year.

The UPCI is a National Cancer Institute (NCI)-designated comprehensive cancer center, and is one of the top ranked cancer research facilities in the nation. In fact, in 2007, UPCI was ranked 10th nationally in its level of NCI funding for cancer research. During the past two decades, UPCI has recruited some of the world's top scientists.

At UPCI, I am the Hillman Professor of Oncology, Professor of Medicine and Associate Vice Chancellor for Cancer Research at the University of Pittsburgh. I also was the founding Chairman of the Board of Directors, and I currently am the President, of the Pennsylvania Cancer Control Consortium, a state-wide cancer control organization. I am a longstanding member and Chairman of the Research and Clinical Trials Team, of C-Change, a national cancer organization, that has President George H.W. Bush, First Lady Barbara Bush, and Sen. Dianne Feinstein as the honorary co-chairs. For the past few years, C-Change has focused mainly on innovative strategies to reduce smoking and other personal risk factors for cancer, and to facilitate medical interventions to protect people at increased risk for cancer.

I also served from 1999–2001 as the President of the Association of American Cancer Institutes, an organization that includes almost all of the major academic cancer centers in the US. All of the organizations that I am associated with are focused on eliminating cancer as a public health problem, a commitment that I take very seriously.

As a cancer researcher, I have published more than 700 peer-reviewed articles in major biomedical journals, and for two decades my scientific publications placed me as among the 100 most cited biomedical scientists. In addition, I have served as an associate editor on more than 10 major, peer-reviewed journals, including Cancer Research, the Journal of the National Cancer Institute (JNCI), and the Journal of Immunology, and I have been a peer reviewer for over 1,000 manuscripts submitted for publication. For nearly two decades before I was recruited to Pittsburgh to found the UPCI, I led research teams at the NCI that focused mainly on characterizing the cellular basis for human anti-tumor immunity and utilizing the insights derived from those studies to develop innovative approaches to use immunotherapy to improve the treatment of cancer. The work of my research team at NCI resulted in the initial identification and then extensive characterization of natural killer (NK) cells. Research by my team at NCI and then at UPCI, along with other leading researchers around the world, have shown that NK cells are a key component of our natural defense against the development and metastatic spread of cancer.

In addition to world class studies in cancer immunology and immunotherapy at UPCI, other programs at our institute are developing prognostic indicators of response to treatment. UPCI also includes experts working on strategies for cancer prevention, early detection, and treatment and approaches for cancer control. Through our innovative Center for Environmental Oncology, we are carrying out studies to better define the role of environmental exposures on cancer risk, coupled with measures to reduce cancer risk by reducing exposure to environmental carcinogens, or using nutritional and other interventions to protect people who have been exposed to environmental hazards.

As part of our overall efforts, we are also working to identify important policy changes that should be developed to reduce the burden of cancer. After years of protracted delays, our nation has finally made progress against smoking by getting individuals to stop smoking. But, smoking control policies proved difficult to implement for

Herberman, Ronald B. From statement before the Domestic Policy Subcommittee of the Oversight and Government Reform Committee, U.S. House of Representatives, September 25, 2008.

many years, because of complex strategies to manipulate information on its dangers. Analogous efforts to identify and then effectively implement actions for other controllable causes of cancer have been fairly limited.

Now, to turn to the issues of direct interest to this committee, I first want to point out that, in contrast to several of the other speakers at this important hearing, who are longstanding experts on some aspects of radiofrequency (RF) radiation associated with cell phones or on the design and implementation of population-based studies, I have only recently become involved in the issue of the possible health risks of cell phones, by issuing a precautionary message to the faculty and staff of the UPCI and the UPMC Cancer Centers. For you to understand why a non-expert in the field took this action, I believe it is important to explain the process that led up to the issuance of the advisory to reduce direct cell phone exposures to the head and body.

Last year, as she was finalizing her well-researched book, The Secret History of the War on Cancer, my colleague, Dr. Devra Davis, Director of the UPCI's Center for Environmental Oncology and an internationally acclaimed expert in environmentally-induced health risks, shared with me the growing scientific literature on the possible association between extensive cell phone and increased risk of malignant and benign brain tumors. My attention was directed to a large body of evidence, including expert analyses showing absorption of RF into the brain and the comprehensive Bioinitiative Report, review of experimental and public health studies pointing to potential adverse biologic effects of RF signals, including brain tumors, associated with long-term and frequent use of cell phones held to the ear. I also learned of a recent series of similar precautionary advisories from international experts and various governments in Europe and Canada. I reacted to this information in the same fashion as I do with other reports of claims of biologically and/or clinically important findings, namely I first carefully reviewed the reports and consulted with a variety of relevant experts.

My evaluation of the scientific and technical information indicating the potential hazards of cell phones was built on the foundation of my extensive experience in cancer research and critical evaluations of reports being submitted for peer-reviewed publications. I recognized that there was sufficient evidence to justify the precautionary advisories that had been issued in other countries, to alert people about the possibility of harm from long-term, frequent cell phone use, especially by young children. Then, Dr. Davis and I consulted with international experts in the biology of radiofrequency (RF) effects and the epidemiology of brain tumors, and with experts in neurology, oncology

and neurosurgery at UPCI. Without exception, all of the experts contacted confirmed my impression that there was a sound basis to make the case for precaution, especially since there are simple and practical measures that can be taken, to be able to continue to use cell phones while substantially reducing the potential hazards.

Another factor influencing my decision was my growing conviction that substantially more attention should be devoted to promoting a range of strategies to reduce the future burden of cancer. Of course, I appreciate the tremendous progress that the US has made in treating cancer, some of which was achieved by studies at the University of Pittsburgh, on melanoma, breast, brain, and colorectal cancer. I also recognize that approaches that aim to prevent new cases from occurring are the most likely ways to more effectively and efficiently reduce the overall burden of cancer. Accordingly, I decided to act, consistent with my responsibilities as the leader of a major US cancer institute, by informing my colleagues about my concerns that cell phone use may be a substantial risk to public health. I also wanted to stimulate broader awareness and discussion of the evidence that I came to be familiar with, and to encourage changes in the behavior of some of my colleagues and by extension, also their families and friends.

Summary of Review of the Published Scientific Evidence for an Association Between Cell Phone Use and Brain Tumors

Obviously, scientific research plays a central role in identifying exposures that may affect our health. In public health research, scientists generally rely on two major types of evidence to evaluate potential risks. First, a combination of laboratory-based experimental studies using animals, cell cultures, and computer models can be used to examine mechanisms, identify biological effects and predict the potential impact for humans. Then, population-based human studies can also be used to determine if observed patterns of disease can be correlated with specific exposures, and other more detailed studies of people with a particular disease in comparison with healthy controls, so-called case-control studies, can be carried out to determine if there are different health patterns in those with and without certain exposures.

Although in some cases a clear association between an exposure and health effect can be demonstrated, often methodological differences among studies can introduce subtle differences in the way data are evaluated, and in some cases can lead to very different conclusions. This is especially true for human population-based cancer epidemiology studies where it is sometimes very difficult to select non-exposed controls, where the critical timing of exposure is not precisely known, where the mechanism by which an exposure might cause cancer is not well defined or understood, or where the characteristics of the exposure change over time. A critical review of the literature on the biological effects of cell phones exemplifies this point. Despite the lack of consistency in outcomes in all the cell phone publications, there are several well-designed studies that suggest that long-term (10 years or more) use of wireless phone devices is associated with a significant increase in risk for glioblastoma (glioma), a very aggressive and fatal brain tumor, and acoustic neuroma, a benign tumor of the auditory nerve that is responsible for our hearing.

For more than eight years, the World Health Organization has been conducting a combined effort to study cell phones and brain cancer in thirteen countries, called the Interphone study. No results synthesizing this overall effort have been published yet. But, several reports from countries participating in the Interphone study have appeared. Some analyses have found no increased risk of cell phones, while others, from countries where study participants used cell phones for a decade or longer, have found increased risks for brain tumors. But, even in these negative studies, when the subset of long-term users are examined separately, there is evidence of increased risk of brain tumors.

Clearly, not all of the published cell phone studies have reached the same conclusion. What are some of the characteristics of study design that can explain the differences among cell phone use studies generally and between the Interphone-related studies and the independent, non-Interphone-related studies?

To address this question, in 2008, Dr. Lennart Hardell, a distinguished oncologist and senior author on several cell phone studies in Sweden that have shown increases in brain tumor risk with long-term use, published a combined analysis (also called a meta-analysis) of published case-control studies that evaluated the effects of cell phone use on brain tumor risk. For gliomas, a malignant tumor of the supporting tissue of the brain, he and his colleagues found 10 studies; 7 were part of the Interphone Study, one was partly based on Interphone participation and partly independent, and 2 were not part of Interphone (one was a Swedish study from Hardell's team, and the second was a Finnish study). In contrast to the Interphone-related studies which found no increased risk for glioma, both of the independent studies found an increased risk of 40–50%. Since

8 of these 10 studies were Interphone-related, and these studies all showed no effect of cell phone use on glioma risk, the combined data result (meta-analysis) also showed no effect. It should be noted, however, that most of these studies included as cell phone users those who only made a single phone call a week and did so over a limited duration.

In contrast, focusing on those who had used cell phones for a decade provided a different story. Of these 10 studies, 6 evaluated long-term exposure effects, resulting from 10 or more years of cell phone use. Of these 6 studies, all showed an increase risk for developing a glioma on the same side of the head where the phone was used, and this increased risk ranged from a low of 20% increased risk for low grade (less aggressive) glioma to more than 400% increase risk of high grade (very aggressive) glioma. The meta-analysis for the combined data indicated that those who regularly used cell phones had twice the risk of malignant brain tumors overall, and four times the risk if they were high users of phones.

For acoustic neuroma, 9 case-control studies have been published that have compared the reported history of cell phone use of persons with and without this benign tumor on the hearing nerve. Eight of these studies are Interphone study-related and one, by Hardell's group, was independent. Whereas six of the 7 Interphone studies showed that no increased risk with regular cell phone use, Hardell found that regular cell phone users had a 70% greater risk. What struck me as especially relevant, and to possibly account for the divergent reports, is one simple fact: all three studies that looked at cell phone users for at least a decade, found a significantly increased risk. In long term users, acoustic neuromas are twice as frequent in regular, long-term users.

Within the last month, as also noted by Dr. David Carpenter in this hearing, Dr. Hardell reported at a meeting of the Royal Society of London that very frequent and long term users of cell phones by teenagers that started before age 20, resulted in a five times higher rate of brain cancer by the age of 29, when compared with non-cell phone users.

Brain cancer, which is one of the health effects of very serious concern, is believed to develop in adults over a period of at least one decade and in some cases, up to several decades. Among the known causes of brain cancer is ionizing radiation, such as x-rays. RF radiation is not ionizing, but it is absorbed into the brain, according to modeling studies that have been produced by the cell phone industry, in particular by French Telecom. There is no debate that radiation emitted by cell phones is absorbed into the brain—dramatically more so in children than in adults.

In summary, my review of the literature suggests that most studies claiming that there is no link between cell phones and brain tumors are outdated, had methodological concerns, and did not include sufficient numbers of long-term cell phone users to find an effect, since most of these negative studies primarily examined people with only a few years of phone use and did not inquire about cordless phone use. In addition, many studies defined regular cell phone use as "once a week."

One major negative study, published by the Danish Cancer Society and supported by the cell phone industry, started with nearly three quarters of a million cell phone users during the period between 1982 and 1995. This study excluded more than 200,000 business users, who were most likely to be the most frequent users during that time period. Recall bias was a problem with all of these studies as solid data such as cell phone records were not used to document usage and people were simply asked, often the day after surgery, whether or not they had used a cell phone and for how long.

Scientists appreciate that diseases like brain cancer can take decades to develop. This means that even well conducted studies of those who have used phones for only a few years, as most of us have, cannot tell us whether or not there are hazards from long-term use.

In contrast, some recent studies in Nordic countries, where phones have been used longest, find that persons who have used cell phones for at least a decade have 30% to more than 200% more brain tumors than do those without such use, and only on the side of the head where the user holds his or her phone. To put these numbers in context, this is at least as high an increase as the added risk of breast cancer that women face from long-term use of hormone replacement therapy. Based on these findings and the increased absorption into the brains of the young, the French Ministry of Health advised that children should be discouraged from using cell phones, a position also taken by British, German and other authorities.

Precautionary Advisory Based on Review of the Published Reports and Consideration of the Precautionary Advisories from Several Countries in Europe and Elsewhere

While those issues are being debated and resolved, and as we eagerly await the results, my review of the available published evidence suggesting some increased brain tumor risk following long-term cell phone use, combined with the current near ubiquity of exposure to cell phones and cordless phone RF fields (more than 90% of the population in the Western European countries and about 90% of the population in the USA use cellular phones), led me to work with both international experts and experts at UPCI to develop a set of prudent and simple precautions that I felt could reduce potential risk, while awaiting more definitive evidence. Certainly, if it turns out that long-term use of cell phones does increase brain tumor risk, the public health implications of *not* taking action are obvious.

On July 21, 2008, I issued the advisory on the safe use of cell phones to the physicians, researchers and staff at UPCI and UPMC Cancer Centers. Before its issuance, this document was reviewed by UPCI experts in neuro-oncology, epidemiology, environmental oncology, and neurosurgery as well as national and international scientific and engineering experts. A copy can be found at the end of my testimony. My sole goal in issuing the cell phone advisory was to suggest simple precautions that would reduce exposure to cell phone electromagnetic radiation. The advisory clearly indicated that the human evidence on the potential hazard of cell phones is still evolving, but it pointed out that there are some studies using experimental and population-based approaches that suggest an association between long-term cell phone use and development of brain tumors. It also pointed out that modeling studies suggest the possibility that there may be additional differences in susceptibility between young children and adults. Based on my review of the data, I felt that there was sufficient evidence for possible human health risks, to warrant providing precautionary advice on cell phone use, especially by children.

What are the main points of the advisory? Adults can reduce direct exposure of the head and bone marrow to radiofrequency radiation by using ear pieces or the speaker phone mode whenever possible. Cell phone use by children should be restricted. Here we advised, as do a number of governments, that cell phone use by children be limited to emergency calls and for older children, text messaging. In circulating this warning, I joined with an international expert panel of pathologists, oncologists and public health specialists, who recently declared that RF radiation emitted by cell phones should be considered a potential human health risk.[1] In fact, shortly before I sent my precautionary message to faculty and staff at UPCI and UPMC Cancer Centers, a number of countries including France, Germany and India, and the province of Ontario, Canada, issued similar advice, suggesting that exposure to RF radiation from cell phones be limited. Very soon after the UPCI advisory was issued, Israel's Health Ministry endorsed my recommendations, and Toronto's Department of Public Health advised that teenagers and young children limit their use of cell phones, to avoid potential health risks.

I appreciate the interest of this committee in exploring the current state of the scientific evidence on the potential hazards of cell phones. I have provided appendices that include links and references to reviews and advisories that have been issued within the past few years by other authorities. In addition, the web site for UPCI's Center for Environmental Oncology (www.preventingcancernow .org) includes the actual papers as pdf files for all major studies published over the past two years. In addition, the Bioinitatives Report (www.bioinitiativereport.org) provides comprehensive, critical review, that includes references to the more than 4,000 relevant studies that have been published to date on this subject.

Most people throughout the developed world are using cell phones. Cell phones save lives and have revolutionized our world in many positive ways. Without doubt, the most immediate danger from the use of cell phones is that of traffic crashes. But, the longer term spectre of harm cannot easily be dismissed at this point. The absence of definitive positive studies should not be confused with proof that there is no association. Rather, it reflects the difficulties of assembling definitive proof and the absence of well-conducted, large-scale independent studies on the problem.

Throughout my career I have witnessed the tremendously important discoveries that have improved cancer care. I also recognize that cancer professionals and physicians in general have failed to pay adequate attention to the need to identify and then promptly and effectively control avoidable causes of cancer. Nowhere is our failure more evident than in the protracted and prolonged debate that played out over the hazards of tobacco. By all accounts, we have also missed the boat with respect to our national policies on known workplace cancer causes such as exposure to asbestos, and we waited far too long before acting to reduce dangers associated with hormone replacement therapy.

It is worth noting that in the case of tobacco and lung cancer, debates over whether there was a true increase in lung cancer associated with smoking raged far longer than they should have, fomented by an active disinformation campaign of which this Congress is well aware. The dilemma of public policy when it comes to controlling and identifying the causes of cancer is profound. If we insist we must be certain of human harm and wait for definitive evidence of such damage, we are

effectively saying that we can only act to prevent future cancers, once past ones have become evident. Recalling the 70 years that it took to remove lead from paint and gasoline and the 50 years that it took to convincingly establish the link between smoking and lung cancer, I argue that we must learn from our past to do a better job of interpreting evidence of potential risk. In failing to act quickly, we subject ourselves, our children and our grandchildren to the possibility of grave harm and to living with the knowledge that with more rapid action that harm could have been averted.

I do not envy policy makers and regulators as they do not always have adequate solid data on which to base standards. In the present case, the link between cell phones and health effects is suggestive but not solidly established. From my careful review of the evidence, I cannot tell you conclusively that phones cause cancer or other diseases. But, I can tell you that there are published peer reviewed studies that have led me to suspect that long term cell phone use may cause cancer. It should be noted in this regard that worldwide, there are three billion regular cell phone users, including a rapidly growing number of children. If we wait until the human evidence is irrefutable and then act, an extraordinarily large number of people will have been exposed to a technology that has never really been shown to be safe. In my opinion, for public health, when there is some evidence of harm and the exposed group is very large, it makes sense to urge caution. This is why I issued advice to our faculty and staff, especially to take precautions to reduce cell phone RF exposures to children.

Now that the issue of a possible association of long-term cell phone with increased brain tumor risk has reached national and international attention, the central question is where we go from here. Should we simply wait and watch? Or, should we take some actions now? I am not sufficiently expert to comment on possible new regulations to affect cell phone usage. Rather, from my perspective as a scientist and cancer center director, I want to do all that I can to see that the matter of cell phones and our health is resolved. I believe that we should undertake additional, more definitive research that will tell the whole story. Many of my colleagues at UPCI, Rutgers University, University of California, San Francisco and a number of senior faculty at M.D. Anderson Cancer Institute are joining with me in calling for an independent scientific investigation, avoiding as many of the limitations of the prior studies as possible, to determine if long-term, frequent use of cell phones and cordless phones increases brain tumor risk. We will urge that these studies engage both university and NIH experts and also the full cooperation of the cell phone industry, which will be asked to provide solid usage data in the form of access to billing records and substantial contribution to the funding of the study but without any direct review or control of the results, in order to clearly settle this issue in the not too distant future.

In the meantime, while we continue to conduct progressively better research on this question, I believe it makes sense to urge caution: it's better to be safe than sorry.

Note

1. *The Case for Precaution in the Use of Cell Phones Advice from University of Pittsburgh Cancer Institute Based on Advice from an International Expert Panel,* available at www.preventingcancernow.org

RONALD B. HERBERMAN is a physician and the director of the Pittsburgh Cancer Institute, Pittsburgh, Pennsylvania.

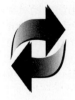

Bernard Leikind

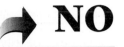 **NO**

Do Cell Phones Cause Cancer?

News reports threaten that our cell phones may cause cancer—brain cancer, eye cancer, and others. We are told that fragile children's developing brains are at risk. Concerned epidemiologists collect their data and warn that they cannot rule out the possibility of harm from cell phone radiation and that they must do more research. Medical professionals assert, as a precaution and in the absence of definitive data, that we should place our phones at arm's length. News accounts fill us with alarm. Danger lurks.

Fears that cell phones cause cancer are groundless. There is not a shred of evidence that the electromagnetic radiation from your cell phones causes harm, much less that from the wiring in the walls of your house, your hair dryer, electric blanket, or the power distribution wires nearby.

We know exactly what happens to energy from any of these sources when it meets the atoms and molecules in your body, and that energy cannot cause cancer. There is no known way that this energy can cause any cancer, nor is there any unknown way that this energy can cause any cancer.

There is a link between some forms of electromagnetic radiation and some cancers. These forms of electromagnetic radiation are ultraviolet radiation, X-rays, and gamma rays. They are dangerous because they may break covalent chemical bonds in your body. Breakage of certain covalent bonds in key molecules leads to an increased cancer risk. For example, there is a link between ultraviolet light from the sun and skin cancers.

All other forms of electromagnetic radiation other than these may add to molecules' or atoms' thermal agitation, but can do nothing else. Visible light has sufficient energy to affect chemical bonds. When light strikes the cones and rods in our retinas rhodopsin bends from its resting state to another, but it does not break. When visible light strikes the chlorophyll molecules in plants, electrons shift about but the chlorophyll does not break. Visible light does not cause cancer.

Electromagnetic radiation transfers its energy to atoms and molecules in chunks called *photons*. The energy of a single photon is proportional to the photon's frequency. The photons of high frequency radiation, such as ultraviolet light, X-rays, and gamma rays, carry relatively large amounts of energy compared to those of lower frequency radiation. That is why high-energy photons can break covalent chemical bonds while the photon energy of all other forms of electromagnetic radiation, including visible light, infrared light, microwave, TV and radio waves, and AC power cannot.

Figure 1 shows a range of energy that is important for life and for the science of biochemistry. The figure displays an energy scale to help you place relevant energy states or processes in context. Horizontal positions indicate the energy range.

Look at the area covered by the long bracket in the middle. It shows the general energy range of the major strong chemical bonds—covalent bonds—which are significant for all of life's molecules. Below to the right you can see where the energy of an important organic covalent bond—that which occurs between two carbon atoms—falls on the scale. Further up the scale, on the upper right, is the energy range of carcinogenic electromagnetic radiation. Notice where the call out for green light falls on this scale. Visible light does not cause cancer.

Notice that the energy of cell phone radiation and AC power radiation in this scale is very low. Cell phone radiation cannot break, damage, or weaken any covalent bond.

Figure 2 shows the lowest energy part of Figure 1's energy scale. Figure 1 ranges from 0 kJ/mole to 600 kJ/mole. Figure 2 ranges from 0 kJ/mole to 30 kJ/mole.

Notice the bracket that shows the range of weak bonds in each figure. These are hydrogen bonds, van der Waals bonds, electrostatic bonds, and various other effects, such as hydrophobic or hydrophilic forces. In the complex molecules of life, these bonds play critical roles holding strands together and creating the three-dimensional shapes of molecules.

Covalent bonds hold together the single strands of DNA. Hydrogen bonds connect one strand to its mate. Enzymes fold and twist to create the forms they require as they perform their role as catalysts. The various weak bonds maintain the shapes of these folds and twists.

Figure 1

The units of this scale are familiar to chemists. Chemists like to think about test-tube-sized quantities of stuff. A mole is a unit that measures how much stuff you have. It is a count of objects: atoms, molecules, photons, chemical bonds. One mole of any object contains 6.023×10^{23} of those objects. Physicists prefer to state the energy in one bond or in one photon. A physicist would divide all the numbers in this figure by the number of objects in a mole to show the energy in Joules in a single object. An (old) physicist might prefer to express this energy in units of electron volts. Measured in electron volts, the energy in one green light photon is about 2.5 electron volts. The energy in one banana is 150 to 200 Calories, which corresponds to 600 or 800 kJ/banana; that is, one banana, not a mole of bananas.

Biochemistry's Energy World

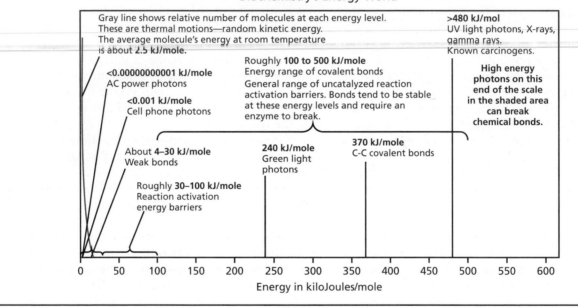

Drawn in both figures is a graph that suggests the energy of molecular thermal motions at body temperature. Everything in our bodies partakes in these thermal motions. The molecules jostle one another. They twist and vibrate. The thick gray line on the graph shows how energy distributes itself among these various motions. The motion's average energy is about 2.5 kJ/mole. Some molecules, but not many, have much more energy.

If energy transfers of 2.5 kJ/mole, more or less, were sufficient to damage life's molecules, life would be impossible because random thermal motions would quickly break most of them. Fortunately, covalent bonds require ten to fifty times this amount of energy transfer before they break. Thermal jostling does not interfere with them. Weak biochemical bonds, however, live within the upper range of thermal bonds and shakes. That is why they do not enter into life's structure as single bonds, but always as groups. In the long double helices of DNA, the hydrogen bonds are like the individual teeth

of a long zipper. Together they withstand what any single one of them could not.

These collisions are electromagnetic interactions. The molecules' outer electrons sense the presence of their neighbors though electromagnetic forces. These electrons resist oncoming neighbors, pushing them away, and pushing upon their own molecules as well. Electromagnetic forces transmit these pushes. All of the molecules of biology must be able to withstand these electromagnetic forces to maintain their shapes and their functions. The forces that electromagnetic fields from cell phones exert on life's molecules are no different from any of these molecular pushes, except that they are much, much smaller.

Cancer is a disease of the heredity of individual cells. Something must cause a cell to begin transferring mistakes to its progeny. One cell goes haywire, replicating wildly, transmitting the mistaken instructions—the damaged DNA—to each of its daughters. If the damage is too great, the cell will die. If the damage is not sufficient, it

Figure 2

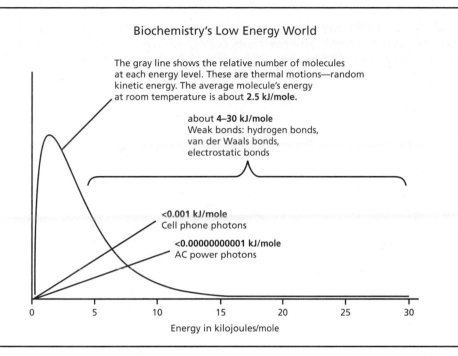

Biochemistry's Low Energy World

The gray line shows the relative number of molecules at each energy level. These are thermal motions—random kinetic energy. The average molecule's energy at room temperature is about **2.5 kJ/mole.**

about **4–30 kJ/mole**
Weak bonds: hydrogen bonds, van der Waals bonds, electrostatic bonds

<0.001 kJ/mole
Cell phone photons

<0.00000000001 kJ/mole
AC power photons

Energy in kilojoules/mole

is not cancer. The damaged cell and its damaged progeny must continue to function in their crippled, uncontrolled states. Cancer generally requires more than one mutation in a single cell.

It is worth understanding how chemical changes occur, why life's molecules are stable in the cytoplasm, and how life controls its chemical reactions, turning them on or off. Consider Figure 3.

This famous diagram appears in all biochemistry books. It is a schematic representation of a reaction. Consider this reaction A + B → C + D, where A and B are reactants and C and D are products. In the diagram and the equation, the reaction begins on the left and moves to the right. The vertical scale is energy. Don't worry about the technical details. Begin with the upper solid black line with the label *Reaction Energy Barrier without an Enzyme.* For this reaction, the molecules A and B must assemble sufficient energy to carry them over the hill. This energy may come from the incessant thermal collisions, from some other molecule's internal energy, from an incoming photon of electromagnetic radiation, or other sources. The total energy of the entire system, including the surroundings, is a constant.

Through the continual random exchange of energy between the molecules A and B and their surroundings, if A and B happen to meet when they have sufficient energy to

make it over the top of the hill, then they will react, forming C and D. These products appear on the diagram's right.

This diagram is illustrative. The actual diagram of even a simple reaction might have several dimensions in place of the single horizontal axis. The hills would be complicated surfaces with mountains and valleys. The diagram would have to take into account factors such as the orientation of the reactant molecules, and much else. It is the case, however, that all of life's stable molecules live in a well—a valley—similar to the left side of the diagram. They will require an injection of energy from their surroundings to escape. Biological molecules have many possible reactions in which they might take part. Remove an atom and replace it with another. Switch any molecular piece with another molecular piece. Natural selection has designed all of the molecules of life so that they are stable in chemical composition, form, and function. High activation energy barriers in all directions make all possible reactions rare. If this were not the case, then the molecules of life would not be stable.

When life requires a particular reaction to take place, there will be an enzyme to facilitate it. An enzyme is a biological catalyst. Consider the lower dashed line in Figure 3. This line has the label *Reaction Energy Barrier with an Enzyme.* This depicts the same reaction A + B → C + D, but this time there is an enzyme to facilitate the reaction.

Figure 3

The symbol E_a is the activation energy, the amount of energy the reactants must have to react. This energy is available to the products on the right. The reactants collect energy E_a from their surroundings. The products have returned it and a little extra ΔE to the surroundings. The surroundings, in this case, are warmer than before the reaction.

Reaction energy barrier with and without an enzyme

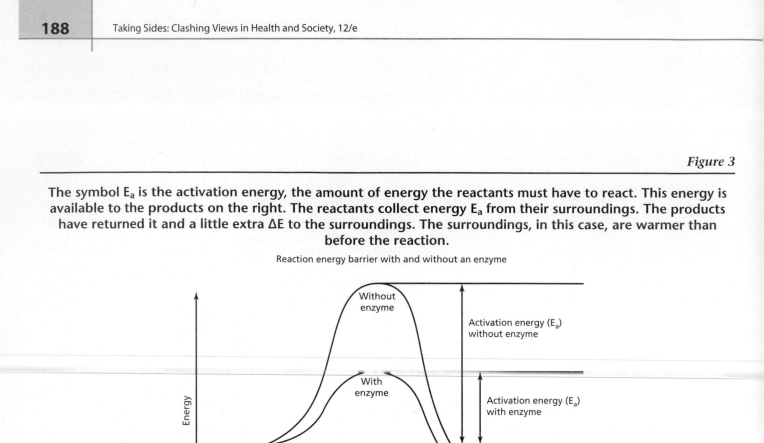

Without going into the remarkable details of enzymatic function, we can say that the enzyme has the effect of lowering the activation energy barrier for the reaction. With lower activation energy, the thermal jostling or other sources of reaction energy have a much easier time pushing the reactants over the hill. The reaction rate goes from nearly zero to some reasonable value.

There are no enzymes for unwanted reactions. Enzymes have and maintain the proper constitution and form to work correctly. For a mutation to occur or an enzyme to change, the energy for the chemical reaction must come from some place. An X-ray photon—from a cosmic ray, from the earth's radioactivity, or from an X-ray machine—may provide the required energy. Photons from any other form of electromagnetic radiation cannot.

Glance at Figure 1 again. All of those chemical bonds across the middle of the diagram are stable. They do not break and reform, unless there is an enzyme to do it. On the left of the diagram is the graph showing the energy available from ordinary thermal motions to break these bonds. Also on the left is a bracket showing the range of typical activation energies. Thermal motions are insufficient to take molecules over the activation energy barrier for any

reaction. Far to the right, however, you can see the photons of ultraviolet light, X-rays, and gamma rays. These photons may break bonds. They may cause mutations directly. They may damage individual enzyme molecules. Even green visible light photons in the middle of this range do not have enough energy to break bonds and take molecules over any activation energy barrier.

Now find the photons of cell phone radiation and of AC power. They are at the far left of this diagram. No photon from a cell phone can ever break a chemical bond. Making the radiation more intense does not make the photons stronger. It just means that there are more of them. The photons cannot gang up. Lots of them cannot do what one of them cannot.

When those weak photons disappear into a molecule, the molecule shifts and quivers a tiny bit. Its energy is a bit larger and the photon is gone. The molecule adjusts itself to its new slightly higher energy, and in subsequent collisions with its neighbors, it may transfer some of that energy to them. The temperature of the biological soup—the cytoplasm—is then a bit higher. The amount of heating due to cell phone radiation is small compared to your microwave, or standing in the sunshine, or wearing a scarf around your neck. This small increase in temperature does not cause cancer.

If cell phone photons or AC power photons, far to the left of Figure 1, were able to cause cancer by any mechanism, known or unknown, then those thermal vibrations also shown to the left side of the diagram would also cause cancer. So would all the forms of electromagnetic radiation that have more energetic photons than cell phone radiation.

Some of the concern over cell phone radiation may have originated from the normal statistical fluctuations that occur when studies are conducted. In recent years, epidemiologists have found significant environmental hazards, such as smoking and asbestos. They are now searching for hazards among much weaker effects. Some studies of a supposed hazard will show a small risk. Other studies of the same hazard will show no risk. In fact, some studies of the same potential hazard will show a benefit. This is the sign that there is no hazard, only statistical fluctuations. But only the studies that suggest risks, even small risks, will make news.

We can all be confident that any epidemiological study that purports to show that cell phone radiation causes any cancer must have at least one mistake. We can be certain because there is no plausible—or even implausible—mechanism by which cell phone radiation can cause any cancer.

When asked for a physicist's advice about cell phone safety, I explain that the radiation cannot cause cancer by any mechanism, known or unknown. If I am further pressed for comment I respond, "don't text while you drive, and don't eat your cell phone."

Acknowledgment: I thank physicists Dr. Arthur West and Dr. Craig Bohren, and biochemists Dr. Joseph H. Guth and Dr. Jill Ferguson, for their careful review of this paper and for their suggestions.

Bernard Leikind is a physicist and board member of *Skeptic* magazine.

EXPLORING THE ISSUE

Do Cell Phones Cause Cancer?

Critical Thinking and Reflection

1. Why do you think so many studies investigating health risks of cell phones are inconclusive and contradictory?
2. Describe some of the reasons researchers believe cell phone pose a risk.
3. What are health concerns related to cell phone use other than cancer?
4. Describe the type of radiation used by cell phones.

Is There Common Ground?

In May 2010, the largest cell phone cancer study, the Interphone Study, conducted by the World Health Organization, proved to be inconclusive (*International Journal of Epidemiology*, May 2010). Over 6,000 people with brain tumors and a similar number of healthy people were asked about their cell phone usage. The hypothesis was that cell phones increase the risk of brain tumors and there would be greater use in the cancer group compared with the healthy population. The study found the opposite to be true initially. However, when the researchers contacted healthy people who declined to take part in the initial investigation, they found that these individuals were less likely to regularly use cell phones than the healthy people who took part in the study. This indicates that the "benefit" that cell phones seemed to offer could be based on an over-representation of individuals who were healthy and regular mobile phone users. It might also mean that any negative effects might have been hidden. The researchers then compared frequent mobile phone users with infrequent ones and found that the level of use seemed to increase the risk of two different types of brain tumors by 40 and 15 percent, respectively.

While the results of the study are intriguing, they are certainly not conclusive. The study relied on people's memories regarding their cell phone use. It may be that people with brain tumors tend to have different memories of cell usage than those who are healthy. Several other studies are in progress, and the final verdict is not yet out. In "Jury Still Out on Cell Phone-Cancer Connection" (*Cancer*, January 5, 2010), author Michael Thun indicates that further research is needed. Since cell phones are a fairly recent phenomenon, it may be several years before any conclusive evidence surfaces relative to their safety.

Additional Resources

Anderson, S. (2011). Are cell phones safe until the FCC tells us they are not? A preemption analysis in the context of cell phone radiation emissions standards. *Journal of Technology Law & Policy, 16*(2), 307–341.

Boice, J. D., & Tarone, R. E. (2011). Cell phones, cancer, and children. *JNCI: Journal of the National Cancer Institute, 103*(16), 1211–1213.

De Vocht, F. (2014). The case of acoustic neuroma: Comment on: Mobile phone use and risk of brain neoplasms and other cancers. *International Journal of Epidemiology, 43*(1), 273–274.

Gultekin, D. H., & Moeller, L. (2013). NMR imaging of cell phone radiation absorption in brain tissue. *Proceedings of the National Academy of Sciences of the United States of America, 110*(1), 58–63.

Holland, C., & Rathod, V. (2013). Influence of personal mobile phone ringing and usual intention to answer on driver error. *Accident Analysis & Prevention, 50*, 793–800.

Internet References . . .

American Cancer Society—Cell Phones and Cancer

www.cancer.org/Cancer/CancerCauses
/OtherCarcinogens/AtHome/cellular-phones

Environmental Protection Agency

www.epa.gov

Federal Communications Commission (FCC)

www.fcc.gov/

Selected, Edited, and with Issue Framing Material by:
Eileen L. Daniel, *SUNY College at Brockport*

ISSUE

Will Hydraulic Fracturing (Fracking) Negatively Affect Human Health and the Environment?

YES: John Rumpler, from "Fracking: Pro and Con," *Tufts Now* (2013)

NO: Bruce McKenzie Everett, from "Fracking: Pro and Con," *Tufts Now* (2013)

Learning Outcomes

After reading this issue, you will be able to:

- Understand the environmental impact of fracking.
- Discuss the health concerns of fracking.
- Discuss the impact that fracking has on the economy and oil dependence.

ISSUE SUMMARY

YES: Environmentalist and senior attorney for Environment America John Rumpler argues that fracking is not worth the damage to health and the environment.

NO: Energy researcher and Adjunct Professor Bruce McKenzie Everett claims fracking provides substantial economic benefits and its health and environmental problems are relatively small.

Hydraulic fracturing, or fracking, is a process that extracts natural gas from rock beneath the earth's surface. Many rocks such as shale, sandstones, and limestone deep in the ground contain natural gas, which was formed as dead organisms in the rock decomposed. This gas can be released and captured at the surface for energy use, when the rocks in which it is trapped are drilled. To enhance the flow of released gas, the rocks are broken apart, or fractured. In the past, drillers often detonated small explosions in the wells to increase flow. Starting about 70 years ago, oil and gas drilling companies began fracking rock by pumping pressurized water into it.

Since the 1940s, about 1 million American wells have been fracked. The majority of these are vertical wells that tap into porous sandstone or limestone. During the past 20 years, however, energy companies have had the ability to capture the gas still stuck in the original shale source.

Fracking shale is achieved by drilling level wells that expand from their vertical well shafts along thin, horizontal shale layers. Drilling of this nature has allowed engineers to insert millions of gallons of high-pressure water directly into layers of shale to generate the fractures that release the gas. Chemicals added to the water dissolve minerals, destroy bacteria that might block the well, and add sand to hold open the fractures.

While the process offers inexpensive energy options, there are many opponents of the process. The majority of these opponents concentrate on possible local environmental outcomes. Some of these consequences are specific to the more recent fracking technology, while others are more relevant to the overall processes of natural gas extraction. The mixture of chemicals used in fracking processes includes acids, detergents, and toxins that are not controlled by federal laws but can cause problems if they leak into drinking water. Since the 1990s, the fracking process has employed increased amounts of chemical-laden water, injected at higher pressures. This causes the escape of methane gas into the environment out of gas wells, producing the real, though slight, chance of hazardous explosions. In general, water from all gas wells often returns to the surface containing very low but measurable concentrations of radioactive elements and large salt concentration. Salts or brine can be harmful if not treated properly. Small earthquakes have been triggered in rare instances after the introduction of brine into deep wells.

Along with these regional consequences, natural gas extraction has worldwide environmental impacts, because both the methane gas that is retrieved through extraction and the carbon dioxide liberated during methane burning are greenhouse gases that add to global climate change. Recent fracking technologies foster the extraction of higher quantities of gas, which adds more to climate change than former natural gas extraction processes.

In Pennsylvania, there has been rapid development of the Marcellus Shale, a geological formation that could contain nearly 500 trillion cubic feet of gas. This amount of natural gas is considered enough to power all U.S. residences for 50 years at current rates of usage. The experience in Pennsylvania with water and soil contamination, however, is of concern. Shale gas in Pennsylvania is accessed at depths of thousands of feet, while water for drinking is removed from depths of only hundreds of feet. Nowhere in the state have fracking chemicals injected at depth been shown to contaminate drinking water. In a research study of 200 private drinking water wells in Pennsylvania fracking regions, water quality was the same before and shortly after drilling in all wells except one. Unfortunately, however, trucking and storage accidents have spilled fracking chemicals and brines, leading to contamination of water and soils that required decontamination. Also, many gas companies do not consistently reveal the composition of all fracking and drilling compounds, which makes it challenging to check for injected chemicals in surface and groundwater.

Instances of methane leaking into aquifers in regions where shale-gas drilling is ongoing have also occurred in Pennsylvania. A portion of this gas is "drift gas" that forms naturally in deposits left behind by the most recent glaciers. But occasionally methane seeps out of gas wells because linings are not structurally sound, which occurs in about 1–2 percent of the wells. The linings can be repaired to address these slight leaks, and the risk of such methane leaks could further decrease if linings were designed specifically for each geological area.

The disposal of shale gas salt/brine was originally addressed in Pennsylvania by permitting the gas industry to use municipal water treatment plants that were not equipped to manage the toxic substances. In 2011 new regulations were enacted and Pennsylvania energy companies now recycle 90 percent of the salty water by using it to frack more shale.

Overall, the experience of fracking in Pennsylvania has led to industry changes that alleviate the impact of drilling and fracking on the local environment. Though the natural gas produced by fracking does increase greenhouse gases in the atmosphere through leakage during gas extraction and carbon dioxide emitted during burning, it does hold an important environmental benefit over coal mining. Gases released from shale contain 50 percent of the carbon dioxide per unit of energy as does coal, and coal burning also releases metals such as mercury into the atmosphere that ultimately settle back into water and soil.

In Europe, there is currently an increase in reliance on coal while discouraging or restricting fracking. If Americans are going to get our energy needs mostly from fossil fuels, banning fracking while mining and burning coal appears to be a negative environmental trade-off. The question is: Should Europe and the United States support fracking or prohibit it? Many regional effects of fracking and drilling have received a lot of press but actually generated a small amount of problems, while others are more serious. Economic interests in the short term favor fracking. The Pennsylvania experience caused natural gas prices to fall and jobs were created both directly in the gas industry and indirectly as local and national economies benefit from reduced energy costs. If, however, fracked gas shifts efforts to develop cleaner energy sources without decreasing reliance on coal, the consequences of accelerated global climate change will occur.

Overall, there are both advantages and disadvantages to hydraulic fracturing. The environmental impact could be lessened as well as the risk to human health via water contamination and the increase in greenhouse gases by utilizing lessons learned from Pennsylvania. In the YES and NO selections, John Rumpler argues that we are making a mistake in thinking that fracking is worth the damage to the environment. Bruce McKenzie Everett disagrees and claims that fracking offers substantial economic benefits and its problems are relatively minor compared to the advantages.

YES ↵

John Rumpler

Fracking: Pro and Con

For some Americans, it is our energy dreams come true. To others, it is an environmental nightmare. Ever since a new drilling technology, called hydraulic fracturing or fracking, made it possible to extract natural gas from shale deposits about a mile underground, a new gold rush has been under way.

While fracking has created jobs and contributed to record-low natural gas prices, it comes with another kind of potential cost: risks to our environment and health that some say are far too high.

The fracking process begins with a bore hole drilled some 6,000 feet below ground, cutting through many geological layers and aquifers, which tend to be no more than a few hundred feet below the surface. The shaft is then lined with steel and cement casing. Monitors above ground signal when drilling should shift horizontally, boring sideways to pierce long running sections of shale bedrock.

Millions of gallons of water mixed with sand and chemicals are then blasted into the bedrock, the pressure creating cracks that release trapped natural gas from the shale. The gas and water mixture then flows back up to the surface, where the gas is separated from the water. While most of the water stays in the well bore, up to 20 percent is either reused for more fracking or injected into disposal wells thousands of feet underground.

The wellpad and related infrastructure take up to eight to nine acres of land, according to the Nature Conservancy. Fracking is currently occurring in Texas and Pennsylvania, the two largest gas-producing states, as well as in North Dakota, Arkansas, California, Colorado and New Mexico. And the oil and gas industry is eager to expand its fracking operations into New York, North Carolina, Maryland and Illinois. . . .

John Rumpler . . . argues that we are making a mistake in thinking that fracking is worth the damage to the environment. He is a senior attorney at Environment America, which is leading a national effort to restrict, regulate and ultimately end the practice of fracking. He has fought for clean air in Ohio and advocated to protect the Great Lakes and the Chesapeake Bay. This fall he is teaching the Experimental College course Fracked Out: Understanding the New Gas Rush.

Tufts Now: Is Fracking Safe?

John Rumpler: Fracking presents a staggering array of threats to our environment and our health. These range from contaminating drinking water and making families living near well sites sick to turning pristine landscapes into industrial wastelands. There are air pollution problems and earthquakes from the deep-well injections of the wastewater into the gas-producing shale, as well as significant global warming emissions.

When the industry says there has not been a single case of groundwater contamination, they mean there is not a verified instance of the fracking fluid traveling up through a mile of bedrock into the water table. What they cannot dispute is that fluid and chemicals have leached into groundwater at 421 fracking waste pits in New Mexico. What they cannot dispute is that a peer-reviewed study by Duke University linked methane in people's drinking water wells to gas-drilling operations in surrounding areas. What they cannot dispute is a University of Colorado study published earlier this year documenting that people living within a half mile of fracking and other gas-drilling operations have an increased risk of health problems, including cancer from benzene emissions.

Are There Sufficient Regulations Now in Place to Ensure Safety?

Rumpler: Is it conceivable to imagine regulatory fixes for all the various problems caused by fracking? Theoretically, perhaps. But imagine trying to implement the hundreds of different rules and regulations at thousands of oil- and gas-drilling sites across the country, and you realize there is no practical likelihood that fracking will ever be made safe.

And there are consequences that we don't even know how to regulate yet. Geologists are just beginning to think about the long-term implications of drilling down a mile and then drilling horizontally through shale rock for another mile. We don't know what happens to the structural integrity of that bedrock once you withdraw all of the gas and liquid from it. No one has the definitive answer. There's been some recent modeling that indicates a loss of stability that goes all the way up to the water table. The U.S. Geological Survey took a look at some earthquakes that occurred in the vicinity of Youngstown, Ohio, in proximity to deep-well fracking. They found that the seismic activity was most certainly manmade—and there was no manmade activity in the area except fracking.

So when you look at the whole picture—from contaminated wells to health problems to earthquakes—[you quickly come] to see that the best defense against fracking is no fracking at all.

As for the current state of regulations, it is worth noting that fracking is exempt from key provisions of our nation's environmental laws, including the Safe Drinking Water Act, the Clean Air Act, the Clean Water Act, and the Resource Conservation Recovery Act. The reason we have national environmental laws is to prevent states from "racing to the bottom of the barrel" to appease powerful industries. . . .

What Are the Economic Benefits of Fracking?

. . .

Rumpler: First of all, any discussion of economics needs to deal with costs as well as benefits. This fall, our *Costs of Fracking* report detailed the dollars drained by dirty drilling—from property damage to health-care costs to roads ruined by heavy machinery. In Pennsylvania's last extractive boom, the state was stuck with a $5 billion bill to clean up pollution from abandoned mines. What happens when the fracking boom is long gone and communities are stuck with the bill?

In contrast, energy efficiency, wind and solar all provide great economic benefits with no hidden costs. But the oversupply of cheap gas is driving wind and solar out of the market. It's long been fashionable to say that natural gas can be a bridge to clean energy, but in fact it's become a wall to clean energy, because investors don't want to put money into wind and solar when gas is so cheap.

What Danger to the Environment or the Economy Is Caused by the Billions of Gallons of Fresh Water Each Year That Are "Consumed" by Fracking Operations? How Might This Affect the Economic Benefits or Environmental Concerns?

. . .

Rumpler: Each fracking well uses millions of gallons of water. And that water mostly winds up either staying down in the well or being injected deep into the earth as wastewater. So unlike other sectors that use much more water by volume, including agriculture and residential, the water used for fracking is mostly consumed, gone to us for ever.

Does the Current Low Price of Natural Gas Affect Fracking or Conventional Gas Production?

Rumpler: Take a look at Chesapeake Energy, which is one of the biggest fracking operators out there. By the accounts of some analysts, they are massively overextended, with too much land and too many drilling leases. With the price at $2 per million BTU, there was some risk that Chesapeake could at some point lose enough money to risk bankruptcy—and then what would happen to these communities where fracking has taken place? If not Chesapeake, it will be another driller—probably one of the smaller ones—that goes under, and the communities will be left holding the bag. And gas companies don't tell landowners leasing property that oil and gas operations are violations of most standard mortgage agreements, because that is not a risk that the lender is willing to take. Likewise, homeowners' insurance may not cover damages from fracking. Nationwide insurance announced just this summer that their standard policy does not cover damage from fracking. That tells you something. The risk analysts who did the math figured out this is not a safety winner for them. . . .

What If We Halted All Fracking Right Now?

. . .

Rumpler: There's a difference between not starting fracking in new areas and halting it everywhere immediately. If we don't open new places to fracking in New York, Pennsylvania and Texas—just stop where we are now—the impact would be minimal. As Bruce notes, there is so much gas being produced right now that some gas companies are aggressively seeking export licenses, because they want to get rid of the excess and earn a profit. We don't need it to fill energy needs.

In North Dakota they are flaring off the gas, just wasting it into the air. If we need this gas to meet our energy needs, then they should make gas flaring a federal crime and should immediately ban any and all exports of natural gas. The industry would fight tooth and nail against this.

Until we know more, the risks to our health and environment far outweigh any possible benefit to our economy or energy future.

JOHN RUMPLER is an environmentalist and attorney.

Bruce McKenzie Everett 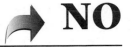 **NO**

Fracking: Pro and Con

For some Americans, it is our energy dreams come true. To others, it is an environmental nightmare. Ever since a new drilling technology, called hydraulic fracturing or fracking, made it possible to extract natural gas from shale deposits about a mile underground, a new gold rush has been under way.

The fracking process begins with a bore hole drilled some 6,000 feet below ground, cutting through many geological layers and aquifers, which tend to be no more than a few hundred feet below the surface. The shaft is then lined with steel and cement casing. Monitors above ground signal when drilling should shift horizontally, boring sideways to pierce long running sections of shale bedrock.

Millions of gallons of water mixed with sand and chemicals are then blasted into the bedrock, the pressure creating cracks that release trapped natural gas from the shale. The gas and water mixture then flows back up to the surface, where the gas is separated from the water. While most of the water stays in the well bore, up to 20 percent is either reused for more fracking or injected into disposal wells thousands of feet underground. . . .

Bruce McKenzie Everett, F70, F72, F80, an adjunct associate professor of international business at the Fletcher School, says fracking provides substantial economic benefits and its problems are relatively small compared to those benefits. He worked at the U.S. Department of Energy from 1974 to 1980 before beginning a 20-year career with ExxonMobil, working in Hong Kong, the Middle East, Africa and Latin America. His research has included gas-to-liquid conversion technology as well as the economics of oil, gas and coal production and use. . . .

Tufts Now: Is Fracking Safe?

Bruce McKenzie Everett: Nothing in the world is entirely safe, but by the standards of industrial activity in the United States, fracking is very, very safe. Think about the airline industry. Lots of things can go wrong with airplanes, but we work very hard to make sure they don't,

and as a result, flying is one of the safest activities we've got. Now, that does not mean that things can't happen. It just means that with proper attention, mistakes can be kept to an extremely low level.

The question about fracking that gets the most attention is contamination of drinking water. Aquifers, the underground rivers that provide our drinking water, are about 100 to 200 feet below the surface. The gas-producing shale rock formations tend to be 5,000 to 6,000 feet below the surface. So you need to make sure that the well you drill to pump the water and chemicals through the shale to fracture it and release the gas is sealed properly, and that's not a hard thing to do. . . .

Are There Sufficient Regulations Now in Place to Ensure Safety?

. . .

Everett: There are a lot of regulations currently in place. The question is whether they should be done at the federal or state level. For example, the state government of Pennsylvania understood that the economic activity from fracking could be very, very positive for the state. So they worked with the fracking industry and enacted numerous regulations to try to make sure that two things happened: that they eliminated the dangers to the extent that you can, but that they allowed fracking sites to go forward because the jobs and tax revenue were so positive.

In New York State, they've put a moratorium on fracking, basically saying, "I don't know what to do, so I'll study it and see what happens." I think that's unfortunate, because most of New York is quite economically depressed, and they are denying people economic opportunities.

I have taken a very strong position that it's a bad idea to federalize regulations. If you leave it at the state level, local governments will tend to strike a balance between the economic benefits and the environmental safety issues. If it is left to the federal government, you'll have the same problem you had with the Keystone oil pipeline: people who are not impacted, who will not enjoy the economic benefits, will be allowed to come in and say they don't like it.

What Are the Economic Benefits of Fracking?

Everett: It creates jobs, but that's not the most important way to measure its economic effect. The cost of everything we purchase has an energy component to it, either in its manufacture or its shipping or its packaging. So it is very important to the economy to have energy prices that are relatively low.

Natural gas has become incredibly inexpensive, way beyond what we ever thought possible. We're talking about prices going from $10 or $11 per thousand cubic feet 10 years ago down to $3.77 now, because the supply that has been released by this innovative fracking production technique is just so large. It is a simple consequence of supply and demand. These natural gas prices are the equivalent of oil prices falling to $21 per barrel from their current $86 per-barrel price. . . .

What Danger to the Environment or the Economy Is Caused by the Billions of Gallons of Fresh Water Each Year That Are "Consumed" By Fracking Operations? How Might This Affect the Economic Benefits or Environmental Concerns?

Everett: The water from fracking can be handled in one of several ways: storing, reinjecting and recycling. The real problem we have is that water is not properly priced. As a landowner, you are entitled to draw water from underground aquifers at whatever rate you wish, even if that water is only flowing through your land. We therefore tend to treat water as a free good. Putting a price on it or, alternatively, finding a way to assign property rights would probably fix this problem. As a third alternative, government could regulate it. In any case, it's a solvable problem. . . .

Does the Current Low Price of Natural Gas Affect Fracking or Conventional Gas Production?

. . .

Everett: The price of natural gas has now gotten so low that some are saying they can't produce it economically— but this is a *good* thing for all of us, because it will force

them to explore new markets and uses. The United States has an open economy and is a large global trading player. Americans pay the global price for the many things we buy and sell, and energy is one. There are several directions that natural gas production, both fracking and conventional, can take.

One is that people just stop producing it at the current rates, and the price returns to a more stable level and just stays there, likely at the $10-to-$12-dollar level of a decade ago. We could also start exporting. The world price for natural gas is $15 to $16 per thousand cubic feet. By selling it on the global market, that money would come into the U.S. economy. It would require some expensive infrastructure to support it, but the profit margin is so huge, some $12 per thousand cubic feet, that it would be well worth it and a positive impact on our economy.

We could also begin to shut down older coal-fired power plants and replace them with cleaner natural gas plants, and natural gas could find its way into the transportation sector. With engine modifications, it could be used as fuel for cars, or it could be used to produce the battery power for electric cars.

What If We Halted All Fracking Right Now?

Everett: If we stopped right now, or placed a moratorium on new fracking, the price of natural gas would go up to the previous $10 to $11, or worse case, to the global price of $15 to $16. This means electricity prices would go up, heating prices would go up, and we'd lose the economic activity the industry is generating through jobs and lower prices. Basically we would be giving up an opportunity.

Hazards can be controlled through solid regulations that include monitoring and quick responses to problems that arise. Any risks are outweighed by economic benefits. It's not even a close call. . . .

Bruce McKenzie Everett is an energy researcher and adjunct professor.

EXPLORING THE ISSUE

Will Hydraulic Fracturing (Fracking) Negatively Affect Human Health and the Environment?

Critical Thinking and Reflection

1. What are the major economic advantages to fracking?
2. What impact will fracking have on the quality of drinking water?
3. What effect will increased fracking have on the incentive to develop other cleaner energy sources including renewable?
4. What are the health implications of fracking?

Is There Common Ground?

In the spring of 2008, filmmaker Josh Fox received an offer from a natural gas company to lease his family's land in Milanville, Pennsylvania, for $100,000 to drill for gas. Fox then set out to see how communities are being affected in the West where a natural gas drilling boom has been underway for the last 10 years. He spent time with people in their homes and on their land as they relayed their stories of natural gas drilling in Colorado, Wyoming, Utah, and Texas. Fox spoke with residents who experienced a variety of chronic health problems they claim were directly traceable to contamination of their air, of their water wells, or of surface water. In some cases, the residents report that they obtained a court injunction or settlement monies from gas companies to replace the affected water supplies with drinkable water.

The result of Fox's research was the documentary film *Gasland*. During the making of the film, Fox connected with scientists, politicians, and gas industry executives and ultimately found himself in Washington as a subcommittee was discussing the Fracturing Responsibility and Awareness of Chemicals Act, a proposed exemption for hydraulic fracturing from the Safe Drinking Water Act. While the film has both supporters and critics, it did bring publicity to the issues surrounding fracking and raised the question: Is the process safe for the environment and human health and do the economic benefits outweigh any actual or potential problems?

As the United States and Europe seek ways to reduce energy costs and reliance on imported fuels, fracking may be an opportunity to achieve these goals. It's a domestic resource that can be extracted around the country and offers jobs and cheaper energy. On the other hand, there are concerns that the fracking processes needed to extract gas may contaminate ground and surface water with toxic chemicals that could impact health and the environment.

Additional Resources

Arnowitt, M. (2012). Pennsylvania's fracking land grab: Threats and opportunities. *Journal of Appalachian Studies, 18*(1/2), 44–47.

Grealy, N. (2013). Fracking is one of the best things to happen to onshore gas exploration for a century. *Engineering & Technology (17509637), 8*(1), 24.

Herman, A. (2015). The liberal war on American energy independence. *Commentary*, 17–24.

Ratcliffe, I. (2013). Fracking is dangerous to environment and throws good energy after bad. *Engineering & Technology (17509637), 8*(1), 25.

Weinhold, B. (2012). The future of fracking. *Environmental Health Perspectives, 120*(7), A272–A279.

Internet References . . .

Environmental Protection Agency

www.epa.gov

Natural Gas.org

www.naturalgas.org

Hydraulic Fracturing—AmericanRivers.org

www.americanrivers.org/fracking

Selected, Edited, and with Issue Framing Material by:
Eileen L. Daniel, *SUNY College at Brockport*

ISSUE

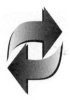

Is There a Valid Link Between Saturated Fat and Heart Disease?

YES: **Henry Blackburn**, from "In Defense of U Research: The Ancel Keys Legacy," *startribune.com* (2014)

NO: **Jon White**, from "Fat or Fiction?" *New Scientist* (2014)

Learning Outcomes

After reading this issue, you will be able to:

- Understand the different types of fat in the diet.
- Discuss the relationship between saturated fat and heart disease researched by Dr. Ancel Keys and his team.
- Understand the possible link between refined carbohydrates and heart disease.

ISSUE SUMMARY

YES: Professor emeritus and researcher Henry Blackburn contends that valid research by Dr. Ancel Keys and his team established a strong link between saturated fat and heart disease.

NO: Opinion editor at *New Scientist* magazine Jon White argues that the science behind the saturated fat–heart disease link was flawed and that carbohydrates, not fats, are the real culprits.

Eating foods that contain saturated fats has long been thought to raise the blood levels of cholesterol, a risk factor for heart disease and stroke. From a chemical standpoint, saturated fats are fat molecules that have no double bonds between carbon molecules because they are saturated with hydrogen molecules. Saturated fats are typically solid at room temperature and occur naturally in many foods. The majority are found in animal products such as beef, lamb, pork, butter, cheese, and other dairy products which contain fat. In addition, many baked goods and fried foods can contain high levels of saturated fats from plant-based oils such as palm oil, palm kernel oil, and coconut oil. Most mainstream organizations including the American Heart Association maintain that eating these foods that contain saturated fats raises the level of serum cholesterol, a risk for cardiovascular disease (CVD).

However, recent research published in respectable medical journals seems to contradict the advice to eat less saturated fat and replace it with unsaturated oils. A 2014 article published in the *Annals of Internal Medicine* concluded that "Current evidence does not clearly support cardiovascular guidelines that encourage high consumption of polyunsaturated fatty acids and low consumption of total saturated fats." Consumers have long been warned of the link between saturated fat and heart disease. But this large and exhaustive new analysis by a team of international scientists found no evidence that eating saturated fat increased heart attacks and other cardiac events. The new findings are part of a growing body of research that has challenged the accepted wisdom that saturated fat is inherently bad for you and will continue the debate about what foods are best to eat. But the new research did not find that individuals who ate higher levels of saturated fat had more heart disease than those who ate less. Nor did it find less disease in those eating higher amounts of unsaturated fat, including monounsaturated fat such as olive oil or corn oil or other polyunsaturated fats.

Scientists claim that looking at individual fats and other nutrient groups in isolation could be misleading, because when people cut down on fats they tend to eat more bread, cold cereal, and other refined carbohydrates that can also be bad for cardiovascular health. Consumers would likely be better off to eat foods that are typical of the Mediterranean diet, like nuts, fish, avocado, high-fiber grains, and olive oil. A recent study showed that a Mediterranean diet with more nuts and extra virgin olive oil reduced heart attacks and strokes when compared with a lower fat diet with more starches.

In the new research, researchers reviewed and evaluated the most relevant evidence to date from 80 studies involving more than a half million people. They looked not only at what people reportedly ate, but also at the composition of fatty acids in their bloodstreams and in their fat tissue. The scientists also reviewed evidence from 27 randomized controlled trials—the gold standard in scientific research—that assessed whether taking polyunsaturated fat supplements such as fish oil promoted heart health. They did determine there was a link between trans fats, partially hydrogenated oils that had long been added to processed foods, and heart disease. But they found no evidence of dangers from saturated fat, or benefits from other kinds of fats.

The primary reason saturated fat has historically had a bad reputation is that it increases low-density lipoprotein cholesterol, or LDL, which raises the risk for heart attacks. But the relationship between saturated fat and LDL is complex. In addition to raising LDL cholesterol, saturated fat also increases high-density lipoprotein, or HDL, the so-called good cholesterol. And the LDL that it raises is a subtype of big, fluffy particles that are generally benign. Doctors refer to a preponderance of these particles as LDL pattern A. The smallest and densest form of LDL is more dangerous. These particles are easily oxidized and are more likely to set off inflammation and contribute to the buildup of artery-narrowing plaque. An LDL profile that consists mostly of these particles, known as pattern B, usually coincides with high triglycerides and low levels of HDL, both risk factors for heart attacks and stroke. The smaller, more artery-clogging particles are increased not by saturated fat, but by sugary foods and an excess of carbohydrates. It appears that a high carbohydrate or sugary diet should be the focus of dietary guidelines.

Although the new research showed no relationship overall between saturated or polyunsaturated fat intake and cardiac events, there are numerous unique fatty acids within these two groups, and there was some indication that they are not all equal. When the researchers looked at fatty acids in the bloodstream, for example, they found that a type of saturated fat found in milk and dairy products was associated with lower cardiovascular risk. Two types of polyunsaturated fats found in fish also appeared protective. But a number of fatty acids commonly found in vegetable oils and processed foods may pose risks, the findings suggested.

The researchers then looked at data from the randomized trials to see if taking supplements like fish oil produced any cardiovascular benefits. It did not. An explanation for this discrepancy might be that the studies involved people who had preexisting heart disease or were at high risk of developing it, while the other studies involved generally healthy populations. So it is possible that the benefits of eating fish or taking fish oils lie in preventing heart disease, rather than treating or reversing it. At least two large clinical trials designed to see if this is the case are currently underway.

While the evidence against restricting saturated fats seems clear, Professor Walter Willett, chair of the Department of Nutrition at Harvard School of Public Health, is concerned that the conclusions may be misleading. A recent World Health Organization (WHO) and Food and Agricultural Organization (FAO) expert consultation report concluded that "intake of saturated fatty acids is directly related to cardiovascular risk. The traditional target is to restrict the intake of saturated fatty acids to less than 10% of daily energy intake and less than 7% for high-risk groups." The Dietary Guidelines for Americans, 2010 produced by the United States Department of Agriculture (USDA) indicates that the human body makes more than enough saturated fats to meet its needs and does not require more from dietary sources. Higher levels of saturated fats are associated with higher levels of total cholesterol and low-density lipoprotein "bad" cholesterol and recommends reduced saturated fat intake. While many other organizations support this, others disagree. Gary Taubes, a science writer, states that "Dietary fat, whether saturated or not, is not a cause of obesity, heart disease, or any other chronic disease of civilization." Author and journalist Michael Pollan states, "The amount of saturated fat in the diet probably may have little if any bearing on the risk of heart disease, and evidence that increasing polyunsaturated fats in the diet will reduce risk is slim to nil."

YES ↵

Henry Blackburn

In Defense of U Research: The Ancel Keys Legacy

Recently, a number of writers identifying themselves as "health-science journalists" have been calling on Americans to "end the war on fat" as they promote a high-fat, low-carbohydrate diet ("Chocolate milk in the schools and other products of expert opinion," June 22). What's puzzling is that they draw attention to their arguments by using personal attacks on one of Minnesota's premier scientists, Ancel Keys.

Keys was a University of Minnesota physiologist who spent most of his career conducting wide-ranging studies on the relationship of lifestyle—especially the foods we eat—to heart disease. He worked at the university from the late 1930s until his death at age 100 in 2004, and he carried out classic experiments of diet effects on blood-cholesterol levels in the laboratory and of diet associations with heart attacks among cultures with contrasting traditional eating patterns. "Contrasting" is the operative word here.

Keys' most influential work is the Seven Countries Study. Begun in 1958 and still in progress, it compares diet, risk factors, and rates of heart attack and stroke among regions of Greece, Italy, the former Yugoslavia, the Netherlands, Finland, the United States and Japan. Some recent (nonscientist) interpreters of the study have accused Keys of "cherry-picking" the countries with "preconceived" ideas about what he would find. Demonstrating a lack of understanding of how scientists approach new questions, they suggest he should have chosen specific other countries or should have chosen his sites "randomly." Any savvy scientist at an early phase of questioning knows to look first not randomly but across wide variations of the cause under consideration, in this case diet.

Keys chose the study areas because of their apparent differences in traditional diet, between the extremes of the rice- and vegetable-based diets of Japanese farmers and fishermen and the fatty meat, cheese and butter lunches of Finnish loggers. Another criterion was the availability of collaborators who understood the cultures and could provide logistical support and access to communities.

After years of observations among these regions, Keys and colleagues found major, five- to tenfold differences in heart-attack rates in relation to diet, an association compatible with the hypothesis that diet influences heart-attack risk and one congruent with their findings in feeding experiments back home. They also showed that the lowest heart-attack rates and longest survival occurred in both Japan, with its low-fat diet, and Greece, where the diet was relatively high in fat, mostly from olive oil. Their common factor was not the amount of fat people ate but the type of fat, with both areas consuming very little saturated fat.

The critics also accuse Keys of suppressing evidence collected during the studies in Crete. They claim that he rejected the results of hundreds of individual diet questionnaires and that his characterization of the diet was inaccurate because it was based on a survey that took place during Lent. Both charges are false and misleading.

Keys determined early that occasional questionnaires about foods we eat were unreliable, useful only for detecting significant departures from a population's typical eating habits. Although individual questionnaires were recorded, the study did not rely on them for the regional comparisons. Instead, Keys collected actual foods eaten for a full week among randomly selected families and chemically analyzed their nutrient content in the standardized laboratory in Minnesota. Repeat food collections were scheduled in different seasons during different years to provide a valid estimate of the nutrients consumed by an entire population. Events such as religious holidays and crop failures have an effect on what people eat at a given time and are part of the bigger picture of a community's eating pattern. Avoiding variations in eating at different parts of the yearly cycle would have been the real "cherry-picking."

The eating pattern that came out of these international comparisons is being referred to by critics as "low-fat" or "extreme low-fat," even though it includes leaner meats and lower-fat dairy foods as well as many types of vegetable oils. In fact, only Keys' saturated-fat recommendation—less than 10 percent of calories—might be considered "low." In the popular cookbooks written with his wife, Margaret, Keys called the pattern "eating well" and, later, "eating well the Mediterranean way."

In the most bizarre accusation of all, several writers are laying the blame on Keys for our modern epidemics of obesity and diabetes. It all started in the 1950s, they say, with Keys' undue influence on the American Heart Association and the later U.S. government dietary guidelines. The idea that one person could hold such sway for years over these notoriously skeptical bodies strains credulity. It was the strength of the evidence, plus a pragmatic decision how best to reduce saturated-fat consumption, not Keys' "force of will," that inspired the dietary policies.

In the meantime, social and cultural changes already underway truly did set the nation on the path to obesity. Restaurants increased portion sizes and people consumed more calories. Suburbs were built without sidewalks, and schools installed pop machines and served fast food. The food industry, already expert at marketing high-fat packaged foods, saw a new marketing opportunity and developed companion product lines in which fats were replaced by sugar and other simple carbohydrates or substitutes—something Keys never advised nor supported. Industry and advertisers, not Keys, led shoppers to believe that these "reduced-fat" foods were the healthier choices.

In addition to finding—and exploiting for profit—a common villain in Keys, these writers use a number of devices to promote what Nina Teicholz, author of "The Big Fat Surprise," advocates as a return to "tallow and lard." Innuendo, distortions and accusations may be good for media attention and book sales, but they can do real damage—not only to the reputation of a pioneering researcher, but to public understanding of the scientific method and the evolving science of nutrition. It's time to end the war on Ancel Keys.

HENRY BLACKBURN is a physician and professor emeritus of epidemiology at the University of Minnesota School of Public Health.

Jon White

→ **NO**

Fat or Fiction?

Can decades of health warnings about steak, butter and cream really be wrong?

There's a famous scene in Woody Allen's film *Sleeper* in which two scientists in the year 2173 are discussing the dietary advice of the late 20th century.

"You mean there was no deep fat, no steak or cream pies or hot fudge?" asks one, incredulous. "Those were thought to be unhealthy," replies the other. "Precisely the opposite of what we now know to be true."

We're not quite in Woody Allen territory yet, but steak and cream pies are starting to look a lot less unhealthy than they once did. After 35 years as dietary gospel, the idea that saturated fat is bad for your heart appears to be melting away like a lump of butter in a hot pan.

So is it OK to eat more red meat and cheese? Will the current advice to limit saturated fat be overturned? If it is, how did we get it so wrong for so long?

The answers matter. According to the World Health Organization, cardiovascular disease is the world's leading cause of death, killing more than 17 million people annually, about a third of all deaths. It predicts that by 2030, 23 million will succumb each year. In the US, an estimated 81 million people are living with cardiovascular disease. The healthcare bill is a small fortune.

The idea that eating saturated fat—found in high levels in animal products such as meat and dairy—directly raises the risk of a heart attack has been a mainstay of nutrition science since the 1970s. Instead, we are urged to favour the "healthy" fats found in vegetable oils and foods such as fish, nuts and seeds.

In the US the official guidance for adults is that no more than 30 per cent of total calories should come from fat, and no more than 10 per cent from saturated fat. UK advice is roughly the same. That is by no means an unattainable target: an average man could eat a whole 12-inch pepperoni pizza and still have room for an ice cream before busting the limit. Nonetheless, adults in the UK and US manage to eat more saturated fat than recommended.

We used to eat even more. From the 1950s to the late 1970s, fat accounted for more than 40 per cent of dietary calories in the UK. It was a similar story in the US. But as warnings began to circulate, people trimmed back on foods such as butter and beef. The food industry responded, filling the shelves with low-fat cookies, cakes and spreads.

So the message got through, at least partially. Deaths from heart disease have gone down in Western nations. In the UK in 1961 more than half of all deaths were from coronary heart disease; in 2009 less than a third were. But medical treatment and prevention have improved so dramatically it's impossible to tell what role, if any, changes in diet played. And even though fat consumption has gone down, obesity and its associated diseases have not.

To appreciate how saturated fat in food affects our health we need to understand how it is handled by the body, and how it differs from other types of fat.

When you eat fat, it travels to the small intestine where it is broken down into its constituent parts—fatty acids and glycerol and absorbed into cells lining the gut. There they are packaged up with cholesterol and proteins and posted into the bloodstream. These small, spherical packages are called lipoproteins, and they are what allow water-insoluble fats and cholesterol (together known as lipids) to get to where they are needed.

The more fat you eat, the higher the levels of lipoprotein in your blood. And that, according to conventional wisdom, is where the health problems begin.

Good and Bad Cholesterol

Lipoproteins come in two main types, high density and low density. Low-density lipoproteins (LDLs) are often simply known as "bad cholesterol" despite the fact that they contain more than just cholesterol. LDLs are bad because they can stick to the insides of artery walls, resulting in deposits called plaques that narrow and harden the vessels, raising the risk that a blood clot could cause a blockage. Of all types of fat in the diet, saturated fats have been shown to raise bad cholesterol levels the most. (Consuming cholesterol has surprisingly little influence: the reason it has a bad name is that it is found in animal foods that also tend to be high in saturated fat.)

High-density lipoproteins (HDLs), or "good cholesterol," on the other hand, help guard against arterial plaques. Conventional wisdom has it that HDL is raised by eating foods rich in unsaturated fats or soluble fibre such as whole grains, fruits and vegetables. This, in a nutshell, is the lipid hypothesis, possibly the most influential idea in the history of human nutrition.

The hypothesis traces its origins back to the 1940s when a rising tide of heart attacks among middle-aged men was spreading alarm in the US. At the time this was explained as a consequence of ageing. But Ancel Keys, a physiologist at the University of Minnesota, had other ideas.

Keys noted that heart attacks were rare in some Mediterranean countries and in Japan, where people ate a diet lower in fat. Convinced that there was a causal link, he launched the pioneering Seven Countries Study in 1958. In all, he recruited 12,763 men aged 40 to 59 in the US, Finland, The Netherlands, Italy, Yugoslavia, Greece and Japan. The participants' diet and heart health were checked five and 10 years after enrolling.

Keys concluded that there was a correlation between saturated fat in food, raised levels of blood lipids and the risk of heart attacks and strokes. The lipid hypothesis was born.

The finding was supported by other research, notably the Framingham Heart Study, which tracked diet and heart health in a town in Massachusetts. In light of this research and the rising toll—by the 1980s nearly a million Americans a year were dying from heart attacks—health authorities decided to officially push for a reduction in fat, and saturated fat in particular. Official guidelines first appeared in 1980 in the US and 1991 in the UK, and have stood firm ever since.

Yet the voices of doubt have been growing for some time. In 2010, scientists pooled the results of 21 studies that had followed 348,000 people for many years. This meta-analysis found "no significant evidence" in support of the idea that saturated fat raises the risk of heart disease (*American Journal of Clinical Nutrition*, vol. 91, p. 535).

The doubters were given a further boost by another meta-analysis published in March (*Annals of Internal Medicine*, vol. 160, p. 398). It revisited the results of 72 studies involving 640,000 people in 18 countries.

To the surprise of many, it did not find backing for the existing dietary advice. "Current evidence does not clearly support guidelines that encourage high consumption of polyunsaturated fatty acids and low consumption of total saturated fats," it concluded. "Nutritional guidelines may require reappraisal."

In essence, the study found that people at the extreme ends of the spectrum—that is, those who ate the most or least saturated fat—had the same chance of developing heart disease. High consumption of unsaturated fat seemed to offer no protection.

The analysis has been strongly criticised for containing methodological errors and omitting studies that should have been included. But the authors stand by their general conclusions and say the paper has already had the intended effect of breaking the taboo around saturated fat.

Green Light

Outside of academia, its conclusion was greeted with gusto. Many commentators interpreted it as a green light to resume eating saturated fat. But is it? Did Keys really get it wrong? Or is there some other explanation for the conflict between his work and the many studies that supported it, and the two recent meta-analyses?

Even as Keys's research was starting to influence health advice, critics were pointing out flaws in it. One common complaint was that he cherry-picked data to support his hypothesis, ignoring countries such as France which had high-fat diets but low rates of heart disease. The strongest evidence in favour of a low-fat diet came from Crete, but it transpired that Keys had recorded some food intake data there during Lent, a time when Greek people traditionally avoid meat and cheese, so he may have underestimated their normal fat intake.

The Framingham research, too, has its detractors. Critics say that it followed an unrepresentative group of predominantly white men and women who were at high risk for heart disease for non-dietary reasons such as smoking.

More recently, it has also become clear that the impact of saturated fat is more complex than was understood back then.

Ronald Krauss of the University of California, San Francisco, has long researched the links between lipoprotein and heart disease. He was involved in the 2010 meta-analysis and is convinced there is room for at least a partial rethink of the lipid hypothesis.

He points to studies suggesting that not all LDL is the same, and that casting it all as bad was wrong. It is now widely accepted that LDL comes in two types—big, fluffy particles and smaller, compact ones. It is the latter, Krauss says, that are strongly linked to heart-disease risk, while the fluffy ones appear a lot less risky. Crucially, Krauss says, eating saturated fat boosts fluffy LDL. What's more, there is some research suggesting small LDL gets a boost from a low-fat, high-carbohydrate diet, especially one rich in sugars.

Why might smaller LDL particles be riskier?

In their journey around the bloodstream, LDL particles bind to cells and are pulled out of circulation. Krauss says smaller LDLs don't bind as easily, so remain in the blood for longer—and the longer they are there, the greater their chance of causing damage. They are also more easily converted into an oxidised form that is considered more damaging. Finally, there are simply more of them for the same overall cholesterol level. And more LDLs equate to greater risk of arterial damage, Krauss says. He thinks that the evidence is strong enough for the health advice to change.

But Susan Jebb, professor of diet and population health at the University of Oxford, says it is too early to buy into this alternative model of LDLs and health. "The jury has to be out because relatively few of the studies have subdivided LDL. It may well be worth exploring, but right now I am not persuaded."

Jeremy Pearson, a vascular biologist and associate medical director at the British Heart Foundation, which part-funded the 2014 meta-analysis, agrees. He says the original idea that a diet high in saturated fat raises the risk of heart disease remains persuasive, and that there are other meta-analyses that support this. He also points to hard evidence from studies in animals, where dietary control is possible to a degree that it is not in people. They repeatedly show high saturated fat leads to high LDL and hardened arteries, he says.

So how does he explain the meta-analyses that cast doubt on the orthodoxy? "I guess what that means is that in free living humans there are other things that are usually more important regarding whether you have a heart attack or not than the balance of saturated and unsaturated fat in your diet," Pearson says. Factors such as lack of exercise, alcohol intake and body weight may simply overshadow the impact of fat.

Certainly, the debate cannot be divorced from the issue of overall calorie intake, which rose in the three decades from the 1970s in the US and many other countries. The result was rising numbers of overweight people. And being overweight or obese raises the risk of heart disease.

Another key factor might be what people now eat instead of saturated fat. "The effect of reducing saturated fat depends on what replaces it," says Walter Willett of the Harvard School of Public Health. "We consciously or unconsciously replace a large reduction in calories with something else."

The problem, as some see it, is that the something else is usually refined carbohydrates, especially sugars, added to foods to take the place of fat. A review in 2009 showed that if carbohydrates were raised while saturated fat cut, the outcome was a raised heart-disease risk. This plays to the emerging idea that sugar is the real villain.

Then there are trans fats. Created by food chemists to replace animal fats such as lard, they are made by chemically modifying vegetable oils to make them solid. Because they are unsaturated, and so "healthy" the food industry piled them into products such as cakes and spreads. But it later turned out that trans fats cause heart disease. All told, it is possible that the meta-analyses simply show that the benefits of switching away from saturated fat were cancelled out by replacing them with sugar and trans fats.

Meanwhile, science continues to unravel some intricacies of fat metabolism which could also help to account for the confusing results. One promising avenue is that not all types of saturated fat are the same. The 2014 meta-analysis, for example, found clear indications that different saturated fatty acids in blood are associated with different coronary risk. Some saturated fats appear to lower the risk; some unsaturated ones increase it.

Meat vs. Dairy

Although further big studies are needed to confirm these findings, lead author Rajiv Chowdhury, an epidemiologist at the University of Cambridge, says this is an avenue that might be worth exploring.

There is other evidence that not all saturated fats are the same. A study from 2012 found that while eating lots of saturated fat from meat increased the risk of heart disease, equivalent amounts from dairy actually reduced it. The researchers calculated that cutting calories from meaty saturated fat by just 2 per cent and replacing them with saturated fat from dairy reduces the risk of a heart attack or stroke by 25 per cent.

Krauss also cites studies showing that eating cheese does not raise bad cholesterol as much as eating butter, even when both have identical levels of saturated fat.

So could future advice say that saturated fat from dairy sources is less risky than that from meat, for example? Or urge us to favour cheese over butter? It's too early to say. Jebb is aware that the idea that some saturated fatty acids may be worse than others is gaining credence, but says it is far from being ready to guide eating habits.

Nonetheless, there is a growing feeling that we need to reappraise our thinking on fat.

Marion Nestle, professor of nutrition at New York University, says that studies of single nutrients have a fundamental flaw. "People do not eat saturated fat," she says. "They eat foods containing fats and oils that are mixtures of saturated, unsaturated and polyunsaturated fats, and many other nutrients that affect health and also vary in calories. So teasing saturated fat out of all that is not simple."

The only way to rigorously test the various hypotheses would be to put some people on one kind of diet and others on another for 20 years or more. "Doable? Fundable? I don't think so," says Nestle.

So where does that leave us? Is it time to reverse 35 years of dietary advice and stop worrying about fuzzing up our arteries?

Some nutritionists say yes. Krauss advocates a rethink of guidelines on saturated fat when a new version of the Dietary Guidelines for Americans is put together next year. He certainly believes that the even stricter limit on saturated fat recommended by the American Heart Association—that it constitute no more than 7 per cent of daily calorie intake—should be relaxed.

Others, though, strike a note of caution. Nestle says that the answer depends on context. "If calories are balanced and diets contain plenty of vegetables, foods richer in saturated fat should not be a problem. But that's not how most people eat," she says.

Jebb and Pearson see no reason to shift the guidance just yet, although Jebb says it may be time for a review of fat by the UK's Scientific Advisory Committee on Nutrition, which last visited the issue in 1991.

So while dietary libertarians may be gleefully slapping a big fat steak on the griddle and lining up a cream pie with hot fudge for dessert, the dietary advice of the 1970s still stands—for now. In other words, steak and butter can be part of a healthy diet. Just don't overdo them.

JON WHITE is opinion editor of *New Scientist* magazine.

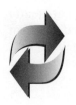

EXPLORING THE ISSUE

Is There a Valid Link Between Saturated Fat and Heart Disease?

Critical Thinking and Reflection

1. Is it better to eat more carbohydrates and less fat? Explain.
2. Why do so many organizations support restricting saturated fats?
3. Why has saturated fat traditionally had a bad reputation?

Is There Common Ground?

In 1955 Dr. Ancel Keys began research that came to be known as the Seven Countries Study. His interest in diet and cardiovascular disease (CVD) was based on seemingly paradoxical data. Well nourished American business executives had high rates of heart disease, while in Europe after World War II, CVD rates had decreased sharply despite limited food supplies. Dr. Keys hypothesized there was a correlation between cholesterol levels and CVD and began a study of Minnesota businessmen. At a 1955 expert meeting at the World Health Organization in Geneva, Keys presented his diet–lipid–heart disease hypothesis.

Following that presentation, Dr. Keys observed that southern Italy had the highest rate of centenarians in the world and theorized that a Mediterranean-style diet low in animal fat protected against heart disease while a high-fat diet increased the risk. The results of what later became known as the Seven Countries Study seemed to indicate that serum cholesterol was strongly correlated to coronary heart disease mortality at both the population and individual levels. Following this, the American Heart Association and the U.S. government began educating the public that a diet which included large amounts of butter, lard, eggs, and beef would lead to coronary heart disease and that these foods should be replaced by fish, oils, and fat-free dairy products.

The conclusion Keys reached was that saturated fats have negative effects as opposed to the beneficial impact of unsaturated fats. For the next 20-year period all dietary fats were considered unhealthy, driven by the hypothesis that all dietary fats cause obesity and cancer. Recent studies question cardiovascular guidelines that encourage high consumption of polyunsaturated fatty acids and low consumption of total saturated fats. Overall, it appears that researchers are questioning Dr. Keys' research, though no final conclusions have been drawn.

Additional Resources

Chowdhury, R., Warnakula, S., Kunutsor, S., Crowe, F., Ward, H. A., Johnson, L.,. . . Di Angelantonio, E. (2014). Association of dietary, circulating, and supplement fatty acids with coronary risk. *Annals of Internal Medicine*, *160*(6), 398–407.

Myers, E. F. (2015). New insights or confusion—is butter really back? *Nutrition Today*, *50*(1), 12–27.

Puaschitz, N. G., Strand, E., Norekvål, T. M., Dierkes, J., Dahl, L., Svingen, G. T., . . . Nygård, O. (2015). Dietary intake of saturated fat is not associated with risk of coronary events or mortality in patients with established coronary artery disease. *Journal of Nutrition*, *145*(2), 299–305.

Ravnskov, U., DiNicolantonio, J. J., Harcombe, Z., Kummerow, F. A., Harumi, O., & Worm, N. (2014). The questionable benefits of exchanging saturated fat with polyunsaturated fat. *Mayo Clinic Proceedings*, *89*(4), 451–453.

Walsh, B. (2014). Don't blame fat. *Time*, *183*(24), 28–35.

Internet References . . .

Academy of Nutrition and Dietetics

www.eatright.org

American Heart Association

www.heart.org

Center for Science in the Public Interest

www.cspinet.org

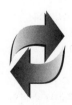

Selected, Edited, and with Issue Framing Material by:
Eileen L. Daniel, *SUNY College at Brockport*

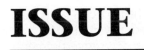

ISSUE

Are Restrictions on Sugar and Sugary Beverages Justified?

YES: Gary Taubes and Cristin Kearns Couzens, from "Sweet Little Lies," *Mother Jones* (2012)

NO: Kenneth W. Krause, from "Saving Us from Sweets: This Is Science and Government on Sugar," *Skeptical Inquirer* (2012)

Learning Outcomes

After reading this issue, you will be able to:

- Discuss the nutritional risk factors associated with the consumption of sugar and sugary beverages.
- Understand the role sugar and sugary beverages may play in the current obesity epidemic.
- Assess the need for government restrictions on the sale of sugary and sugar beverages.

ISSUE SUMMARY

YES: Writers Gary Taubes and Cristin Kearns Couzens maintain that added sugars and sweeteners pose dangers to health and that the sugar industry continually campaigns to enhance its image.

NO: Journalist Kenneth W. Krause argues that individuals have the ability to make decisions about sugar consumption themselves and that government should not restrict our access to sugar and sugar-containing food products.

The per capita consumption of refined sugar in the United States has varied between 60 and 100 pounds in the last 40 years. In 2008, American per capita total consumption of sugar and sweeteners, exclusive of artificial sweeteners, equaled 136 pounds per year. This consisted of 65.4 pounds of refined sugar and 68.3 pounds of corn-derived sweeteners per person. Granulated sugars are used at the table to sprinkle on foods and to sweeten hot drinks and in home baking to add sweetness and texture to cooked products. From a dietary perspective, the top five contributors to added sugars in our food supply are sugar-sweetened sodas, grain-based desserts and snacks such as cakes and cookies, fruit drinks, dairy-based desserts including ice cream, and puddings and candy.

There are numerous studies linking sugar to a variety of health concerns including diabetes and obesity. Studies on the relationship between sugars and diabetes are inconsistent since some propose that consuming large quantities of sugar does not directly increase the risk of diabetes. The extra calories, however, from eating excessive amounts of sugar can lead to obesity, which may itself increase the risk of developing this diabetes. Other studies show a relationship between refined sugar consumption and the onset of diabetes. These included a 2010 analysis of 11 studies involving over 300,000 participants. Researchers found that sugar-sweetened beverages may increase the risk of developing type 2 diabetes through obesity and other metabolic abnormalities linked to sugar consumption.

To address the increasing rates of obesity and its link to diabetes and other diseases, the New York City Board of Health approved a ban on the sale of large sodas and other sugary drinks at restaurants, street carts, and movie theaters, the first restriction of its kind in the country, in the fall of 2012. The measure, promoted by Mayor Michael R. Bloomberg, is likely to strengthen a growing national debate about soft drinks and obesity, and it could prompt other cities to follow suit, despite the fact that many New

Yorkers appear uncomfortable with the ban. The measure, which bars the sale of many sweetened drinks in containers larger than 16 ounces, was to take effect in March 2013. The vote by the Board of Health was the only regulatory approval needed to make the ban binding in the city, but the American soft drink industry has campaigned strongly against the measure and promised to fight it through other means, possibly in the courts. The soft drink industry argued that to single out one food item and claim it is the cause of obesity is inappropriate. While a state judge blocked the law in March 2013, the mayor vowed to continue his fight against mounting obesity by encouraging a ban on super large sized soft drinks.

Soft drink and other food manufacturers, like all companies, advertise and promote their products in order to maximize sales. Many non-nutritious foods are presented to the public in a misleading way for that purpose. For instance, low fiber, high sugar breakfast cereals may be sprinkled with vitamins and marketed as a low fat, nutritious breakfast. Some school districts, working with food manufacturers and producers, sell fast food items in school cafeterias. Soft drink companies have provided monies and other support to schools who promote their products. Non-nutritious foods including sugary breakfast cereals, fast food, and candy are heavily advertised on television shows catering to children.

Ethical and legal standards for the food industry, mandated by the government, could address some of these concerns. For instance, clearer food labels, which allow consumers to better understand what they're eating, might help reduce excessive consumption of calories, fat, and sugar. Many non-nutritious food labels seem to have incredibly small or unrealistic serving sizes. A more accurate serving size might be beneficial to consumers. A ban on the advertising of junk foods in public schools,

specifically soft drinks, candy, and other items with high sugar content, could also be enacted as well as increased taxes on these foods. Alcohol and tobacco advertisements are not allowed on children's television, so it would seem reasonable to ban the promotion of foods that encourage overeating and obesity. In addition, non-nutritious foods could have health warnings similar to the warnings on cigarette packs or bottles of alcoholic beverages.

On the other hand, the proposed ban on the sale of large containers of soft drinks, while well intentioned, is controversial as some consumers wonder just how far the government should go to protect us from ourselves. To promote public health, New York City currently restricts smoking in public parks and bans trans fats from food served in restaurants. But Mayor Bloomberg's proposal raises questions about government's role in shaping and restricting individual choices. If government officials can limit the size of sodas, next it could decide to restrict portion sizes of restaurant food or the size of pre-made meals sold at supermarkets. If government is within its rights to restrict behavior to protect health, many other limits could be imposed in the name of health promotion. As many ponder the role of government in restricting the individual freedom to eat what one wants in whatever quantity, the rate of obesity in this country remains a serious health issue.

In addressing the question of whether or not restrictions on sugar and sugary beverages are justified, Gary Taubes and Cristin Kearns Couzens believe that added sugars and sweeteners pose a threat to health by increasing the risk for diabetes and heart disease. In countering with a NO answer, Kenneth W. Krause argues that individuals have the ability to make decisions about sugar consumption themselves and that government should not restrict our access to sugar or sugar-containing foods.

YES ↵

Gary Taubes and Cristin Kearns Couzens

Sweet Little Lies

Inside an industry's campaign to frost its image, hold regulators at bay, and keep scientists from asking: **Does sugar kill?**

On a brisk spring Tuesday in 1976, a pair of executives from the Sugar Association stepped up to the podium of a Chicago ballroom to accept the Oscar of the public relations world, the Silver Anvil award for excellence in "the forging of public opinion." The trade group had recently pulled off one of the greatest turnarounds in PR history. For nearly a decade, the sugar industry had been buffeted by crisis after crisis as the media and the public soured on sugar and scientists began to view it as a likely cause of obesity, diabetes, and heart disease. Industry ads claiming that eating sugar helped you lose weight had been called out by the Federal Trade Commission, and the Food and Drug Administration had launched a review of whether sugar was even safe to eat. Consumption had declined 12 percent in just two years, and producers could see where that trend might lead. As John "JW" Tatem Jr. and Jack O'Connell Jr., the Sugar Association's president and director of public relations, posed that day with their trophies, their smiles only hinted at the coup they'd just pulled off.

Their winning campaign, crafted with the help of the prestigious public relations firm Carl Byoir & Associates, had been prompted by a poll showing that consumers had come to see sugar as fattening, and that most doctors suspected it might exacerbate, if not cause, heart disease and diabetes. With an initial annual budget of nearly $800,000 ($3.4 million today) collected from the makers of Dixie Crystals, Domino, C&H, Great Western, and other sugar brands, the association recruited a stable of medical and nutritional professionals to allay the public's fears, brought snack and beverage companies into the fold, and bankrolled scientific papers that contributed to a "highly supportive" FDA ruling, which, the Silver Anvil application boasted, made it "unlikely that sugar will be subject to legislative restriction in coming years."

The story of sugar, as Tatem told it, was one of a harmless product under attack by "opportunists dedicated to exploiting the consuming public." Over the subsequent decades, it would be transformed from what the *New York Times* in 1977 had deemed "a villain in disguise" into a nutrient so seemingly innocuous that even the American Heart Association and the American Diabetes Association approved it as part of a healthy diet. Research on the suspected links between sugar and chronic disease largely ground to a halt by the late 1980s, and scientists came to view such pursuits as a career dead end. So effective were the Sugar Association's efforts that, to this day, no consensus exists about sugar's potential dangers. The industry's PR campaign corresponded roughly with a significant rise in Americans' consumption of "caloric sweeteners," including table sugar (sucrose) and high-fructose corn syrup (HFCS). This increase was accompanied, in turn, by a surge in the chronic diseases increasingly linked to sugar. (See chart below.) Since 1970, obesity rates in the United States have more than doubled, while the incidence of diabetes has more than tripled.

Precisely how did the sugar industry engineer its turnaround? The answer is found in more than 1,500 pages of internal memos, letters, and company board reports we discovered buried in the archives of now-defunct sugar companies as well as in the recently released papers of deceased researchers and consultants who played key roles in the industry's strategy. They show how Big Sugar used Big Tobacco-style tactics to ensure that government agencies would dismiss troubling health claims against their products. Compared to the tobacco companies, which knew for a fact that their wares were deadly and spent billions of dollars trying to cover up that reality, the sugar industry had a relatively easy task. With the jury still out on sugar's health effects, producers simply needed to make sure that the uncertainty lingered. But the goal was the same: to safeguard sales by creating a body of evidence companies could deploy to counter any unfavorable research.

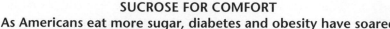

SUCROSE FOR COMFORT
As Americans eat more sugar, diabetes and obesity have soared

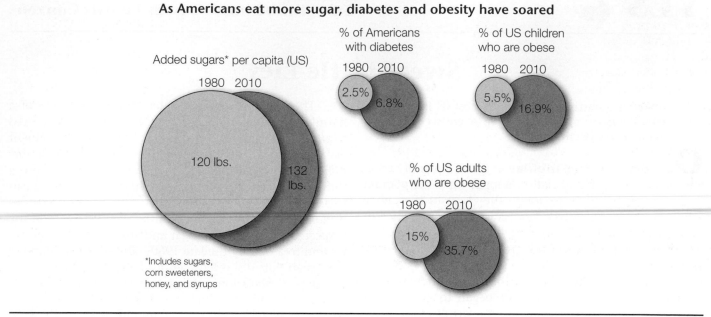

Added sugars* per capita (US)

1980   2010

120 lbs.   132 lbs.

*Includes sugars, corn sweeteners, honey, and syrups

% of Americans with diabetes

1980 2010

2.5%   6.8%

% of US children who are obese

1980 2010

5.5%   16.9%

% of US adults who are obese

1980   2010

15%   35.7%

Sources: USDA, CDC, US Census Bureau

This decades-long effort to stack the scientific deck is why, today, the USDA's dietary guidelines only speak of sugar in vague generalities. ("Reduce the intake of calories from solid fats and added sugars.") It's why the FDA insists that sugar is "generally recognized as safe" despite considerable evidence suggesting otherwise. It's why some scientists' urgent calls for regulation of sugary products have been dead on arrival, and it's why—absent any federal leadership—New York City Mayor Michael Bloomberg felt compelled to propose a ban on oversized sugary drinks that passed in September.

In fact, a growing body of research suggests that sugar and its nearly chemically identical cousin, HFCS, may very well cause diseases that kill hundreds of thousands of Americans every year, and that these chronic conditions would be far less prevalent if we significantly dialed back our consumption of added sugars. Robert Lustig, a leading authority on pediatric obesity at the University of California-San Francisco (whose arguments Gary explored in a 2011 *New York Times Magazine* cover story), made this case last February in the prestigious journal *Nature*. In an article titled "The Toxic Truth About Sugar," Lustig and two colleagues observed that sucrose and HFCS are addictive in much the same way as cigarettes and alcohol, and that overconsumption of them is driving worldwide epidemics of obesity and type 2 diabetes (the type associated with obesity). Sugar-related diseases are costing America

around $150 billion a year, the authors estimated, so federal health officials need to step up and consider regulating the stuff.

The Sugar Association dusted off what has become its stock response: The Lustig paper, it said, "lacks the scientific evidence or consensus" to support its claims, and its authors were irresponsible not to point out that the full body of science "is inconclusive at best." This inconclusiveness, of course, is precisely what the Sugar Association has worked so assiduously to maintain. "In confronting our critics," Tatem explained to his board of directors back in 1976, "we try never to lose sight of the fact that no confirmed scientific evidence links sugar to the death-dealing diseases. This crucial point is the lifeblood of the association."

The Sugar Association's earliest incarnation dates back to 1943, when growers and refiners created the Sugar Research Foundation to counter World War II sugar-rationing propaganda—"How Much Sugar Do You Need? None!" declared one government pamphlet. In 1947, producers rechristened their group the Sugar Association and launched a new PR division, Sugar Information Inc., which before long was touting sugar as a "sensible new approach to weight control." In 1968, in the hope of enlisting foreign sugar companies to help defray costs, the Sugar Association spun off its research division as the International Sugar Research Foundation. "Misconceptions concerning the causes of tooth decay, diabetes, and heart problems exist on a worldwide basis," explained a 1969 ISRF recruiting brochure.

As early as 1962, internal Sugar Association memos had acknowledged the potential links between sugar and chronic diseases, but at the time sugar executives had a more pressing problem: Weight-conscious Americans were switching in droves to diet sodas—particularly Diet Rite and Tab—sweetened with cyclamate and saccharin. From 1963 through 1968, diet soda's share of the soft-drink market shot from 4 percent to 15 percent. "A dollar's worth of sugar," ISRF vice president and research director John Hickson warned in an internal review, "could be replaced with a dime's worth" of sugar alternatives. "If anyone can undersell you nine cents out of 10," Hickson told the *New York Times* in 1969, "you'd better find some brickbat you can throw at him."

By then, the sugar industry had doled out more than $600,000 (about $4 million today) to study every conceivable harmful effect of cyclamate sweeteners, which are still sold around the world under names like Sugar Twin and Sucaryl. In 1969, the FDA banned cyclamates in the United States based on a study suggesting they could cause bladder cancer in rats. Not long after, Hickson left the ISRF to work for the Cigar Research Council. He was described in a confidential tobacco industry memo as a "supreme scientific politician who had been successful in condemning cyclamates, on behalf of the [sugar industry], on somewhat shaky evidence." It later emerged that the evidence suggesting that cyclamates caused cancer in rodents was not relevant to humans, but by then the case was officially closed. In 1977, saccharin, too, was nearly banned on the basis of animal results that would turn out to be meaningless in people.

Meanwhile, researchers had been reporting that blood lipids—cholesterol and triglycerides in particular—were a risk factor in heart disease. Some people had high cholesterol but normal triglycerides, prompting health experts to recommend that they avoid animal fats. Other people were deemed "carbohydrate sensitive," with normal cholesterol but markedly increased triglyceride levels. In these individuals, even moderate sugar consumption could cause a spike in triglycerides. John Yudkin, the United Kingdom's leading nutritionist, was making headlines with claims that sugar, not fat, was the primary cause of heart disease.

In 1967, the Sugar Association's research division began considering "the rising tide of implications of sucrose in atherosclerosis." Before long, according to a confidential 1970 review of industry-funded studies, the

newly formed ISRF was spending 10 percent of its research budget on the link between diet and heart disease. Hickson, the ISRF's vice president, urged his member corporations to keep the results of the review under wraps. Of particular concern was the work of a University of Pennsylvania researcher on "sucrose sensitivity," which sugar executives feared was "likely to reveal evidence of harmful effects." One ISRF consultant recommended that sugar companies get to the truth of the matter by sponsoring a full-on study. In what would become a pattern, the ISRF opted not to follow his advice. Another ISRF-sponsored study, by biochemist Walter Pover of the University of Birmingham, in England, had uncovered a possible mechanism to explain how sugar raises triglyceride levels. Pover believed he was on the verge of demonstrating this mechanism "conclusively" and that 18 more weeks of work would nail it down. But instead of providing the funds, the ISRF nixed the project, assessing its value as "nil."

The industry followed a similar strategy when it came to diabetes. By 1973, links between sugar, diabetes, and heart disease were sufficiently troubling that Sen. George McGovern of South Dakota convened a hearing of his Select Committee on Nutrition and Human Needs to address the issue. An international panel of experts—including Yudkin and Walter Mertz, head of the Human Nutrition Institute at the Department of Agriculture—testified that variations in sugar consumption were the best explanation for the differences in diabetes rates between populations, and that research by the USDA and others supported the notion that eating too much sugar promotes dramatic population-wide increases in the disease. One panelist, South African diabetes specialist George Campbell, suggested that anything more than 70 pounds per person per year—about half of what is sold in America today—would spark epidemics.

In the face of such hostile news from independent scientists, the ISRF hosted its own conference the following March, focusing exclusively on the work of researchers who were skeptical of a sugar/diabetes connection. "All those present agreed that a large amount of research is still necessary before a firm conclusion can be arrived at," according to a conference review published in a prominent diabetes journal. In 1975, the foundation reconvened in Montreal to discuss research priorities with its consulting scientists. Sales were sinking, Tatem reminded the gathered sugar execs, and a major factor was "the impact of consumer advocates who link sugar consumption with certain diseases."

Following the Montreal conference, the ISRF disseminated a memo quoting Errol Marliss, a University of

Toronto diabetes specialist, recommending that the industry pursue "well-designed research programs" to establish sugar's role in the course of diabetes and other diseases. "Such research programs *might* produce an answer that sucrose is bad in certain individuals," he warned. But the studies "should be undertaken in a sufficiently comprehensive way as to produce results. A gesture rather than full support is unlikely to produce the sought-after answers."

A gesture, however, is what the industry would offer. Rather than approve a serious investigation of the purported links between sucrose and disease, American sugar companies quit supporting the ISRF's research projects. Instead, via the Sugar Association proper, they would spend roughly $655,000 between 1975 and 1980 on 17 studies designed, as internal documents put it, "to maintain research as a main prop of the industry's defense." Each proposal was vetted by a panel of industry-friendly scientists and a second committee staffed by representatives from sugar companies and "contributing research members" such as Coca-Cola, Hershey's, General Mills, and Nabisco. Most of the cash was awarded to researchers whose studies seemed explicitly designed to exonerate sugar. One even proposed to explore whether sugar could be shown to boost serotonin levels in rats' brains, and thus "prove of therapeutic value, as in the relief of depression," an internal document noted.

At best, the studies seemed a token effort. Harvard Medical School professor Ron Arky, for example, received money from the Sugar Association to determine whether sucrose has a different effect on blood sugar and other diabetes indicators if eaten alongside complex carbohydrates like pectin and psyllium. The project went nowhere, Arky told us recently. But the Sugar Association "didn't care."

In short, rather than do definitive research to learn the truth about its product, good or bad, the association stuck to a PR scheme designed to "establish with the broadest possible audience—virtually everyone is a consumer—the safety of sugar as a food." One of its first acts was to establish a Food & Nutrition Advisory Council consisting of a half-dozen physicians and two dentists willing to defend sugar's place in a healthy diet, and set aside roughly $60,000 per year (more than $220,000 today) to cover its cost.

Working to the industry's recruiting advantage was the rising notion that cholesterol and dietary fat—especially saturated fat—were the likely causes of heart disease. (Tatem even suggested, in a letter to the *Times Magazine,* that some "sugar critics" were motivated merely by wanting "to keep the heat off saturated fats.") This was

the brainchild of nutritionist Ancel Keys, whose University of Minnesota laboratory had received financial support from the sugar industry as early as 1944. From the 1950s through the 1980s, Keys remained the most outspoken proponent of the fat hypothesis, often clashing publicly with Yudkin, the most vocal supporter of the sugar hypothesis—the two men "shared a good deal of loathing," recalled one of Yudkin's colleagues.

So when the Sugar Association needed a heart disease expert for its Food & Nutrition Advisory Council, it approached Francisco Grande, one of Keys' closest colleagues. Another panelist was University of Oregon nutritionist William Connor, the leading purveyor of the notion that it is dietary cholesterol that causes heart disease. As its top diabetes expert, the industry recruited Edwin Bierman of the University of Washington, who believed that diabetics need not pay strict attention to their sugar intake so long as they maintained a healthy weight by burning off the calories they consumed. Bierman also professed an apparently unconditional faith that it was dietary fat (and *being* fat) that caused heart disease, with sugar having no meaningful effect.

It is hard to overestimate Bierman's role in shifting the diabetes conversation away from sugar. It was primarily Bierman who convinced the American Diabetes Association to liberalize the amount of carbohydrates (including sugar) it recommended in the diets of diabetics, and focus more on urging diabetics to lower their fat intake, since diabetics are particularly likely to die from heart disease. Bierman also presented industry-funded studies when he coauthored a section on potential causes for a National Commission on Diabetes report in 1976; the document influences the federal diabetes research agenda to this day. Some researchers, he acknowledged, had "argued eloquently" that consumption of refined carbohydrates (such as sugar) is a precipitating factor in diabetes. But then Bierman cited five studies—two of them bankrolled by the ISRF—that were "inconsistent" with that hypothesis. "A review of all available laboratory and epidemiologic evidence," he concluded, "suggests that the most important dietary factor in increasing the risk of diabetes is total calorie intake, irrespective of source."

The point man on the industry's food and nutrition panel was Frederick Stare, founder and chairman of the department of nutrition at the Harvard School of Public Health. Stare and his department had a long history of ties to Big Sugar. An ISRF internal research review credited the sugar industry with funding some 30 papers in his department from 1952 through 1956 alone. In 1960, the department broke ground on a new $5 million building funded largely by private donations, including a $1 million gift from General Foods, the maker of Kool-Aid and Tang.

By the early 1970s, Stare ranked among the industry's most reliable advocates, testifying in Congress about the wholesomeness of sugar even as his department kept raking in funding from sugar producers and food and beverage giants such as Carnation, Coca-Cola, Gerber, Kellogg, and Oscar Mayer. His name also appears in tobacco documents, which show that he procured industry funding for a study aimed at exonerating cigarettes as a cause of heart disease.

The first act of the Food & Nutrition Advisory Council was to compile "Sugar in the Diet of Man," an 88-page white paper edited by Stare and published in 1975 to "organize existing scientific facts concerning sugar." It was a compilation of historical evidence and arguments that sugar companies could use to counter the claims of Yudkin, Stare's Harvard colleague Jean Mayer, and other researchers whom Tatem called "enemies of sugar." The document was sent to reporters—the Sugar Association circulated 25,000 copies—along with a press release headlined "Scientists dispel sugar fears." The report neglected to mention that it was funded by the sugar industry, but internal documents confirm that it was.

The Sugar Association also relied on Stare to take its message to the people: "Place Dr. Stare on the AM America Show" and "Do a 3½ minute interview with Dr. Stare for 200 radio stations," note the association's meeting minutes. Using Stare as a proxy, internal documents explained, would help the association "make friends with the networks" and "keep the sugar industry in the background." By the time Stare's copious conflicts of interest were finally revealed—in "Professors on the Take," a 1976 exposé by the Center for Science in the Public Interest—Big Sugar no longer needed his assistance. The industry could turn to an FDA document to continue where he'd left off.

While Stare and his colleagues had been drafting "Sugar in the Diet of Man," the FDA was launching its first review of whether sugar was, in the official jargon, generally recognized as safe (GRAS), part of a series of food-additive reviews the Nixon administration had requested of the agency. The FDA subcontracted the task to the Federation of American Societies of Experimental Biology, which created an 11-member committee to vet hundreds of food additives from acacia to zinc sulfate. While the mission of the GRAS committee was to conduct unbiased reviews of the existing science for each additive, it was led by biochemist George W. Irving Jr., who had previously served two years as chairman of the scientific advisory board of the International Sugar Research Foundation.

Industry documents show that another committee member, Samuel Fomon, had received sugar-industry funding for three of the five years prior to the sugar review.

The FDA's instructions were clear: To label a substance as a potential health hazard, there had to be "credible evidence of, or reasonable grounds to suspect, adverse biological effects"—which certainly existed for sugar at the time. But the GRAS committee's review would depend heavily on "Sugar in the Diet of Man" and other work by its authors. In the section on heart disease, committee members cited 14 studies whose results were "conflicting," but 6 of those bore industry fingerprints, including Francisco Grande's chapter from "Sugar in the Diet of Man" and 5 others that came from Grande's lab or were otherwise funded by the sugar industry.

The diabetes chapter of the review acknowledged studies suggesting that "long term consumption of sucrose can result in a functional change in the capacity to metabolize carbohydrates and thus lead to diabetes mellitus," but it went on to cite five reports contradicting that notion. All had industry ties, and three were authored by Ed Bierman, including his chapter in "Sugar in the Diet of Man."

In January 1976, the GRAS committee published its preliminary conclusions, noting that while sugar probably contributed to tooth decay, it was not a "hazard to the public." The draft review dismissed the diabetes link as "circumstantial" and called the connection to cardiovascular disease "less than clear," with fat playing a greater role. The only cautionary note, besides cavities, was that all bets were off if sugar consumption were to increase significantly. The committee then thanked the Sugar Association for contributing "information and data." (Tatem would later remark that while he was "proud of the credit line . . . we would probably be better off without it.")

The committee's perspective was shared by many researchers, but certainly not all. For a public hearing on the draft review, scientists from the USDA's Carbohydrate Nutrition Laboratory submitted what they considered "abundant evidence that sucrose is one of the dietary factors responsible for obesity, diabetes, and heart disease." As they later explained in the *American Journal of Clinical Nutrition,* some portion of the public—perhaps 15 million Americans at that time—clearly could not tolerate a diet rich in sugar and other carbohydrates. Sugar consumption, they said, should come down by "a minimum of 60 percent," and the government should launch a national campaign "to inform the populace of the hazards of excessive sugar consumption." But the committee stood by its conclusions in the final version of its report presented to the FDA in October 1976.

For the sugar industry, the report was gospel. The findings "should be memorized" by the staff of every company associated with the sugar industry, Tatem told his membership. "In the long run," he said, the document "cannot be sidetracked, and you may be sure we will push its exposure to all comers of the country."

The association promptly produced an ad for newspapers and magazines exclaiming "Sugar is Safe!" It "does not cause death-dealing diseases," the ad declared, and "there is no substantiated scientific evidence indicating that sugar causes diabetes, heart disease or any other malady. . . . The next time you hear a promoter attacking sugar, beware the ripoff. Remember he can't substantiate his charges. Ask yourself what he's promoting or what he is seeking to cover up. If you get a chance, ask him about the GRAS Review Report. Odds are you won't get an answer. Nothing stings a nutritional liar like scientific facts."

The Sugar Association would soon get its chance to put the committee's sugar review to the test. In 1977, McGovern's select committee—the one that had held the 1973 hearings on sugar and diabetes—blindsided the industry with a report titled "Dietary Goals for the United States," recommending that Americans lower their sugar intake by 40 percent. The association "hammered away" at the McGovern report using the GRAS review "as our scientific Bible," Tatem told sugar executives.

McGovern held fast, but Big Sugar would prevail in the end. In 1980, when the USDA first published its own set of dietary guidelines, it relied heavily on a review written for the American Society of Clinical Nutrition by none other than Bierman, who used the GRAS committee's findings to bolster his own. "Contrary to widespread opinion, too much sugar does not seem to cause diabetes," the USDA guidelines concluded. They went on to counsel that people should "avoid too much sugar," without bothering to explain what that meant.

In 1982, the FDA once again took up the GRAS committee's conclusion that sugar was safe, proposing to make it official. The announcement resulted in a swarm of public criticism, prompting the agency to reopen its case. Four years later, an agency task force concluded, again leaning on industry-sponsored studies, that "there is no conclusive evidence . . . that demonstrates a hazard to the general public when sugars are consumed at the levels that are now current." (Walter Glinsmann, the task force's lead administrator, would later become a consultant to the Corn Refiners Association, which represents producers of high-fructose corn syrup.)

The USDA, meanwhile, had updated its own dietary guidelines. With Fred Stare now on the advisory committee,

the 1985 guidelines retained the previous edition's vague recommendation to "avoid too much" sugar but stated unambiguously that "too much sugar in your diet does not cause diabetes." At the time, the USDA's own Carbohydrate Nutrition Laboratory was still generating evidence to the contrary and supporting the notion that "even low sucrose intake" might be contributing to heart disease in 10 percent of Americans.

By the early 1990s, the USDA's research into sugar's health effects had ceased, and the FDA's take on sugar had become conventional wisdom, influencing a generation's worth of key publications on diet and health. Reports from the surgeon general and the National Academy of Sciences repeated the mantra that the evidence linking sugar to chronic disease was inconclusive, and then went on to equate "inconclusive" with "nonexistent." They also ignored a crucial caveat: The FDA reviewers had deemed added sugars—those in excess of what occurs naturally in our diets—safe at "current" 1986 consumption levels. But the FDA's consumption estimate was 43 percent lower than that of its sister agency, the USDA. By 1999, the average American would be eating more than double the amount the FDA had deemed safe—although we have cut back by 13 percent since then.

Asked to comment on some of the documents described in this article, a Sugar Association spokeswoman responded that they are "at this point historical in nature and do not necessarily reflect the current mission or function" of the association. But it is clear enough that the industry still operates behind the scenes to make sure regulators never officially set a limit on the amount of sugar Americans can safely consume. The authors of the 2010 USDA dietary guidelines, for instance, cited two scientific reviews as evidence that sugary drinks don't make adults fat. The first was written by Sigrid Gibson, a nutrition consultant whose clients included the Sugar Bureau (England's version of the Sugar Association) and the World Sugar Research Organization (formerly the ISRF). The second review was authored by Carrie Ruxton, who served as research manager of the Sugar Bureau from 1995 to 2000.

The Sugar Association has also worked its connections to assure that the government panels making dietary recommendations—the USDA's Dietary Guidelines Advisory Committee, for instance—include researchers sympathetic to its position. One internal newsletter boasted in 2003 that for the USDA panel, the association had "worked diligently to achieve the nomination of another expert wholly through third-party endorsements."

In the few instances when governmental authorities have sought to reduce people's sugar consumption, the industry has attacked openly. In 2003, after an expert panel convened by the World Health Organization recommended that no more than 10 percent of all calories in people's diets should come from added sugars—nearly 40 percent less than the USDA's estimate for the average American—current Sugar Association president Andrew Briscoe wrote the WHO's director general warning that the association would "exercise every avenue available to expose the dubious nature" of the report and urge "congressional appropriators to challenge future funding" for the WHO. Larry Craig (R-Idaho, sugar beets) and John Breaux (D-La., sugarcane), then co-chairs of the Senate Sweetener Caucus, wrote a letter to Secretary of Health and Human Services Tommy Thompson, urging his "prompt and favorable attention" to prevent the report from becoming official WHO policy. (Craig had received more than $36,000 in sugar industry contributions in the previous election cycle.) Thompson's people responded with a 28-page letter detailing "where the US Government's policy recommendations and interpretation of the science differ" with the WHO report. Not surprisingly, the organization left its experts' recommendation on sugar intake out of its official dietary strategy.

In recent years, the scientific tide has begun to turn against sugar. Despite the industry's best efforts, researchers and public health authorities have come to accept that the primary risk factor for both heart disease and type 2 diabetes is a condition called metabolic syndrome, which now affects more than 75 million Americans, according to the Centers for Disease Control and Prevention. Metabolic syndrome is characterized by a cluster of abnormalities—some of which Yudkin and others associated with sugar almost 50 years ago—including weight gain, increased insulin levels, and elevated triglycerides. It also has been linked to cancer and Alzheimer's disease. "Scientists have now established causation," Lustig said recently. "Sugar causes metabolic syndrome."

Newer studies from the University of California-Davis have even reported that LDL cholesterol, the classic risk factor for heart disease, can be raised significantly in just *two weeks* by drinking sugary beverages at a rate well within the upper range of what Americans consume—four 12-ounce glasses a day of beverages like soda, Snapple, or Red Bull. The result is a new wave of researchers coming out publicly against Big Sugar.

During the battle over the 2005 USDA guidelines, an internal Sugar Association newsletter described its strategy toward anyone who had the temerity to link sugar consumption with chronic disease and premature death: "Any disparagement of sugar," it read, "will be met with forceful, strategic public comments and the supporting science." But since the latest science is anything but supportive of the industry, what happens next?

"At present," Lustig ventures, "they have absolutely no reason to alter any of their practices. The science is in—the medical and economic problems with excessive sugar consumption are clear. But the industry is going to fight tooth and nail to prevent that science from translating into public policy."

Like the tobacco industry before it, the sugar industry may be facing the inexorable exposure of its product as a killer—science will ultimately settle the matter one way or the other—but as Big Tobacco learned a long time ago, even the inexorable can be held up for a very long time.

GARY TAUBES is a science writer and journalist.

CRISTIN KEARNS COUZENS is a senior consultant at the University of Colorado Center for Health Administration and an acting instructor at the University of Washington School of Dentistry.

Kenneth W. Krause

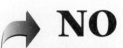 **NO**

Saving Us from Sweets: This Is Science and Government on Sugar

I've carried an intense personal grudge against "sugar" for decades. No, not the mostly benign, unrefined types packed into blueberries, green beans, and pumpernickels, for example. And no, not *only* the sickly sweet stuff shamelessly dumped into sodas, pastries, and swirling coffee froths either. I truly despise every pale-ish, pure and innocent looking slice of bread, wedge of potato, and grain of rice, and, I promise you, no pasta noodle, cracker, or corn flake will ever again bamboozle its way into my ever-shriveling food pantry.

At emotionally critical moments, my well-intentioned mother told me I was "husky" or "big-boned," which, by the way, is never true if it needs to be said. I was just plain F-A-T—obese, actually, just like more than a third of Americans today—until my junior year of high school. At that fateful point, I got fed up and decided to take matters into my own ignorant yet determined hands. Thanks to vigorous exercise and a dramatically reformed diet, I dropped seventy pounds in about three months. From then on, my world just got bigger and brighter.

Even now, at age forty-seven, I can relish every exhilaration my aging body will tolerate. In fact, I've recently given up weight lifting and jogging for power lifting, plyometrics, and high-intensity intervals. Last month, I look up mountain biking (the initial wounds should heal well before publication) because road cycling just wasn't exciting enough anymore.

I'm not bragging. Truth he told, I'm not particularly good at any of it. The point, rather, is that I love it all, and that I should have enjoyed an even richer physical life as a kid. In some tragic measure, I squandered the most dynamic years of my life guzzling and gobbling the same general strain of refuse that farmers use every day to fatten their cattle for slaughter. Yes, I'm a little bitter about sugar.

And I'm clearly not alone. "Clean-eating" advocates now dominate the nutrition world, and most of us agree generally with food guru Michael Pollan that we should eat less and that our diets should consist of mostly plants. Nevertheless, others in our ranks have lately embraced a more militant and less scientifically defensible approach to the problem.

Take, for example, Robert Lustig, Laura Schmidt, and Claire Brindis, three public health experts from the University or California, San Francisco. In a recent issue of *Nature*, they compared the "deadly effect" of added sugars (high-fructose corn syrup and sucrose) to that of alcohol. When consumed to excess, they observe, both substances cause a host of dreadful maladies, including hypertension, myocardial infarction, dyslipidemia, pancreatitis, obesity, malnutrition, hepatic dysfunction, and habituation (if not addiction).[1]

Far from mere "empty calories," they add, sugar is potentially "toxic." It alters metabolism, raises blood pressure, causes hormonal chaos, and damages our livers. Like both tobacco and alcohol (a distillation of sugar), it affects our brains, encouraging us to increase consumption. Indeed, they say, worldwide sugar consumption has tripled in the last fifty years.

Thus, Lustig et al. infer that sugar is at least partly responsible tor thirty-five million deaths every year from chronic, non-communicable diseases, which according to the United Nations now pose a greater health risk worldwide than their infectious counterparts. The authors also point out that Americans waste $65 billion in lost productivity and $150 billion on health-care related resources annually vis-à-vis illnesses linked to sugar-induced metabolic syndrome.

At the risk of piling on, I should emphasise that 17 percent of U.S. children are now obese too, and that the average American consumes more than forty pounds of high-fructose corn syrup per year. Recent investigations suggest that sugar might also impair our cognition. For example, in a new study from the University of California, Los Angeles, physiologist Fernando Gomez-Pinilla concludes that dicts consistently high in fructose can slow brain functions and weaken memory and learning in rats.

All of this reinforces my already firm personal resolve. But apparently many accomplished scientists lack not only confidence in our abilities as individuals to educate or control ourselves, but also respect for our rights to disagree or to make informed but less than perfectly rational decisions regarding our private consumption habits. As such, Lustig et al. urge Americans especially to support restrictions on their own liberty in the form of government-imposed regulation of sugar.

To support their cause, Lustig et al. rely on four criteria, "now largely accepted by the public health community," originally offered by social psychologist Thomas Babor in 2003 to justify the regulation of alcohol. The target substance must be toxic and unavoidable (or pervasive), and it must have a negative impact on society and a potential for abuse. Sugar satisfies each requirement, they contend, and is thus analogous to alcohol in terms of demanding bureaucratic imposition.

In a letter to me, Gomez-Pinilla echoed their concerns. Diabetes and obesity, he specified, come with greatly increased risks of several neurological and psychiatric disorders. In light of both the human and economic costs, he opined broadly, "it is in the general public concern to regulate high-sugar products as well as other unhealthy aspects of diet and lifestyle."

Unsurprisingly, the *Nature* paper inspired a flurry of defiant correspondences. Observers close to the sugar industry quickly took issue with both the researchers' facts and their logic. Richard Cottrell from the World Sugar Research Organisation in London first disputed the San Franciscans' calculation of worldwide sugar consumption. Because global population has more than doubled since 1960, he corrected, intake has increased only by 60 percent, not 300 percent. Moreover, he added, consumption in the United States, the United Kingdom, and Canada has risen only marginally as a proportion of total food-energy intake.

Judging metabolic syndrome a "controversial concept" in itself, Cottrell then cited analyses from the United Nations, the United States, and Europe that found no evidence of typical sugar consumption's contribution to any non-dental disease. On the other hand, he chided, "Overconsumption of anything is harmful, including water and air."

Ron Boswell, a senator from Queensland, Australia, noted that while the overweight population in his country has doubled and the incidence of diabetes has tripled since 1980, sugar consumption has actually dropped 23 percent during the same period. To describe sugar as "toxic," he continued, "is extreme, as is its ludicrous comparison with alcohol." The senator then scolded Lustig et al. for risking "damage to the livelihoods of thousands of people working in the sugar industry worldwide."

Other writers were no less reproachful. Christiani Jeyakumar Henry, a nutrition researcher in Singapore,

criticized the *Nature* piece for its exclusive emphasis on sugar. Several foods with high glycemic indices, he noted, including wheat, rice, and potatoes, also contribute to both obesity and diabetes. Finally, writing from the University of Vermont, Burlington, Saleem Ali criticized the San Franciscans' "misleading" comparison of sugar to alcohol and tobacco, the former of which causes neither behavioral intoxication nor second-hand contamination.

But David Katz, MD, renowned nutritionist and founding director of the Yale University Prevention Research Center, has long contested Lustig's claims. Last spring, for example, Katz characterized the researcher's dualistic, good vs. evil attacks on sugar as fanatical "humbug." "It is the overall quality and quantity of our diet that matters," he reasoned, "not just one villainous or virtuous nutrient du jour."

Refreshingly, Katz reassessed the subject from a broader, more reliable perspective based on evolutionary science. "We like sweet," he appreciated, "because mammals who like sweet are more apt to survive than mammals who don't. Period." Why should it shock and abhor so many of us that sugar is addictive? The real surprise, Katz answered, is not that high-energy food is habit-forming, "but rather that anything else is."

Katz's subsequent response to the *Nature* article, however, sends a frustratingly abstruse and well-mixed message. On the one hand, he recognizes that "Regulating nutrients, *per se*, is a slippery slope." Good intentions, he wisely if somewhat vaguely counsels, "could bog us down in conflict that forestalls all progress, distort the relative importance of just one nutrient relative to overall nutrition," and lead us to "unintended consequences."

On the other hand, Katz expressly defends some of Lustig et al.'s proposed governmental intrusions, Most reasonably, he favors restrictions on the sale of sugary products to kids where their attendance is officially compelled. "There is no reason," he argues, "why schools should be propagating the consumption of solid or liquid candy by students." Many locales have already seen fit to install such policies.

Far less noble, however, is the good doctor's support for punitive taxes on sugary drinks. "There is no inalienable right to afford soda in the Constitution," he observes. Those of lesser means, Katz resolves, "should perhaps consider that they can't afford to squander such limited funds on the empty calories of soda." Indeed they should, but Katz never explains how people can make decisions already made on their behalf.

But—in the name of science, most regrettably—Lustig et al. advocate considerably more intrusive schemes decorously styled "gentle, supply-side" controls.

Unsatisfied with a soda tax, they favor a similar penalty on "processed foods that contain any form of added sugars." That means ketchup, salsa, jam, deli meat, frozen fruit, many breads, and chocolate milk (now highly rated as a recovery drink following intense exercise). Ideally, the trio adds, such tariffs would be accompanied by an outright "ban" on television advertisements.

The San Franciscans would like to "limit availability" as well, by "reducing the hours that retailers are open, controlling the location and density of retail markets and limiting who can legally purchase the products." Alluding to a cadre of parents in South Philadelphia who recently blocked children from entering nearby convenience stores for snacks, Lustig et al. inquired, "Why couldn't a public health directive do the same?"

In late May of this year, New York City Mayor Michael Bloomberg announced the first plan in U.S. history to outlaw the sale of large sugary drinks—anything over sixteen fluid ounces—in all restaurants, movie theaters, sports arenas, and even from street carts. If approved by the Bloomberg-appointed Board of Health, the ban could take effect next March.

Sugar can be bad; most of us get that. But even the most impassioned personal grudge against potentially harmful food is just that—personal. Science, like government, is valued beyond calculation insofar as it expands personal choice. But the appropriate boundaries of science are almost always exceeded when it attempts to join with government to first judge the masses incompetent and then restrict their personal choices.

I grow particularly nervous when even the most distinguished researchers transcend their callings to campaign for product taxes and bans or, most egregiously, to vaguely advocate for the regulation of "unhealthy aspects of diet and lifestyle." Science's time-tested authority springs vibrantly from its practitioners' exacting and impartial roles as explorers, skeptics, and even teachers. But never has it spawned from the deluded cravings of some to act as our parents or priests.

Notes

1. The authors dispute the common assertion that these diseases are caused by obesity. Rather, they argue, obesity is merely "a marker for metabolic dysfunction, which is even more prevalent." In support, they cite statistics showing that 20 percent of obese people have normal metabolism and that 40 percent of normal-weight people develop metabolic syndrome.
2. Neither "inalienable" nor "unalienable" rights are listed in the Constitution, of course. But three of the latter—life, liberty, and the pursuit of happiness—are enshrined in the Declaration of Independence. Katz and others might wish to reexamine their historical and philosophical significance.

KENNETH W. KRAUSE is a contributing editor, book editor, and "The Good Book" columnist for *The Humanist* and a contributing editor and columnist for *Skeptical Inquirer*.

EXPLORING THE ISSUE

Are Restrictions on Sugar and Sugary Beverages Justified?

Critical Thinking and Reflection

1. What impact would restriction of sugar and sugary beverages have on our right to make individual choices?
2. Do the health risks of sugar warrant bans on the sale of large sized sugary beverages?
3. Describe the role government should play in regard to prevention of obesity.

Is There Common Ground?

Jacob Sullum, in "The War on Fat: Is the Size of Your Butt the Government's Business?" (*Reason*, August/September 2004), grants that while obesity is a health problem, it should not be a government issue. Despite Sullum's views, Americans have been steadily gaining weight over the past 30 years. Children, in particular, have grown heavier for a variety of reasons including less physical activity, more eating away from home, and increased portion sizes. Food manufacturers advertise an increasing array of non-nutritious foods to children while schools offer these foods in the cafeteria. With the success of the antismoking forces, some nutritionists see the government as the answer to the obesity problem. Increased taxes on junk food, warning labels on non-nutritious food packages, and restrictions on advertising have all been discussed as a means of improving the nation's nutritional status. In "The Perils of Ignoring History: Big Tobacco Played Dirty and Millions Died. How Similar Is Big Food?" (*Milbank Quarterly*, March 2009), the authors discussed how in 1954 the tobacco industry paid to publish the "Frank Statement to Cigarette Smokers" in hundreds of U.S. newspapers. It stated that the public's health was the industry's concern above all others and promised a variety of good-faith changes. What followed were years of lies and actions that cost countless lives. The tobacco industry had a script that focused on personal responsibility, paying scientists who delivered research that instilled doubt, criticizing the "junk" science that found risks associated with smoking, making self-regulatory pledges, lobbying with massive resources to stifle government action, introducing "safer" products, and simultaneously manipulating and denying both the addictive nature of their products and their marketing to children. The script of the food industry is both similar to and different from the tobacco industry script. Food is quite different from tobacco, and the food industry differs from tobacco companies in other ways, but there are also major similarities in the actions that these two industries have taken in response to concern that their products cause disease. Because obesity is now a major global problem, the world cannot afford a repeat of the tobacco history. If sugary food advertisements were banned from children's television, less might be consumed.

Other proposals to improve Americans' diets include levying a tax on sugary foods such as soft drinks, candy, and sugared cereals and the ban on trans fats in New York City. While many states already tax these items if purchased in a restaurant or grocery store, proponents argue that these foods should be taxed regardless of where purchased. While this may seem to be a reasonable approach to address the problem, it is not approved by all. The food industry, understandably, is not in favor of any of these measures.

Additional Resources

Grynbaum, M. M. (2012, July 24). Fighting ban on big sodas with appeals to patriotism. *New York Times*, p. 18.

Jacobson, M. E., & Lusk, J. L. (2014). At issue: Should the government tax sugary soda? *CQ Researcher*, *24*(35), 833.

Jacobson, M. F. (2014). Time to rein in "big soda." *Nutrition Action Health Letter*, *41*(5), 2.

Lustig, R. H., Schmidt, L. A., & Brindis, C. D. (2012). The toxic truth about sugar. *Nature*, *482*, 27–29.

Sullum, J. (2012). Bloomberg's big beverage ban. *Reason*, *44*(5), 8.

Internet References . . .

The American Dietetic Association

www.eatright.org

Center for Science in the Public Interest (CSPI)

www.cspinet.org

Food and Nutrition Information Center

http://fnic.nal.usda.gov/

The Sugar Association, Inc.

www.sugar.org

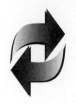

Unit 6

UNIT

Consumer Health Issues

A shift is occurring in medical care toward informed self-care. People are starting to reclaim their autonomy, and the relationship between doctor and patient is changing. Many patients are asking more questions of their physicians, considering a wider range of medical options, accessing medical information online, focusing on prevention, and in general, becoming more educated about what determines their health. They are also concerned about the quality of numerous consumer health products, prescription and over-the-counter drugs, and services available to them. This section addresses consumer issues and initiatives that empower consumers to make decisions and take actions that improve personal, family, and community health.

Selected, Edited, and with Issue Framing Material by:
Eileen L. Daniel, *SUNY College at Brockport*

ISSUE

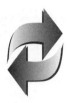

Is Weight-Loss Maintenance Possible?

YES: Barbara Berkeley, from "The Fat Trap: My Response," *refusetoregain.com* (2011)

NO: Tara Parker-Pope, from "The Fat Trap," *The New York Times Magazine* (2011)

Learning Outcomes

After reading this issue, you will be able to:

- Discuss why it is so difficult for many people to maintain weight loss.
- Discuss the argument that weight-loss maintenance is not possible for most people.
- Discuss the risk factors associated with obesity and overweight.

ISSUE SUMMARY

YES: Physician Barbara Berkeley believes that weight maintenance is not easy but possible as long as people separate themselves from the world of typical American eating. She also claims that some individuals are heavy because they are susceptible to the modern diet or because they use food for comfort.

NO: Journalist Tara Parker-Pope disagrees and maintains that there are biological imperatives that cause people to regain all the weight they lose and for those genetically inclined to obesity, it's almost impossible to maintain weight loss.

While the number of Americans who diet varies, depending on the source, the Boston Medical Center indicates that approximately 45 million Americans diet each year and spend $33 billion on weight-loss products in their pursuit of a trimmer, fitter body. Currently, about two-thirds of American adults are overweight including more than one-third who are classified as obese. This is almost 20 percent more than 20 years ago. Obesity can double mortality and can reduce life expectancy by 10–20 years. If current trends continue, the average American's life expectancy will actually begin to decline by 5 years. Obesity is linked to unhealthy blood fat levels including cholesterol and heart disease. Other health risks associated with obesity include high blood pressure, some cancers, diabetes, gallbladder and kidney disease, sleep disorders, arthritis, and other bone and joint disorders. Obesity is also linked to complications of pregnancy, stress incontinence, and elevated surgical risk. The risks from obesity rise with its severity, and they are much more likely to occur among people more than double their recommended body weight. Obesity can impact psychological as well as physical well-being. Being obese can contribute to psychological problems including depression, anxiety, and low self-esteem.

Since 1990, the prevalence of overweight and obesity has been rising in the United States. Despite public health campaigns, the trend shows little sign of changing. A 2006 campaign conducted by Ogden et al. ("Prevalence of Overweight and Obesity in the US 1999–2004," *JAMA*, vol. 295, 2006) reported that during the 6-year period from 1999 to 2004, the prevalence of overweight in children and adolescents increased significantly, as did the prevalence of obesity in men. Along with these rising rates of obesity come increased rates of obesity-related health issues. There has been a 60 percent rise in type 2 diabetes since 1990. Inactivity and overweight may be responsible for as many as 112,000 premature deaths each year in the United States, second only to smoking-related deaths.

According to the U.S. Department of Agriculture (USDA), the average American has increased his/her caloric intake by more than 500 calories per day while levels of physical activity have decreased. This is related to more meals eaten away from the home, which typically are higher in calories, fat, sugar, and salt. Restaurants also tend to serve larger portions than home-cooked meals. Many Americans are also sleep deprived. Lack of sleep appears to trigger weight gain. Finally, Americans are more engaged in sedentary activities and less likely to engage in physical activity on a regular basis. Whatever the cause of obesity, its incidence and prevalence appear to be rising and it is linked to multiple health concerns.

Because of health and appearance concerns, many Americans attempt to lose weight by dieting and/or exercise. Types of weight-loss diets typically include reduced calories or a reduction of a major nutrient such as fat or carbohydrates. Interestingly, most studies find no difference between the main diet types and subsequent weight loss. However, long-term studies of dieting indicate that the majority of individuals who lose weight regain virtually all of the weight that was lost after dieting, regardless of whether they maintain their diet or exercise program.

The YES and NO selections address whether it is possible to diet, lose weight, and actually maintain that weight loss. Barbara Berkeley maintains that while it's not easy to maintain lost pounds, it is certainly possible. Tara Parker-Pope disagrees and believes that our biological makeup causes us to regain weight and for most people, it's almost impossible to maintain a weight loss.

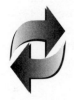

YES ⬅

Barbara Berkeley

The Fat Trap: My Response

Once a month, in a small room off the lobby of Lake West Hospital in Willoughby, Ohio, a special group convenes. For someone observing the group and unaware of its purpose, it might appear to be a simple mix of everyday people . . . young, old, racially diverse. The members would seem to be old friends but with a particular seriousness of purpose, perhaps a community group attending a lecture or learning some new skill together. What a casual observer would not guess is that each of these people was once obese, some having weighed over 100 pounds more than they do today.

Our Refuse to Regain group is an experiment, a safe haven for maintainers who have lost weight in many different ways and now face the reality of reconstructing their lives. We've had people from Weight Watchers, people who've undergone bariatric surgery, people I've treated in my practice and others who simply did it on their own. A weight loss diet is no different than emptying the trash. It doesn't matter which technique you use to toss out the garbage. But learning how to avoid the reaccumulation of unwanted junk is a completely different skill. There are many basics in this process that will be the same for everyone. There are also many specifics that will vary from person to person and which must be individually discovered.

Here's some of what we've learned so far:

1. Weight maintenance is possible. There is nothing in our group experience (or in my personal clinical experience) to suggest that the body "forces" one to regain.
2. Weight maintenance requires a separation from the world of "normal" American eating . . . which is not normal at all.
3. Some people are heavy simply because they are susceptible to the modern diet, no more no less. Others are heavy because they use food for soothing or sedation. Most people are a mix of both. If psychological issues are a *major* part of weight gain—significantly beyond the common enjoyment of food for pleasure, they need to be addressed during the maintenance phase.
4. Weight maintainers are special people who live on a kind of food island. It's really nice to know that the island is inhabited, often with fascinating, determined people just like you. Rarely do maintainers get to meet and talk with one another.

This week, I gave my group a reading assignment. That was a first. I asked everyone to read Tara Parker Pope's article on weight maintenance called *The Fat Trap.* This article is currently online and will appear in Sunday's *New York Times Magazine.* Our group will be discussing it at our January meeting, but I'll give you a preview of my reaction here. Many of you may be reading our blog because you read "The Fat Trap" and discovered Lynn Haraldson, my blogging partner on this site. The fact that you got here likely means that you are interested in knowing whether we are bound to regain the weight we lose, so please, read on . . . leave comments and join the discussion.

For those of you who are new to this blog, you should know that I am a physician who has specialized in weight management since the late 1980s. This is the only thing I do and that's unusual. Why? Because most doctors are not particularly interested in obesity, and certainly weren't back in the 80s. Over the past twenty years, a continuing source of frustration for me has been the willingness of doctors and the general public to accept "truths" about weight loss that are the beliefs of everyone *except* those who actually work with overweight people.

Scientific research needs to square with what we see in clinical practice. If it doesn't, we should question its validity. "The Fat Trap" is an article that starts with a single, small research study and builds around it. Its point? That there are inevitable biological imperatives that cause people to regain all the weight they lose.

I don't buy it.

Here is the opening paragraph of Ms. Parker Pope's article:

> For 15 years, Joseph Proietto has been helping people lose weight. When these obese patients arrive at his weight-loss clinic in Australia, they are determined to slim down. And most of the time, he says, they do just that, sticking to the clinic's program and dropping excess pounds. But then, almost without exception, the weight begins to creep back. In a matter of months or years, the entire effort has come undone, and the patient is fat again.

At one time, this was my experience too. But things have changed. After years of focusing my practice much more on weight maintenance, writing a book about it, and trying to figure out how to teach and encourage it, I no longer see patients with an "entire effort come undone." Instead, I see more and more people learning how to become successfully anchored at their new weight. And these POWs (previous overweight people) are not from my practice alone. They are people like Lynn Haraldson and her friends "The Maintaining Divas." They are the long term POWs who write to me via this blog, on Facebook and on Twitter. They are the people I hear about with increasing frequency every day.

I admire Ms. Parker Pope for acknowledging her own struggles with weight, but as someone who has not yet solved the maintenance problem I would submit that she is not the best person to rationally evaluate evidence that says that regain is inevitable. After talking to a number of scientists who believe that the body fights weight loss, her concluding paragraph says:

> For me, understanding the science of weight loss has helped make sense of my own struggles to lose weight, as well as my mother's endless cycle of dieting, weight gain and despair. I wish she were still here so I could persuade her to finally forgive herself for her dieting failures. While I do, ultimately, blame myself for allowing my weight to get out of control, it has been somewhat liberating to learn that there are factors other than my character at work when it comes to gaining and losing weight.

Those of us who come from families which struggle with obesity can believe one of two things. We can believe that biological and metabolic factors doom us to fatness or we can believe that we come from families who are very sensitive to the current food environment and

perhaps need to live in a new and more creative way. It has been my experience that all successful maintainers have learned how to live a life that exists outside the current food norms. For some, this is a daily and difficult challenge and for others it becomes a simple and treasured way of life, but either way, it is not about some inevitable biological destiny. Rather, these maintainers have come to terms with the fact that they are ancient bodies and souls living in a modern environment and that our food culture is capable of killing them. Controlling that environment is their choice and their challenge.

Where I do agree with "The Fat Trap" is in its assertion that obesity is much more difficult to deal with once it is established. We would do well to focus intense and constant attention on healthful nutrition during pregnancy and in childhood. I believe that we can do this much more easily than we believe, if we would only adopt the idea that we should eat more like we did originally as hunter-gatherers. It has been my clinical experience that elimination (or major curtailment) of starches and sugars (including whole grains and the things that come from them, by the way) simply works. And this clinical observation makes sense, since the ancestors whose genes we carry were not exposed to the large amounts of starch and sugar we now eat. Along with consumption of real food . . . not things in boxes, cans, or packages . . . this easy concept can change lives. We could make things so much easier by teaching this lesson to kids rather than endlessly focusing them on percents of fat, protein and carbs and on counting calories.

But such approaches to weight maintenance are not easily sold. It's far simpler to believe that weight must be regained. I'm fond of using this example for patients: If you were to tell your friends that you are becoming vegetarian and that you will no longer touch a drop of red meat, fish, or poultry, no one would blink an eye. You'd probably be encouraged and congratulated. If, on the other hand, you announced that you were giving up sugar and grain, the same friends would be horrified. "You mean you're never going to have another piece of bread???"

I believe that the resistance to finding the maintenance solution comes from the addictive nature of starch and sugar foods. I also believe that most of America and other SAD (standard American diet) countries are operating "under the influence" of addictive carbs. Life without them, or even with LESS of them, is too awful to contemplate.

But I digress. To return to my original point, I want to forcefully say that we must stop finding reasons we can't maintain and start getting much, much better at teaching people how to do it. Support networks, communication between maintainers, and many more books, advocates, and techniques that focus on maintenance are key.

I believe I may scream if I see yet another book with a catchy title that touts yet another weight loss approach without ever talking about what happens in the after-diet world. January is the month for those glossy little productions.

Time to get serious. Maintenance can be done, and if you want to meet the people who are doing it, hang around this blog.

BARBARA BERKELEY is a physician and diplomate of the American Board of Internal Medicine and the American Board of Obesity Medicine. She has specialized in the care of overweight and obese patients since 1988.

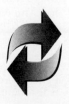

Tara Parker-Pope

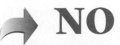 **NO**

The Fat Trap

For 15 years, Joseph Proietto has been helping people lose weight. When these obese patients arrive at his weight-loss clinic in Australia, they are determined to slim down. And most of the time, he says, they do just that, sticking to the clinic's program and dropping excess pounds. But then, almost without exception, the weight begins to creep back. In a matter of months or years, the entire effort has come undone, and the patient is fat again. "It has always seemed strange to me," says Proietto, who is a physician at the University of Melbourne. "These are people who are very motivated to lose weight, who achieve weight loss most of the time without too much trouble and yet, inevitably, gradually, they regain the weight."

Anyone who has ever dieted knows that lost pounds often return, and most of us assume the reason is a lack of discipline or a failure of willpower. But Proietto suspected that there was more to it, and he decided to take a closer look at the biological state of the body after weight loss.

Beginning in 2009, he and his team recruited 50 obese men and women. The men weighed an average of 233 pounds; the women weighed about 200 pounds. Although some people dropped out of the study, most of the patients stuck with the extreme low-calorie diet, which consisted of special shakes called Optifast and two cups of low-starch vegetables, totaling just 500 to 550 calories a day for eight weeks. Ten weeks in, the dieters lost an average of 30 pounds.

At that point, the 34 patients who remained stopped dieting and began working to maintain the new lower weight. Nutritionists counseled them in person and by phone, promoting regular exercise and urging them to eat more vegetables and less fat. But despite the effort, they slowly began to put on weight. After a year, the patients already had regained an average of 11 of the pounds they struggled so hard to lose. They also reported feeling far more hungry and preoccupied with food than before they lost the weight.

While researchers have known for decades that the body undergoes various metabolic and hormonal changes while it's losing weight, the Australian team detected something new. A full year after significant weight loss, these men and women remained in what could be described as a biologically altered state. Their still-plump bodies were acting as if they were starving and were working overtime to regain the pounds they lost. For instance, a gastric hormone called ghrelin, often dubbed the "hunger hormone," was about 20 percent higher than at the start of the study. Another hormone associated with suppressing hunger, peptide YY, was also abnormally low. Levels of leptin, a hormone that suppresses hunger and increases metabolism, also remained lower than expected. A cocktail of other hormones associated with hunger and metabolism all remained significantly changed compared to pre-dieting levels. It was almost as if weight loss had put their bodies into a unique metabolic state, a sort of post-dieting syndrome that set them apart from people who hadn't tried to lose weight in the first place. "What we see here is a coordinated defense mechanism with multiple components all directed toward making us put on weight," Proietto says. "This, I think, explains the high failure rate in obesity treatment."

While the findings from Proietto and colleagues, published this fall in *The New England Journal of Medicine,* are not conclusive—the study was small and the findings need to be replicated—the research has nonetheless caused a stir in the weight-loss community, adding to a growing body of evidence that challenges conventional thinking about obesity, weight loss and willpower. For years, the advice to the overweight and obese has been that we simply need to eat less and exercise more. While there is truth to this guidance, it fails to take into account that the human body continues to fight against weight loss long after dieting has stopped. This translates into a sobering reality: once we become fat, most of us, despite our best efforts, will probably stay fat.

I have always felt perplexed about my inability to keep weight off. I know the medical benefits of weight loss, and I don't drink sugary sodas or eat fast food. I exercise regularly—a few years ago, I even completed a marathon. Yet during the 23 years since graduating from college, I've lost 10 or 20 pounds at a time, maintained it for a little while and then gained it all back and more, to the point where I am now easily 60 pounds overweight.

I wasn't overweight as a child, but I can't remember a time when my mother, whose weight probably fluctuated between 150 and 250 pounds, wasn't either on a diet or, in her words, cheating on her diet. Sometimes we ate healthful, balanced meals; on other days dinner consisted of a bucket of Kentucky Fried Chicken. As a high-school cross-country runner, I never worried about weight, but in college, when my regular training runs were squeezed out by studying and socializing, the numbers on the scale slowly began to move up. As adults, my three sisters and I all struggle with weight, as do many members of my extended family. My mother died of esophageal cancer six years ago. It was her great regret that in the days before she died, the closest medical school turned down her offer to donate her body because she was obese.

It's possible that the biological cards were stacked against me from the start. Researchers know that obesity tends to run in families, and recent science suggests that even the desire to eat higher-calorie foods may be influenced by heredity. But untangling how much is genetic and how much is learned through family eating habits is difficult. What is clear is that some people appear to be prone to accumulating extra fat while others seem to be protected against it.

In a seminal series of experiments published in the 1990s, the Canadian researchers Claude Bouchard and Angelo Tremblay studied 31 pairs of male twins ranging in age from 17 to 29, who were sometimes overfed and sometimes put on diets. (None of the twin pairs were at risk for obesity based on their body mass or their family history.) In one study, 12 sets of the twins were put under 24-hour supervision in a college dormitory. Six days a week they ate 1,000 extra calories a day, and one day they were allowed to eat normally. They could read, play video games, play cards and watch television, but exercise was limited to one 30-minute daily walk. Over the course of the 120-day study, the twins consumed 84,000 extra calories beyond their basic needs.

That experimental binge should have translated into a weight gain of roughly 24 pounds (based on 3,500 calories to a pound). But some gained less than 10 pounds, while others gained as much as 29 pounds. The amount of weight gained and how the fat was distributed around the body closely matched among brothers, but varied considerably among the different sets of twins. Some brothers gained three times as much fat around their abdomens as others, for instance. When the researchers conducted similar exercise studies with the twins, they saw the patterns in reverse, with some twin sets losing more pounds than others on the same exercise regimen. The findings, the researchers wrote, suggest a form of "biological determinism" that can make a person susceptible to weight gain or loss.

But while there is widespread agreement that at least some risk for obesity is inherited, identifying a specific genetic cause has been a challenge. In October 2010, the journal *Nature Genetics* reported that researchers have so far confirmed 32 distinct genetic variations associated with obesity or body-mass index. One of the most common of these variations was identified in April 2007 by a British team studying the genetics of Type 2 diabetes. According to Timothy Frayling at the Institute of Biomedical and Clinical Science at the University of Exeter, people who carried a variant known as FTO faced a much higher risk of obesity—30 percent higher if they had one copy of the variant; 60 percent if they had two.

This FTO variant is surprisingly common; about 65 percent of people of European or African descent and an estimated 27 to 44 percent of Asians are believed to carry at least one copy of it. Scientists don't understand how the FTO variation influences weight gain, but studies in children suggest the trait plays a role in eating habits. In one 2008 study led by Colin Palmer of the University of Dundee in Scotland, Scottish schoolchildren were given snacks of orange drinks and muffins and then allowed to graze on a buffet of grapes, celery, potato chips and chocolate buttons. All the food was carefully monitored so the researchers knew exactly what was consumed. Although all the children ate about the same amount of food, as weighed in grams, children with the FTO variant were more likely to eat foods with higher fat and calorie content. They weren't gorging themselves, but they consumed, on average, about 100 calories more than children who didn't carry the gene. Those who had the gene variant had about four pounds more body fat than noncarriers.

I have been tempted to send in my own saliva sample for a DNA test to find out if my family carries a genetic predisposition for obesity. But even if the test came back negative, it would only mean that my family doesn't carry a known, testable genetic risk for obesity. Recently the British television show "Embarrassing Fat Bodies" asked Frayling's lab to test for fat-promoting genes, and the results showed one very overweight family had a lower-than-average risk for obesity.

A positive result, telling people they are genetically inclined to stay fat, might be self-fulfilling. In February, *The New England Journal of Medicine* published a report on how genetic testing for a variety of diseases affected a person's mood and health habits. Overall, the researchers found no effect from disease-risk testing, but there was a suggestion, though it didn't reach statistical significance, that after testing positive for fat-promoting genes, some people were more likely to eat fatty foods, presumably because they thought being fat was their genetic destiny and saw no sense in fighting it.

While knowing my genetic risk might satisfy my curiosity, I also know that heredity, at best, would explain only part of why I became overweight. I'm much more interested in figuring out what I can do about it now.

The National Weight Control Registry tracks 10,000 people who have lost weight and have kept it off. "We set it up in response to comments that nobody ever succeeds at weight loss," says Rena Wing, a professor of psychiatry and human behavior at Brown University's Alpert Medical School, who helped create the registry with James O. Hill, director of the Center for Human Nutrition at the University of Colorado at Denver. "We had two goals: to prove there were people who did, and to try to learn from them about what they do to achieve this long-term weight loss." Anyone who has lost 30 pounds and kept it off for at least a year is eligible to join the study, though the average member has lost 70 pounds and remained at that weight for six years.

Wing says that she agrees that physiological changes probably do occur that make permanent weight loss difficult, but she says the larger problem is environmental, and that people struggle to keep weight off because they are surrounded by food, inundated with food messages and constantly presented with opportunities to eat. "We live in an environment with food cues all the time," Wing says. "We've taught ourselves over the years that one of the ways to reward yourself is with food. It's hard to change the environment and the behavior."

There is no consistent pattern to how people in the registry lost weight—some did it on Weight Watchers, others with Jenny Craig, some by cutting carbs on the Atkins diet and a very small number lost weight through surgery. But their eating and exercise habits appear to reflect what researchers find in the lab: to lose weight and keep it off, a person must eat fewer calories and exercise far more than a person who maintains the same weight naturally. Registry members exercise about an hour or more each day—the average weight-loser puts in the equivalent of a four-mile daily walk, seven days a week. They get on a scale every day in order to keep their weight within a

narrow range. They eat breakfast regularly. Most watch less than half as much television as the overall population. They eat the same foods and in the same patterns consistently each day and don't "cheat" on weekends or holidays. They also appear to eat less than most people, with estimates ranging from 50 to 300 fewer daily calories.

Kelly Brownell, director of the Rudd Center for Food Policy and Obesity at Yale University, says that while the 10,000 people tracked in the registry are a useful resource, they also represent a tiny percentage of the tens of millions of people who have tried unsuccessfully to lose weight. "All it means is that there are rare individuals who do manage to keep it off," Brownell says. "You find these people are incredibly vigilant about maintaining their weight. Years later they are paying attention to every calorie, spending an hour a day on exercise. They never don't think about their weight."

Janice Bridge, a registry member who has successfully maintained a 135-pound weight loss for about five years, is a perfect example. "It's one of the hardest things there is," she says. "It's something that has to be focused on every minute. I'm not always thinking about food, but I am always aware of food." Bridge, who is 66 and lives in Davis, Calif., was overweight as a child and remembers going on her first diet of 1,400 calories a day at 14. At the time, her slow pace of weight loss prompted her doctor to accuse her of cheating. Friends told her she must not be paying attention to what she was eating. "No one would believe me that I was doing everything I was told," she says. "You can imagine how tremendously depressing it was and what a feeling of rebellion and anger was building up."

After peaking at 330 pounds in 2004, she tried again to lose weight. She managed to drop 30 pounds, but then her weight loss stalled. In 2006, at age 60, she joined a medically supervised weight-loss program with her husband, Adam, who weighed 310 pounds. After nine months on an 800-calorie diet, she slimmed down to 165 pounds. Adam lost about 110 pounds and now weighs about 200.

During the first years after her weight loss, Bridge tried to test the limits of how much she could eat. She used exercise to justify eating more. The death of her mother in 2009 consumed her attention; she lost focus and slowly regained 30 pounds. She has decided to try to maintain this higher weight of 195, which is still 135 pounds [less] than her heaviest weight.

"It doesn't take a lot of variance from my current maintenance for me to pop on another two or three pounds," she says. "It's been a real struggle to stay at this weight, but it's worth it, it's good for me, it makes me feel better. But my body would put on weight almost instantaneously if I ever let up."

So she never lets up. Since October 2006 she has weighed herself every morning and recorded the result in a weight diary. She even carries a scale with her when she travels. In the past six years, she made only one exception to this routine: a two-week, no-weigh vacation in Hawaii.

She also weighs everything in the kitchen. She knows that lettuce is about 5 calories a cup, while flour is about 400. If she goes out to dinner, she conducts a Web search first to look at the menu and calculate calories to help her decide what to order. She avoids anything with sugar or white flour, which she calls her "gateway drugs" for cravings and overeating. She has also found that drinking copious amounts of water seems to help; she carries a 20-ounce water bottle and fills it five times a day. She writes down everything she eats. At night, she transfers all the information to an electronic record. Adam also keeps track but prefers to keep his record with pencil and paper.

"That transfer process is really important; it's my accountability," she says. "It comes up with the total number of calories I've eaten today and the amount of protein. I do a little bit of self-analysis every night."

Bridge and her husband each sought the help of therapists, and in her sessions, Janice learned that she had a tendency to eat when she was bored or stressed. "We are very much aware of how our culture taught us to use food for all kinds of reasons that aren't related to its nutritive value," Bridge says. Bridge supports her careful diet with an equally rigorous regimen of physical activity. She exercises from 100 to 120 minutes a day, six or seven days a week, often by riding her bicycle to the gym, where she takes a water-aerobics class. She also works out on an elliptical trainer at home and uses a recumbent bike to "walk" the dog, who loves to run alongside the low, three-wheeled machine. She enjoys gardening as a hobby but allows herself to count it as exercise on only those occasions when she needs to "garden vigorously." Adam is also a committed exerciser, riding his bike at least two hours a day, five days a week.

Janice Bridge has used years of her exercise and diet data to calculate her own personal fuel efficiency. She knows that her body burns about three calories a minute during gardening, about four calories a minute on the recumbent bike and during water aerobics and about five a minute when she zips around town on her regular bike.

"Practically anyone will tell you someone biking is going to burn 11 calories a minute," she says. "That's not my body. I know it because of the statistics I've kept."

Based on metabolism data she collected from the weight-loss clinic and her own calculations, she has discovered that to keep her current weight of 195 pounds, she can eat 2,000 calories a day as long as she burns 500 calories in exercise. She avoids junk food, bread and pasta and many dairy products and tries to make sure nearly a third of her calories come from protein. The Bridges will occasionally share a dessert, or eat an individual portion of Ben and Jerry's ice cream, so they know exactly how many calories they are ingesting. Because she knows errors can creep in, either because a rainy day cuts exercise short or a mismeasured snack portion adds hidden calories, she allows herself only 1,800 daily calories of food. (The average estimate for a similarly active woman of her age and size is about 2,300 calories.)

Just talking to Bridge about the effort required to maintain her weight is exhausting. I find her story inspiring, but it also makes me wonder whether I have what it takes to be thin. I have tried on several occasions (and as recently as a couple weeks ago) to keep a daily diary of my eating and exercise habits, but it's easy to let it slide. I can't quite imagine how I would ever make time to weigh and measure food when some days it's all I can do to get dinner on the table between finishing my work and carting my daughter to dance class or volleyball practice. And while I enjoy exercising for 30- or 40-minute stretches, I also learned from six months of marathon training that devoting one to two hours a day to exercise takes an impossible toll on my family life.

Bridge concedes that having grown children and being retired make it easier to focus on her weight. "I don't know if I could have done this when I had three kids living at home," she says. "We know how unusual we are. It's pretty easy to get angry with the amount of work and dedication it takes to keep this weight off. But the alternative is to not keep the weight off."

"I think many people who are anxious to lose weight don't fully understand what the consequences are going to be, nor does the medical community fully explain this to people," Rudolph Leibel, an obesity researcher at Columbia University in New York, says. "We don't want to make them feel hopeless, but we do want to make them understand that they are trying to buck a biological system that is going to try to make it hard for them."

Leibel and his colleague Michael Rosenbaum have pioneered much of what we know about the body's response to weight loss. For 25 years, they have meticulously tracked about 130 individuals for six months or longer at a stretch. The subjects reside at their research clinic where every aspect of their bodies is measured. Body fat is determined by bone-scan machines. A special hood monitors oxygen consumption and carbon-dioxide output to precisely measure metabolism. Calories burned during digestion are tracked. Exercise tests measure maximum heart rate, while blood tests measure hormones and brain chemicals. Muscle biopsies are taken to analyze their metabolic efficiency. (Early in the research, even stool samples were collected and tested to make sure no calories went unaccounted for.) For their trouble, participants are paid $5,000 to $8,000.

Eventually, the Columbia subjects are placed on liquid diets of 800 calories a day until they lose 10 percent of their body weight. Once they reach the goal, they are subjected to another round of intensive testing as they try to maintain the new weight. The data generated by these experiments suggest that once a person loses about 10 percent of body weight, he or she is metabolically different than a similar-size person who is naturally the same weight.

The research shows that the changes that occur after weight loss translate to a huge caloric disadvantage of about 250 to 400 calories. For instance, one woman who entered the Columbia studies at 230 pounds was eating about 3,000 calories to maintain that weight. Once she dropped to 190 pounds, losing 17 percent of her body weight, metabolic studies determined that she needed about 2,300 daily calories to maintain the new lower weight. That may sound like plenty, but the typical 30-year-old 190-pound woman can consume about 2,600 calories to maintain her weight—300 more calories than the woman who dieted to get there.

Scientists are still learning why a weight-reduced body behaves so differently from a similar-size body that has not dieted. Muscle biopsies taken before, during and after weight loss show that once a person drops weight, their muscle fibers undergo a transformation, making them more like highly efficient "slow twitch" muscle fibers. A result is that after losing weight, your muscles burn 20 to 25 percent fewer calories during everyday activity and moderate aerobic exercise than those of a person who is naturally at the same weight. That means a dieter who thinks she is burning 200 calories during a brisk half-hour walk is probably using closer to 150 to 160 calories.

Another way that the body seems to fight weight loss is by altering the way the brain responds to food. Rosenbaum and his colleague Joy Hirsch, a neuroscientist also at Columbia, used functional magnetic resonance imaging to track the brain patterns of people before and after weight loss while they looked at objects like grapes, Gummi Bears, chocolate, broccoli, cellphones and yo-yos. After weight loss, when the dieter looked at food, the scans showed a bigger response in the parts of the brain associated with reward and a lower response in the areas associated with control. This suggests that the body, in order to get back to its pre-diet weight, induces

cravings by making the person feel more excited about food and giving him or her less willpower to resist a high-calorie treat.

"After you've lost weight, your brain has a greater emotional response to food," Rosenbaum says. "You want it more, but the areas of the brain involved in restraint are less active." Combine that with a body that is now burning fewer calories than expected, he says, "and you've created the perfect storm for weight regain." How long this state lasts isn't known, but preliminary research at Columbia suggests that for as many as six years after weight loss, the body continues to defend the old, higher weight by burning off far fewer calories than would be expected. The problem could persist indefinitely. (The same phenomenon occurs when a thin person tries to drop about 10 percent of his or her body weight—the body defends the higher weight.) This doesn't mean it's impossible to lose weight and keep it off; it just means it's really, really difficult.

Lynn Haraldson, a 48-year-old woman who lives in Pittsburgh, reached 300 pounds in 2000. She joined Weight Watchers and managed to take her 5-foot-5 body down to 125 pounds for a brief time. Today, she's a member of the National Weight Control Registry and maintains about 140 pounds by devoting her life to weight maintenance. She became a vegetarian, writes down what she eats every day, exercises at least five days a week and blogs about the challenges of weight maintenance. A former journalist and antiques dealer, she returned to school for a two-year program on nutrition and health; she plans to become a dietary counselor. She has also come to accept that she can never stop being "hypervigilant" about what she eats. "Everything has to change," she says. "I've been up and down the scale so many times, always thinking I can go back to 'normal,' but I had to establish a new normal. People don't like hearing that it's not easy."

What's not clear from the research is whether there is a window during which we can gain weight and then lose it without creating biological backlash. Many people experience transient weight gain, putting on a few extra pounds during the holidays or gaining 10 or 20 pounds during the first years of college that they lose again. The actor Robert De Niro lost weight after bulking up for his performance in "Raging Bull." The filmmaker Morgan Spurlock also lost the weight he gained during the making of "Super Size Me." Leibel says that whether these temporary pounds became permanent probably depends on a person's genetic risk for obesity and, perhaps, the length of time a person carried the extra weight before trying to lose it. But researchers don't know how long it takes for the body to reset itself permanently to a higher weight. The good news is that it doesn't seem to happen overnight.

"For a mouse, I know the time period is somewhere around eight months," Leibel says. "Before that time, a fat mouse can come back to being a skinny mouse again without too much adjustment. For a human we don't know, but I'm pretty sure it's not measured in months, but in years."

Nobody wants to be fat. In most modern cultures, even if you are healthy—in my case, my cholesterol and blood pressure are low and I have an extraordinarily healthy heart—to be fat is to be perceived as weak-willed and lazy. It's also just embarrassing. Once, at a party, I met a well-respected writer who knew my work as a health writer. "You're not at all what I expected," she said, eyes widening. The man I was dating, perhaps trying to help, finished the thought. "You thought she'd be thinner, right?" he said. I wanted to disappear, but the woman was gracious. "No," she said, casting a glare at the man and reaching to warmly shake my hand. "I thought you'd be older."

If anything, the emerging science of weight loss teaches us that perhaps we should rethink our biases about people who are overweight. It is true that people who are overweight, including myself, get that way because they eat too many calories relative to what their bodies need. But a number of biological and genetic factors can play a role in determining exactly how much food is too much for any given individual. Clearly, weight loss is an intense struggle, one in which we are not fighting simply hunger or cravings for sweets, but our own bodies.

While the public discussion about weight loss tends to come down to which diet works best (Atkins? Jenny Craig? Plant-based? Mediterranean?), those who have tried and failed at all of these diets know there is no simple answer. Fat, sugar and carbohydrates in processed foods may very well be culprits in the nation's obesity problem. But there is tremendous variation in an individual's response.

The view of obesity as primarily a biological, rather than psychological, disease could also lead to changes in the way we approach its treatment. Scientists at Columbia have conducted several small studies looking at whether injecting people with leptin, the hormone made by body fat, can override the body's resistance to weight loss and help maintain a lower weight. In a few small studies, leptin injections appear to trick the body into thinking it's still fat. After leptin replacement, study subjects burned more calories during activity. And in brain-scan studies, leptin injections appeared to change how the brain responded to food, making it seem less enticing. But such treatments are

still years away from commercial development. For now, those of us who want to lose weight and keep it off are on our own.

One question many researchers think about is whether losing weight more slowly would make it more sustainable than the fast weight loss often used in scientific studies. Leibel says the pace of weight loss is unlikely to make a difference, because the body's warning system is based solely on how much fat a person loses, not how quickly he or she loses it. Even so, Proietto is now conducting a study using a slower weight-loss method and following dieters for three years instead of one.

Given how hard it is to lose weight, it's clear, from a public-health standpoint, that resources would best be focused on preventing weight gain. The research underscores the urgency of national efforts to get children to exercise and eat healthful foods.

But with a third of the U.S. adult population classified as obese, nobody is saying people who already are very overweight should give up on weight loss. Instead, the solution may be to preach a more realistic goal. Studies suggest that even a 5 percent weight loss can lower a person's risk for diabetes, heart disease and other health problems associated with obesity. There is also speculation that the body is more willing to accept small amounts of weight loss.

But an obese person who loses just 5 percent of her body weight will still very likely be obese. For a 250-pound woman, a 5 percent weight loss of about 12 pounds probably won't even change her clothing size. Losing a few pounds may be good for the body, but it does very little for the spirit and is unlikely to change how fat people feel about themselves or how others perceive them.

So where does that leave a person who wants to lose a sizable amount of weight? Weight-loss scientists say they believe that once more people understand the genetic and biological challenges of keeping weight off, doctors and patients will approach weight loss more realistically and more compassionately. At the very least, the science may compel people who are already overweight to work harder to make sure they don't put on additional pounds. Some people, upon learning how hard permanent weight loss can be, may give up entirely and return to overeating. Others may decide to accept themselves at their current weight and try to boost their fitness and overall health rather than changing the number on the scale.

For me, understanding the science of weight loss has helped make sense of my own struggles to lose weight, as well as my mother's endless cycle of dieting, weight gain and despair. I wish she were still here so I could persuade her to finally forgive herself for her dieting failures. While

I do, ultimately, blame myself for allowing my weight to get out of control, it has been somewhat liberating to learn that there are factors other than my character at work when it comes to gaining and losing weight. And even though all the evidence suggests that it's going to be very, very difficult for me to reduce my weight permanently, I'm surprisingly optimistic. I may not be ready to fight this battle this month or even this year. But at least I know what I'm up against.

Tara Parker-Pope is an author of books on health topics and a columnist for *The New York Times,* where she edits the Well blog.

EXPLORING THE ISSUE

Is Weight-Loss Maintenance Possible?

Critical Thinking and Reflection

1. Why is it so difficult for most people to maintain their weight loss?
2. What role does the typical American diet play in overweight and obesity?
3. Describe the biological mechanisms that make weight-loss maintenance so challenging.
4. What role does genetics play in the onset of obesity?

Is There Common Ground?

Although genetics and metabolism may elevate the risk for overweight and obesity, they don't explain the rising rate of obesity seen in the United States. Our genetic background has not changed significantly in the past 40 years, during which time the rate of obesity among Americans has more than doubled. The causes can be linked to changing eating habits and a decline in physical activity.

While dieting is a common means of losing weight, there is an overall belief that even if one loses weight, virtually no one succeeds in long-term maintenance of weight loss. However, research has shown that approximately 20 percent of overweight people are successful at long-term weight loss (defined as losing at least 10 percent of initial body weight and maintaining the loss for at least 1 year). The National Weight Control Registry provides information about the approaches used by successful weight-loss maintainers to attain and sustain long-term weight loss. To maintain their weight loss, the successful report high levels of physical activity, eating a low-calorie, low-fat diet, eating breakfast regularly, self-monitoring weight, and maintaining a consistent eating pattern across weekdays and weekends. In addition, weight-loss maintenance may get less challenging over time. After individuals have successfully maintained their weight loss for over 2 years, the chance of longer-term success greatly increases. Continuing to diet and exercise is also associated with long-term success. National Weight Control Registry members provide evidence that long-term weight-loss maintenance is possible and helps identify the specific approaches associated with long-term success (Wing and Phelan, 2005).

The same tactics that help people lose weight don't necessarily help them keep it off. A recent study, which appears in the August 2011 issue of the *American Journal of Preventive Medicine*, suggests that successful losers need to rethink their eating and exercise practices to maintain their weight loss. Researchers interviewed nearly 1,200 adults about 36 specific behaviors to find out which of these practices were associated with weight loss and, more important, weight-loss maintenance.

From the study results, it appears that different skill sets and behaviors are involved with weight loss and weight maintenance. Participating in a weight-loss program, restricting sugar, eating healthy snacks, and not skipping meals may help people initially lose weight, but these practices don't appear to be effective in maintaining the loss.

Eating low-fat sources of protein, following a consistent exercise routine, and using rewards for maintaining these behaviors were linked to maintaining weight loss.

Additional Resources

Derbyshire, D., Weir, K., Gunther, M., & Weeks, J. (2015). Thinking big about obesity. *Food Technology, 69*(3), 20–31.

8 weight mistakes. (2015). *Nutrition Action Healthletter, 42*(3), 3–6.

Sherwood, N. E., Crain, A., Martinson, B. C., Anderson, C. P., Hayes, M. G., Anderson, J. D., & Jeffery, R. W. (2013). Enhancing long-term weight loss maintenance: 2-Year results from the Keep It Off randomized controlled trial. *Preventive Medicine, 56*(3/4), 171–177.

Stubbs, R. J., & Lavin, J. H. (2013). The challenges of implementing behavior changes that lead to sustained weight management. *Nutrition Bulletin, 38*(1), 5–22.

Wing, R. R., & Phelan, S. (2005). Long-term weight loss maintenance. *American Journal of Clinical Nutrition, 82*, 2225–2255.

Internet References . . .

The American Dietetic Association

www.eatright.org

Center for Science in the Public Interest
(CSPI)

www.cspinet.org

Food and Nutrition Information Center

http://fnic.nal.usda.gov/

National Weight Control Registry

www.nwcr.ws

Shape Up America!

www.shapeup.org

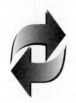

Selected, Edited, and with Issue Framing Material by:
Eileen L. Daniel, *SUNY College at Brockport*

ISSUE

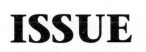

Are Energy Drinks with Alcohol Dangerous Enough to Ban?

YES: Don Troop, from "Four Loko Does Its Job with Efficiency and Economy, Students Say," *The Chronicle of Higher Education* (2010)

NO: Jacob Sullum, from "Loco Over Four Loko," *Reason* (2011)

Learning Outcomes
After reading this issue, you will be able to: • Discuss the health implications of energy drinks.   • Discuss the argument that energy drinks should be banned from sale and distribution.   • Assess the reasons for the drink's popularity among college students.

ISSUE SUMMARY

YES: *Chronicle of Higher Education* journalist Don Troop argues that the combination of caffeine and alcohol is extremely dangerous and should not be sold or marketed to college students and young people.

NO: Journalist and editor of *Reason* magazine Jacob Sullum disagrees and claims that alcoholic energy drinks should not have been targeted and banned since many other products are far more dangerous.

Energy drinks such as Four Loko are alcoholic beverages that originally also contained caffeine and other stimulants. These products have been the object of legal, ethical, and health concerns related to companies supposedly marketing them to underaged consumers and the alleged danger of combining alcohol and caffeine. After the beverage was banned in several states, a product reintroduction in December 2010 removed caffeine and the malt beverage is no longer marketed as an energy drink.

In 2009, companies that produced and sold caffeinated alcohol beverages were investigated, on the grounds that their products were being inappropriately advertised to an underage audience and that the drinks had possible health risks by masking feelings of intoxication due to the caffeine content. Energy drinks came under major fire in 2010, as colleges and universities across the United States began to see injuries and blackouts related to the drink's consumption. Colleges such as the University of Rhode Island banned this product from their campus

that year. The state of Washington banned Four Loko after nine university students, all under 20, from Central Washington University became ill after consuming the beverage at a nearby house party. The Central Washington college students were hospitalized and one student, with extremely high blood alcohol content, nearly died.

Following the hospitalization of 17 students and 6 visitors in 2010, Ramapo College of New Jersey banned the possession and consumption of Four Loko on its campus. Several other colleges also prohibited the sale of the beverages. Many colleges and universities sent out notices informing their students to avoid the drinks because of the risk associated with their consumption.

Other efforts to control the use of energy drinks have been under way. The Pennsylvania Liquor Control Board sent letters to all liquor stores urging distributors to discontinue the sale of the drink. The PLCB also sent letters to all colleges and universities warning them of the dangers of the product. While the board has stopped short of a ban, it has asked retailers to stop selling the drink

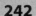

until U.S. Food and Drug Administration (FDA) findings prove the products are safe. Several grocery chains have voluntarily removed energy beverages from their stores. In Oregon, the sale of the restricted products carried a penalty of 30-day suspension of one's liquor license.

The U.S. FDA issued a warning letter in 2010 to four manufacturers of caffeinated alcohol beverages stating that the caffeine added to their malt alcoholic beverages is an "unsafe food additive" and said that further action, including seizure of their products, may occur under federal law. The FDA determined that beverages that combine caffeine with alcohol, such as Four Loco energy drinks, are a "public health concern" and couldn't stay on the market in their current form. The FDA also stated that concerns have been raised that caffeine can mask some of the sensory cues individuals might normally rely on to determine their level of intoxication. Warning letters were issued to each of the four companies requiring them to provide to the FDA in writing within 15 days of the specific steps the firms will be taking. Prior to the FDA ruling, many consumers bought and hoarded large quantities of the beverage. This buying frenzy created a black market for

energy drinks, with some sellers charging inflated prices. A reformulated version of the drink was put on shelves in late 2010. The new product had exactly the same design as the original, but the caffeine had been removed.

Effective February 2013, cans of Four Loko carry an "Alcohol Facts" label. The label change is part of a final settlement between the Federal Trade Commission and Phusion Projects, the manufacturer of Four Loko. The company still disagrees with the commission's allegations, but said in a statement that the agreement provides a practical way for the company to move ahead. The FTC claimed that ads for Four Loko inaccurately claimed that a 23.5-ounce can contain the alcohol equivalent of one to two cans of beer. In fact, the FTC says, it's more like four to five beers. In the YES and NO selections, Don Troop argues that the combination of caffeine and alcohol is extremely dangerous and should not be sold or marketed to college students and young people. Journalist and editor of *Reason Magazine* Jacob Sullum disagrees and claims that alcoholic energy drinks should not have been targeted and banned since many other products are far more dangerous.

YES ↵

Don Troop

Four Loko Does Its Job with Efficiency and Economy, Students Say

It's Friday night in this steep-hilled college town, and if anyone needs an excuse to party, here are two: In 30 minutes the Mountaineers football team will kick off against the UConn Huskies in East Hartford, Conn., and tonight begins the three-day Halloween weekend.

A few blocks from the West Virginia University campus, young people crowd the aisles of Ashebrooke Liquor Outlet, an airy shop that is popular among students. One rack in the chilled-beverage cooler is nearly empty, the one that is usually filled with 23.5-ounce cans of Four Loko, a fruity malt beverage that combines the caffeine of two cups of coffee with the buzz factor of four to six beers.

"That's what everyone's buying these days," says a liquor store employee, "Loko and Burnett's vodka," a line of distilled spirits that are commonly mixed with nonalcoholic energy drinks like Red Bull and Monster to create fruity cocktails with a stimulating kick.

Four Loko's name comes from its four primary ingredients—alcohol (12 percent by volume), caffeine, taurine, and guarana. Although it is among dozens of caffeinated alcoholic drinks on the market, Four Loko has come to symbolize the dangers of such beverages because of its role in binge-drinking incidents this fall involving students at New Jersey's Ramapo College and at Central Washington University. Ramapo and Central Washington have banned Four Loko from their campuses, and several other colleges have sent urgent e-mail messages advising students not to drink it. But whether Four Loko is really "blackout in a can" or just the highest-profile social lubricant of the moment is unclear.

Just uphill from Ashebrooke Liquor Outlet, four young men stand on a porch sipping cans of Four Loko—fruit punch and cranberry-lemonade. All are upperclassmen except for one, Philip Donnachie, who graduated in May. He says most Four Loko drinkers he knows like to guzzle a can of it at home before meeting up with friends, a custom that researchers in the field call "predrinking."

"Everyone that's going to go out for the night, they're going to start with a Four Loko first," Mr. Donnachie says, adding that he generally switches to beer.

A student named Tony says he paid $5.28 at Ashebrooke for two Lokos—a bargain whether the goal is to get tipsy or flat-out drunk. Before the drink became infamous, he says, he would see students bring cans of it into classrooms. "The teachers didn't know what it was," Tony says, and if they asked, the student would casually reply, "It's an energy drink."

Farther uphill, on the sidewalk along Grant Avenue, the Tin Man from *The Wizard of Oz* carries a Loko—watermelon flavor, judging by its color. Down the block a keg party spills out onto the front porch, where guests sprawl on a sofa and flick cigarette ashes over the railing. No one here is drinking Four Loko, but most are eager to talk about the product because they've heard that it could be banned by the federal government as a result of the student illnesses.

Research Gap

That's not likely to happen anytime soon, according to the Food and Drug Administration.

"The FDA's decision regarding the regulatory status of caffeine added to various alcoholic beverages will be a high priority for the agency," Michael L. Herndon, an FDA spokesman, wrote in an e-mail message. "However, a decision regarding the use of caffeine in alcoholic beverages could take some time." The FDA does not consider such drinks to be "generally recognized as safe." A year ago the agency gave 27 manufacturers 30 days to provide evidence to the contrary, if it existed. Only 19 of the companies have responded.

Dennis L. Thombs is chairman of the Department of Social and Behavioral Sciences at the University of North Texas Health Science Center, in Fort Worth. He knows a great deal about the drinking habits of young people.

Last year he was the lead author on a paper submitted to the journal *Addictive Behaviors* that described his team's study of bar patrons' consumption of energy drinks and alcohol in the college town of Gainesville, Fla. After interviewing 802 patrons and testing their blood-alcohol content, Mr. Thombs and his fellow researchers concluded that energy drinks' labels should clearly describe the ingredients, their amounts, and the potential risks involved in using the products.

But Mr. Thombs says the government should have more data before it decides what to do about alcoholic energy drinks.

"There's still a big gap in this research," he says. "We need to get better pharmacological measures in natural drinking environments" like bars.

He says he has submitted a grant application to the National Institutes of Health in hopes of doing just that.

"Liquid Crack"

Back at the keg party in Morgantown, a student wearing Freddy Krueger's brown fedora and razor-blade glove calls Four Loko "liquid crack" and says he prefers not to buy it for his underage friends. "I'll buy them something else," he says, "but not Four Loko."

Dipsy from the *Teletubbies* says the people abusing Four Loko are younger students, mostly 17- and 18-year-olds. He calls the students who became ill at Ramapo and Central Washington "a bunch of kids that don't know how to drink."

Two freshmen at the party, Gabrielle and Meredith, appear to confirm that assertion.

"I like Four Loko because it's cheap and it gets me drunk," says Gabrielle, 19, who seems well on her way to getting drunk tonight, Four Loko or not. "Especially for concerts. I drink two Four Lokos before going, and then I don't have to spend $14 on a couple drinks at the stadium."

Meredith, 18 and equally intoxicated, says that although she drinks Four Loko, she favors a ban. "They're 600 calories, and they're gross."

An interview with Alex, a 19 year old student at a religiously affiliated college in the Pacific Northwest, suggests one reason that the drink might be popular among a younger crowd. In his state and many others, the laws that govern the sale of Four Loko and beer are less stringent than those for hard liquor.

That eases the hassle for older friends who buy for Alex. These days that's not a concern, though. He stopped drinking Four Loko because of how it made him feel the next day.

"Every time I drank it I got, like, a blackout," says Alex. "Now I usually just drink beer."

DON TROOP is a senior editor of the *Chronicles of Higher Education,* which covers state policy, as well as economic development, town-and-gown relations, fund raising and endowments, and other financial issues at the campus level.

Jacob Sullum   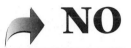 **NO**

Loco Over Four Loko: How a Fruity, Brightly Colored Malt Beverage Drove Politicians to Madness in Two Short Years

In a column at the end of October, *The New York Times* restaurant critic Frank Bruni looked down his nose at Four Loko, a fruity, bubbly, brightly colored malt beverage with a lower alcohol content than Chardonnay and less caffeine per ounce than Red Bull. "It's a malt liquor in confectionery drag," Bruni wrote, "not only raising questions about the marketing strategy behind it but also serving as the clearest possible reminder that many drinkers aren't seeking any particular culinary or aesthetic enjoyment. They're taking a drug. The more festively it's dressed and the more vacuously it goes down, the better."

Less than two weeks after Bruni panned Four Loko and its déclassé drinkers, he wrote admiringly of the "ambition and thought" reflected in hoity-toity coffee cocktails offered by the Randolph at Broome, a boutique bar in downtown Manhattan. He conceded that "there is a long if not entirely glorious history of caffeine and alcohol joining forces, of whiskey or liqueurs poured into after-dinner coffee by adults looking for the same sort of effect that Four Loko fans seek: an extension of the night without a surrender of the buzz."

Like Bruni's distaste for Four Loko, the moral panic that led the Food and Drug Administration (FDA) to ban the beverage and others like it in November, just two years after it was introduced, cannot be explained in pharmacological terms. As Brum admitted and as the drink's Chicago-based manufacturer, Phusion Projects, kept pointing out to no avail, there is nothing new about mixing alcohol with caffeine. What made this particular formulation intolerable—indeed "adulterated," according to the FDA—was not its chemical composition but its class connotations: the wild and crazy name, the garish packaging, the low cost, the eight color-coded flavors, and the drink's popularity among young partiers who see "blackout in a can" as a recommendation. Those attributes made Four Loko offensive to the guardians of public health

and morals in a way that Irish coffee, rum and cola, and even Red Bull and vodka never were.

The FDA itself conceded that the combination of alcohol and caffeine, a feature of many drinks, that remain legal, was not the real issue. Rather, the agency complained that "the marketing of the caffeinated versions of this class of alcoholic beverage appears to be specifically directed to young adults," who are "especially vulnerable" to "combined ingestion of caffeine and alcohol."

Because Four Loko was presumed to be unacceptably hazardous, the FDA did not feel a need to present much in the way of scientific evidence. A grand total of two studies have found that college students who drink alcoholic beverages containing caffeine (typically bar or home-mixed cocktails unaffected by the FDA's ban) tend to drink more and are more prone to risky behavior than college students who drink alcohol by itself. Neither study clarified whether the differences were due to the psychoactive effects of caffeine or to the predispositions of hearty partiers attracted to drinks they believe will help keep them going all night. But that distinction did not matter to panic-promoting politicians and their publicists in the press, who breathlessly advertised Four Loko while marveling at its rising popularity.

This dual function of publicity about an officially condemned intoxicant is familiar to anyone who has witnessed or read about previous scare campaigns against stigmatized substances, ranging from absinthe to *Salvia divinorum*. So is the evidentiary standard employed by Four Loko alarmists: If something bad happens and Four Loko is anywhere in the vicinity, blame Four Loko.

The National Highway Traffic Safety Administration counted 13,800 alcohol-related fatalities in 2008. It did not place crashes involving Four Loko drinkers in a special category. But news organizations around the country, primed to perceive the drink as unusually dangerous, routinely did. Three days before the FDA declared Four Loko illegal, a 14-year-old stole his parents' SUV and crashed it into a guardrail on Interstate 35 in Denton, Texas. His girlfriend, who was not wearing a seat belt, was ejected from the car and killed. Police, who said they found a 12-pack of beer and five cans of Four Loko in the SUV, charged the boy with intoxication manslaughter. Here is how the local Fox station headlined its story: "'Four Loko' Found in Deadly Teen Crash."

Likewise, college students were getting sick after drinking too much long before Four Loko was introduced in August 2008. According to the federal government's Drug Abuse Warning Network, more than 100,000 18-to-20-year-olds make alcohol-related visits to American emergency rooms every year. Yet 15 students at two colleges who were treated for alcohol poisoning after consuming excessive amounts of Four Loko were repeatedly held up as examples of the drink's unique dangers.

If all alcoholic beverages had to satisfy the reckless college student test, all of them would be banned. In a sense, then, we should be grateful for the government's inconsistency. With Four Loko, as with other taboo tipples and illegal drugs, there is little logic to the process by which the scapegoat is selected, but there are noticeable patterns. Once an intoxicant has been identified with a disfavored group—in this case, heedless, hedonistic "young adults"—everything about it is viewed in that light. Soon the wildest charges seem plausible: Four Loko is "a recipe for disaster," "a death wish disguised as an energy drink," a "witch's brew" that drives you mad, makes you shoot yourself in the head, and compels you to steal vehicles and crash them into things.

The timeline that follows shows how quickly a legal product can be transformed into contraband once it becomes the target of such over-the-top opprobrium. Although it's too late for Four Loko, lessons gleaned from the story of its demise could help prevent the next panicky prohibition by scaremongers who criminalize first and ask questions later.

June 2008: Anheuser-Busch, under pressure from 11 attorneys general who are investigating the brewing giant for selling the caffeinated malt beverages Tilt and Bud Extra, agrees to decaffeinate the drinks. "Drinking is not a sport, a race, or an endurance test," says New York Attorney General Andrew Cuomo, who will later be elected governor. "Adding alcohol to energy drinks sends exactly the wrong message about responsible drinking, most especially to young people."

August 2008: Phusion Projects, a Chicago company founded in 2005 by three recent graduates of Ohio State University, introduces Four Loko, which has an alcohol content of up to 12 percent (depending on state

regulations); comes in brightly colored, 23.5-ounce cans; contains the familiar energy-drink ingredients caffeine, guarana, and taurine; and is eventually available in eight fruity, neon-hued varieties.

September 2008: The Center for Science in the Public Interest (CSPI), a pro-regulation group that is proud of being known as "the food police," sues MillerCoors Brewing Company over its malt beverage Sparks, arguing that the caffeine and guarana in the drink are additives that have not been approved by the FDA. "Mix alcohol and stimulants with a young person's sense of invincibility," says CSPI's George Hacker, "and you have a recipe for disaster. Sparks is a drink designed to mask feelings of drunkenness and to encourage people to keep drinking past the point at which they otherwise would have stopped. The end result is more drunk driving, more injuries, and more sexual assaults."

December 2008: In a deal with 13 attorneys general and the city of San Francisco, MillerCoors agrees to reformulate Sparks, removing the caffeine, guarana, taurine, and ginseng. Cuomo says caffeinated alcoholic beverages are "fundamentally dangerous and put drinkers of all ages at risk."

July 2009: *The Wall Street Journal* reports that Cuomo, Connecticut Attorney General Richard Blumenthal (now a U.S. senator), California Attorney General Jerry Brown (now governor), and their counterparts in several other states are investigating Four Loko and Joose, a close competitor. The National Association of Convenience Stores says the two brands are growing fast now that Tilt and Sparks have left the caffeinated malt beverage market.

August 2009: To demonstrate the threat that Four Loko poses to the youth of America, Blumenthal cites an online testimonial from a fan of the drink: "You just gotta drink it and drink it and drink it and drink it and not even worry about it because it's awesome and you're just partying and having fun and getting wild and drinking it." *The Chicago Tribune* cannot locate that particular comment on Phusion Projects' website, but it does find this: "I'm having a weird reaction to Four that makes me want to dance in my bra and panties. Please advise."

September 2009: Eighteen attorneys general ask the FDA to investigate the safety of alcoholic beverages containing caffeine.

November 2009: The FDA sends letters to 27 companies known to sell caffeinated alcoholic beverages, warning them that the combination has never been officially approved and asking them to submit evidence that it is "generally recognized as safe," as required by the Food, Drug, and Cosmetic Act. In addition to Phusion Projects, the recipients include Joose's manufacturer, United Brands;

Charge Beverages, which sells similar products; the PINK Spirits Company, which makes caffeinated vodka, rum, gin, whiskey, and sake; and even the Ithaca Beer Company, which at one point made a special-edition stout brewed with coffee. "I continue to be very concerned that these drinks are extremely dangerous," says Illinois Attorney General Lisa Madigan, "especially in the hands of young people."

February 2010: In a feature story carried by several newspapers under headlines such as "Alcopops Only Look Innocent and Can Hook Kids," Kim Hone-McMahan of the *Akron Beacon Journal* outlines one scenario in which these extremely dangerous drinks might end up in tiny hands: "Intentionally or by accident, a child could grab an alcoholic beverage that looks like an energy drink, and hand it to Mom to pay for at the register. Without taking a closer look at the label, Mom may think it's just another brand of nonalcoholic energy beverage." It does seem like the sort of mistake that Hone-McMahan, who confuses fermented malt beverages with distilled spirits and warns parents about an alcoholic energy drink that was never actually introduced, might make. She explains that the combination of alcohol and caffeine "can confuse the nervous system," producing "wired, wide-awake drunks."

July 12, 2010: Sen. Charles Schumer (D-N.Y.) urges the Federal Trade Commission to investigate Four Loko and products like it. "It is my understanding that caffeine-infused, flavored malt beverages are becoming increasingly popular among teenagers," he writes. "The style and promotion of these products is extremely troubling." Schumer complains that the packaging of Joose and Four Loko is "designed to appear hip with flashy colors and funky designs that could appeal to younger consumers."

July 29, 2010: Schumer, joined by Sens. Dianne Feinstein (D-Calif.), Amy Klobuchar (D-Minn.), and Jeff Merkley (D-Ore.), urges the FDA to complete its investigation. "The FDA needs to determine once and for all if these drinks are safe, and if they're not, they ought to be banned," says Schumer, right before telling the FDA the conclusion it should reach: "Caffeine and alcohol are a dangerous mix, especially for young people."

August 1, 2010: After a crash in St. Petersburg, Florida, that kills four visitors from Orlando, police arrest 20-year-old Demetrius Jordan and charge him with drunk driving and manslaughter. The *St. Petersburg Times* reports that Jordan, who "had been drinking liquor and a caffeinated alcoholic beverage and smoking marijuana prior to the crash," "may have been going in excess of 80 mph when he crashed into the other vehicle." It notes that a "can of Four Loko was found on the floor of the back seat."

August 5, 2010: In a follow-up story, the *St. Petersburg Times* reports that "Four Loko, the caffeine-fueled malt liquor that police say Demetrius Jordan downed before he was accused of driving drunk and killing four people, is part of a new breed of beverages stirring controversy across the country." It quotes Bruce Goldberger, a toxicologist at the University of Florida, who declares, "I don't think there's a place for these beverages in the marketplace." The headline: "Alcohol, Caffeine: A Deadly Combo?"

August 12, 2010: The *Orlando Sentinel*, catching up with the *St. Petersburg Times*, shows it can quote Goldberger too. "It's a very bad combination having alcohol, plus caffeine, plus the brain of a young person," he says. "It's like a perfect storm." The headline: "Did High-Octane Drink Fuel Deadly Crash?"

September 2010: Peter Mercer, president of Ramapo College in Mahwah, New Jersey, bans Four Loko and other caffeinated malt beverages from campus after several incidents in which a total of 23 students were hospitalized for alcohol poisoning. Just six of the students were drinking Four Loko. Mercer later tells the Associated Press, "There's no redeeming social purpose to be served by having the beverage."

October 9, 2010: In a story about nine gang members who tied up and tortured a gay man after luring him to an abandoned building in the Bronx by telling him they were having a party, the *New York Daily News* plays up the detail that they "forced him to guzzle four cans" of the Four Loko he had brought with him. "The sodomized man couldn't give police a clear account of what he'd gone through," the paper reports, "possibly because of the Four Loko he was forced to drink."

October 10, 2010: In a follow-up story, the *Daily News* reports that Four Loko, a "wild drink full of caffeine and booze," "is causing controversy from coast to coast," citing the deadly crash in St. Petersburg.

October 13, 2010: Police in New Port Richey, Florida, arrest Justin Barker, 21, after he breaks into an old woman's home, trashes the place, strips naked, defecates on the floor, and then breaks into another house, where he falls asleep on the couch. Barker says Four Loko made him do it.

October 15, 2010: Calling Four Loko "a quick and intense high that has been dubbed 'blackout in a can,'" the Passaic County, New Jersey, *Herald News* notes the Ramapo College ban and quotes Mahwah Police Chief James Batelli. "The bottom line on the product is it gets you very drunk, very quick," he says. "To me, Four Loko is just a dangerous substance." The "blackout in a can" sobriquet, obviously hyperbolic when applied to a beverage that contains less alcohol per container than a bottle of wine, originated with Four Loko fans who considered it high praise; one of their Facebook pages is titled "four lokos are blackouts in a can and the end of my morals."

October 19, 2010: Bruce Goldberger, who co-authored one of the two studies linking caffeinated alcohol to risky behavior, tells the *Pittsburgh Post-Gazette* "the science is clear that consumption of alcohol with caffeine leads to risky behaviors." Mary Claire O'Brien, the Wake Forest University researcher who co-authored the other study, expresses her anger at the FDA. "I'm mad as a hornet that they didn't do something in the first place," she says, "and I'm mad as a hornet that they haven't done anything yet."

October 20, 2010: Based on a single case of a 19-year-old who came to Temple University Hospital in Philadelphia with chest pains after drinking Four Loko, ABC News warns that the stuff, which contains about one-third as much caffeine per ounce as coffee, can cause fatal heart attacks in perfectly healthy people. "That was the only explanation we had," says the doctor who treated the 19-year-old, before extrapolating further from his sample of one: "This is a dangerous product from what we've seen. It doesn't have to be chronic use. I think it could happen to somebody on a first-time use."

October 25, 2010: Citing the hospitalization of nine Central Washington University students for alcohol poisoning following an October 8 party in Roslyn where they drank Four Loko along with beer, rum, and vodka, Washington Attorney General Rob McKenna calls for a ban on caffeinated malt liquor. "The wide availability of the alcoholic energy drinks means that a single mistake can be deadly," he says. "They're marketed to kids by using fruit flavors that mask the taste of alcohol, and they have such high levels of stimulants that people have no idea how inebriated they really are." McKenna's office cites Ken Briggs, chairman of the university's physical education department, who says Four Loko is known as "liquid cocaine" as well as "blackout in a can," and with good reason, since it is "a binge drinker's dream."

October 26, 2010: McKenna's reaction to college students who drank too much Four Loko, like Peter Mercer's at Ramapo, attracts national attention. A Pennsylvania E.R. doctor quoted by *The New York Times* calls Four Loko "a recipe for disaster" and "one of the most dangerous new alcohol concoctions I have ever seen."

November 1, 2010: The Pennsylvania Liquor Control Board asks retailers to stop selling Four Loko, which is produced at the former Rolling Rock brewery in Latrobe, because it may "pose a significant threat to the health

of all Pennsylvanians." State Rep. Robert Donatucci (D-Philadelphia) says "there is overriding circumstantial evidence that this combination may be very dangerous," and "until we can determine its effect on people and what kind of danger it may present, it should be yanked from the shelves."

November 3, 2010: Two Chicago aldermen propose an ordinance that would ban Four Loko from the city where its manufacturer is based. "I think it is completely irresponsible," says one, "to manufacture and market a product that can make young people so intoxicated so fast."

November 4, 2010: The Michigan Liquor Control Commission bans 55 "alcohol energy drinks," including Four Loko, Joose, a "hard" iced tea that no longer exists, a cola-flavored variety of Jack Daniel's Country Cocktails, and an India pale ale brewed with yerba mate. "With all the things that are happening, it's very alarming," explains commission chairwoman Nida Samona. "It's more serious than any of us ever imagined."

November 8, 2010: Oklahoma's Alcoholic Beverage Laws Enforcement Commission bans Four Loko from the state "in light of the growing scientific evidence against alcohol energy drinks, and the October 8th incident involving Four Loko in Roslyn, Washington."

November 9, 2010: NPR quotes Washington State University student Jarod Franklin as an authority on Four Loko's effects. "We would start to lose those inhibitions," he says, "and then [it would be like], 'How did you get a broken knuckle?' 'Oh, I punched through a three-inch layer of ice [because] you bet me I couldn't.'"

November 10, 2010: The Washington State Liquor Control Board bans beverages that "combine beer, strong beer, or malt liquor with caffeine, guarana, taurine, or other similar substances." Gov. Christine Gregoire, who recommended the ban, explains her reasoning: "I was particularly concerned that these drinks tend to target young people. Reports of inexperienced or underage drinkers consuming them in reckless amounts have given us cause for concern. . . . By taking these drinks off the shelves we are saying 'no' to irresponsible drinking and taking steps to prevent incidents like the one that made these college students so ill."

Sen. Schumer urges the New York State Liquor Authority to "immediately ban caffeinated alcoholic beverages." He says drinks like Four Loko "are a toxic, dangerous mix of caffeine and alcohol, and they are spreading like a plague across the country." Schumer claims "studies have shown that caffeinated alcoholic beverages raise unique and disturbing safety concerns, especially for younger drinkers."

While they "can be extremely hazardous for teens and adults alike," he says, they "pose a unique danger because they target young people" with their "vibrantly colored aluminum can colors and funky designs."

November 12, 2010: A CBS station in Baltimore reports that two cans of Four Loko caused a 21-year-old Maryland woman to "lose her mind," steal a friend's pickup truck, and crash it into a telephone pole, killing herself.

A CBS station in Philadelphia reports that a middle-aged suburban dad "spiraled into a hallucinogenic frenzy" featuring "nightmarish delusions" after drinking a can and a half of Four Loko. "It was like he was stuck inside a horror movie and he couldn't get out and I couldn't get him out," the man's wife says. "In his mind, he had harmed all of our kids and he had to kill me and kill himself so that we could go to heaven to take care of them. Next thing I know, he was having convulsions [and] making gurgling sounds as if someone were choking him, and then he stopped breathing."

Connecticut Attorney General Blumenthal urges the FDA to "impose a nationwide ban on these dangerous and potentially deadly drinks."

November 14, 2010: Under pressure from Gov. David Paterson and the state liquor authority, Phusion Projects agrees to stop shipping Four Loko to New York. "We have an obligation to keep products that are potentially hazardous off the shelves," says the liquor authority's chairman.

Bruce Goldberger tells the *New Haven Register* Four Loko is "a very significant problem" for the "instant gratification generation." The kids today, he says, "text, they have iPhones, and they can access the Internet any minute of their life. And now, they can get drunk for literally less than $5, and they can get drunk very rapidly."

November 15, 2010: WBZ, the CBS affiliate in Boston, reports that the Massachusetts Alcoholic Beverages Control Commission plans to ban Four Loko. According to WBZ, commission officials say the drink—a fermented malt beverage with an alcohol content of 12 percent, compared to 40 percent or more for distilled spirits—"is really not a malt liquor, but a much more potent form of hard liquor, like vodka." The commission's chairman explains that the ban is aimed at protecting consumers who cannot read: "We are concerned that people who are drinking these alcoholic beverages are not aware of the ingredients which are contained in them."

The New York Times reports that Four Loko "has been blamed for several deaths over the last several months," including that of a 20-year-old sophomore at Florida State

University in Tallahassee who "started playing with a gun and fatally shot himself after drinking several cans of Four Loko over a number of hours." Richard Blumenthal tells the *Times* "there's just no excuse for the delay in applying standards that clearly should bar this kind of witch's brew." Mary Claire O'Brien argues that Four Loko is guilty until proven innocent: "The addition of the caffeine impairs the ability of the drinker to tell when they're drunk. What is the level at which it becomes dangerous? We don't know that, and until we can figure it out, the answer is that no level is safe."

November 16, 2010: Phusion Projects says it will reformulate Four Loko, removing the caffeine, guarana, and taurine. "We have repeatedly contended—and still believe, as do many people throughout the country—that the combination of alcohol and caffeine is safe," the company's founders say. "We are taking this step after trying—unsuccessfully—to navigate a difficult and politically charged regulatory environment at both the state and federal levels."

The Arizona Republic reports that an "extremely intoxicated" 18-year-old from Mesa crashed her SUV into a tree after "playing 'beer pong' with the controversial caffeinated alcoholic beverage Four Loko." The headline: "Caffeine, Alcohol Drink Tied to Crash."

Reporting on a lawsuit against Phusion Projects by the parents of the FSU student who shot himself after drinking Four Loko, ABC News quotes Schumer, who avers, "It's almost a death wish disguised as an energy drink."

November 17, 2010: The FDA and the Federal Trade Commission send warning letters to Phusion Projects, United Brands, Charge Beverages, and New Century Brewing Company, which makes a caffeinated lager called Moonshot. The agency says their products are "adulterated," and therefore illegal under the Food, Drug, and Cosmetic Act, because they contain an additive, caffeine, that is not generally recognized as safe in this context. But the FDA does not conclude that all beverages combining alcohol and caffeine are inherently unsafe. It focuses on these particular companies because they "seemingly target the young adult user." Federal drug czar Gil Kerlikowske approves the FDA's marketing-based definition of adulteration, saying "these products are designed, branded, and promoted to encourage binge drinking."

NPR correspondent Tovia Smith reports that "many college students say they agree with the FDA that alcoholic energy drinks do result in more risky behavior, like drunk driving or sexual assaults." Smith presents one such student, Ali Burak of Boston College, who says "it seems like every time someone wakes up in the morning and regrets the night before it's usually because they had Four Loko."

November 20, 2010: In a *Huffington Post* essay, David Katz, director of Yale University's Prevention Research Center, explains why "anyone who is for sanity and safety in marketing" should welcome the FDA's ban. "Combining alcohol and caffeine is—in one word—crazy," he writes. "Don't do it! It has an excellent chance of hurting you, and a fairly good chance of killing you." His evidence: the Maryland car crash in which a woman who had been drinking Four Loko died after colliding with a telephone pole. "It's hard to imagine any argument for such products," Katz concludes. "It's also hard to imagine anyone objecting to a ban of such products."

JACOB SULLUM is a journalist and editor of *Reason* magazine.

EXPLORING THE ISSUE

Are Energy Drinks with Alcohol Dangerous Enough to Ban?

Critical Thinking and Reflection

1. Why were energy drinks with caffeine banned?
2. Why are caffeinated energy drinks so popular among college students?
3. Describe why the drinks are dangerous and how they contributed to deaths among some college students.

Is There Common Ground?

Four Loko and other energy drinks provide the effects of caffeine and sugar, but there is little or no evidence that a wide variety of other ingredients have any impact on the body. A variety of physiological and psychological effects, however, have been blamed on energy drinks and their components. Excess use of energy drinks may produce mild to moderate euphoria primarily due to the stimulant properties of caffeine. The drinks may also cause agitation, anxiety, irritability, and sleeplessness.

Ingestion of a single energy drink will not lead to excessive caffeine intake, but consumption of two or more drinks over the course of a day can. Ginseng, guarana, and other stimulants are often added to energy drinks and may bolster the effects of caffeine. Negative effects associated with caffeine consumption in amounts greater than 400 mg include nervousness, irritability, sleeplessness, increased urination, abnormal heart rhythms, and upset stomach. By comparison, a cup of drip coffee contains about 150 mg of caffeine. Caffeine in energy drinks can cause the excretion of water from the body to dilute high concentrations of sugar entering the blood stream, leading to dehydration.

In the United States, energy drinks have been linked with reports of emergency room visits due to heart palpitations and anxiety. The beverages have been associated with seizures due to the crash following the high energy that occurs after ingestion. In the United States, caffeine dosage is not required to be on the product label for food, unlike drugs, but some advocates are urging the FDA to change this practice.

Drinking one 24-ounce can of Four Loko provides the alcoholic kick of four beers and the caffeine buzz of a strong cup of coffee. Drinking one quickly makes someone pretty drunk and reasonably awake, and able to drink more. As a result, college students seem particularly drawn to it, which has landed some in hospitals. But should Four Loko be banned state-by-state as a result? Banning Four Loko might prevent some people, especially some college students, from hurting themselves or others. But does it improve people's judgment or otherwise empower them to protect themselves?

Additional Resources

The party's over. (2010, November 25). *Nature, 475*.

Esser, M. B., & Siegel, M. (2014). Alcohol facts labels on Four Loko: Will the Federal Trade Commission's order be effective in reducing hazardous drinking among underage youth? *American Journal of Drug & Alcohol Abuse, 40*(6), 424–427.

Siegel, S. (2011). The Four-Loko effect. *Perspectives on Psychological Science, 6*(4), 357–362.

Stoll, J. D., Esterl, M., Robinson, F., Houston-Waesch, M., & Bomsdorf, C. (2014, May 16). Energy drink ban takes bull by horns. *Wall Street Journal— Eastern Edition*. pp. B1–B2.

Wood, D. B. (2010, November 19). Four Loko: Does FDA's caffeinated alcoholic beverage ban go too far? *Christian Science Monitor*, p. N.PAG.

Internet References . . .

Energy Drinks—American Association of Poison Control Centers

www.aapcc.org/alerts/energy-drinks

Food and Drug Administration

www.fda.gov

National Institute on Drug Abuse (NIDA)

www.nida.nih.gov

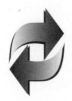

Selected, Edited, and with Issue Framing Material by:
Eileen L. Daniel, *SUNY College at Brockport*

ISSUE

Are Homeopathic Remedies Effective?

YES: Rachel Roberts, from "I Don't Know How, but Homeopathy Really Does Work," *guardian.com* (2010)

NO: Harriet Hall, from "An Introduction to Homeopathy: A Brief Guide to a Popular Alternative System of Remedies Based on a Nineteenth-Century Concept That Has No Scientific Validity," *Skeptical Inquirer* (2014)

Learning Outcomes
After reading this issue, you will be able to: • Understand the basic principles of homeopathy.   • Discuss the relationship between homeopathic dilution and efficacy.   • Explain the popularity of homeopathic therapies.

ISSUE SUMMARY

YES: Homeopathic practitioner Rachel Roberts maintains that homeopathy works and scientific research confirms this.

NO: Retired Air Force physician Harriet Hall counters that scientific knowledge about biology, chemistry, and physics tells us it should not work and careful testing shows that it does not work.

The basic theories of homeopathy were developed by Dr. Samuel Hahnemann, a German physician, in the early nineteenth century. Two central principles form the basic tenets of homeopathy: the law of similars and the law of infinitesimals. The law of similars maintains that a substance able to cause a symptom in healthy individuals can also be used to cure that symptom. The latter principle is based on the belief that therapeutic substances become more potent with dilution as long the dilution is accompanied by a specific type of vigorous shaking. Dr. Hahnemann believed the primary causes of disease were phenomena that he called miasms, and that homeopathic remedies effectively treated these. These remedies are prepared using a process of homeopathic dilution, which involves diluting a chosen substance in alcohol or distilled water, followed by forceful shaking. Dilution usually continues well past the point where no molecules of the original substance remain. Homeopathic practitioners choose remedies by consulting reference books known as repertories, and by considering the totality of the patient's symptoms, personal traits, physical and psychological state, and life history.

Dr. Hahnemann and his followers put together a body of literature based on their scrutiny of the observed effects of the administration of a range of diluted substances on various patients. These key principles and knowledge base of homeopathy have remained basically unchanged since the early 1800s and they form the foundation of current homeopathic practice.

Homeopathy's popularity grew in the 1800s and was introduced to the United States in 1825 by Hans Birch Gram, a student of Hahnemann. Throughout the nineteenth century, dozens of homeopathic institutions appeared in Europe and the United States and by 1900, there were 22 homeopathic colleges and 15,000 practitioners in the United States. In those days, patients of homeopaths often had better outcomes than those of traditional doctors. Medical practice at the time relied on ineffective and often harmful treatments, and homeopathic remedies, even if ineffective, would almost surely cause no harm, making the users of homeopathic remedies less likely to be killed by the treatment that was supposed to be helping them. Another reason for the growing popularity of homeopathy at the time was its apparent success in treating people suffering from infectious disease epidemics. During nineteenth-century epidemics of cholera, death rates in homeopathic hospitals were often lower than in conventional hospitals. This was due to the conventional treatments used at the time which were often harmful and even fatal and did little or nothing to actually treat or cure the disease.

Homeopathy from its beginning, however, was criticized by conventional medicine and it became less popular, especially in the United States, until its recent revival. During World War II, the Nazi regime in Germany was fascinated by homeopathy, and spent large sums of money on researching its mechanisms, but without gaining a positive result. In the United States, despite some early popularity in the nineteenth century, homeopathy never really took off, but remained more deeply established in Europe.

However, by the mid- to late 1970s, homeopathy made a major comeback in the United States and sales of homeopathic companies increased significantly. Some homeopaths give credit for the revival to the New Age movement which began in the late 1960s and favored nontraditional approaches to medicine and health care. Also, the increased popularity of homeopathy in recent times may be due to the comparatively long consultations practitioners are able and willing to give their patients, unlike rushed visits to conventional physicians. In addition, a preference for "natural" products, which people believe are the basis of homeopathic remedies, has also contributed to their acceptance.

While its popularity has grown in the United States, the proposed mechanisms for homeopathy do not appear to have scientific validity based on numerous research studies. The extreme dilutions used in homeopathic preparations usually leave none of the original substance in the final product. Despite this lack of scientific evidence, homeopathic practitioners have promoted a number of theories to counter this. They maintain that dilution produces a therapeutically active remedy, selectively including only the intended remedy. Critics, however, note that water will

have been in contact with millions of different substances throughout its history, and homeopaths have not been able to account for a reason why only the selected homeopathic remedy would become potent in this process. Homeopathic practitioners also claim that higher dilutions, described as being of higher potency, produce stronger therapeutic outcomes. This design is also inconsistent with observed dose–response relationships, where effects are dependent on the concentration of the active ingredient in the body. The dose–response relationship has been confirmed in multiple experiments on diverse organisms including animals and humans.

Researchers propose a variety of explanations for why homeopathy may *appear* to cure illnesses or lessen symptoms even though the remedies themselves are ineffective and inert. These include the placebo effect and the extensive consultation process and expectations for the treatment which cause the desired result. The practitioner's care, concern, and reassurance can have a positive effect on the patient's well-being. In addition, time and the body's ability to heal on its own can eradicate many diseases of their own accord. Some diseases or conditions are also cyclical and symptoms fluctuate over time and patients tend to seek care when distress is greatest. Patients may feel better because of the timing of the visit to the homeopath and attribute improvement to the remedy prescribed. Finally, discontinuing unpleasant conventional treatment which can cause unpleasant side effects appears to reduce symptoms. These improvements are often attributed to homeopathy when the actual cause is the cessation of the treatment causing side effects in the first place. Often homeopaths recommend patients stop getting traditional medical treatment such as surgery or drugs and substitute homeopathic remedies, and unfortunately, the underlying disease remains untreated and still potentially dangerous to the patient. Overall, no individual homeopathic preparation has been shown by legitimate research to be different from a placebo. Despite the lack of scientific validity, the practice continues, though not without controversy.

YES ↵

Rachel Roberts

I Don't Know How, but Homeopathy Really Does Work

More of a mystery is why scientists continue to debunk it despite mounting evidence that homeopathy is effective

I was a dedicated scientist about to begin a PhD in neuroscience when, out of the blue, homeopathy bit me on the proverbial bottom.

Science had been my passion since I began studying biology with Mr Hopkinson at the age of 11, and by the age of 21, when I attended the dinner party that altered the course of my life, I had still barely heard of it. The idea that I would one day become a homeopath would have seemed ludicrous.

That turning point is etched in my mind. A woman I'd known my entire life told me that a homeopath had successfully treated her when many months of conventional treatment had failed. As a sceptic, I scoffed, but was nonetheless a little intrigued.

She confessed that despite thinking homeopathy was a load of rubbish, she'd finally agreed to an appointment, to stop her daughter nagging. But she was genuinely shocked to find that, after one little pill, within days she felt significantly better. A second tablet, she said, "saw it off completely".

I admit I ruined that dinner party. I interrogated her about every detail of her diagnosis, previous treatment, time scales, the lot. I thought it through logically—she was intelligent, she wasn't lying, she had no previous inclination towards alternative medicine, and her reluctance would have diminished any placebo effect.

Scientists are supposed to make unprejudiced observations, then draw conclusions. As I thought about this, I was left with the highly uncomfortable conclusion that homeopathy appeared to have worked. I had to find out more.

So, I started reading about homeopathy, and what I discovered shifted my world for ever. I became convinced enough to hand my coveted PhD studentship over to my best friend and sign on for a three-year, full-time homeopathy training course.

Now, as an experienced homeopath, it is "science" that is biting me on the bottom. I know homeopathy works, not only because I've seen it with my own eyes countless times, but because scientific research confirms it. And yet I keep reading reports in the media saying that homeopathy doesn't work and that this scientific evidence doesn't exist.

The facts, it seems, are being ignored. By the end of 2009, 142 randomised control trials (the gold standard in medical research) comparing homeopathy with placebo or conventional treatment had been published in peer-reviewed journals—74 were able to draw firm conclusions: 63 were positive for homeopathy and 11 were negative. Five major systematic reviews have also been carried out to analyse the balance of evidence from RCTs of homeopathy—four were positive and one was negative. It's usual to get mixed results when you look at a wide range of research results on one subject, and if these results were from trials measuring the efficacy of "normal" conventional drugs, ratios of 63:11 and 4:1 in favour of a treatment working would be considered pretty persuasive.

Of course, the question of how homeopathy works is another matter. And that is where homeopathy courts controversy. It is indeed puzzling that ultra-high dilutions of substances, with few or no measurable molecules of the original substance left in them, should exert biological effects, but exert biological effects they do.

There are experiments showing that homeopathic thyroxine can alter the rate of metamorphosis of tadpoles into frogs, that homeopathic histamine can alter the activity of white blood cells, and that under the right conditions, homeopathic sodium chloride can be made to release light in the same way as normal sodium chloride. The idea that such highly diluted preparations are not only still active, but retain characteristics of the original substances, may seem impossible, but these kinds of results show it's a demonstrable fact.

Surely science should come into its own here—solving the riddles of the world around us, pushing the frontiers of knowledge. At least, that is the science I fell in love with. More of a puzzle to me now is the blinkered approach of those who continue, despite increasing evidence, to deny what is in front of them.

In the last few years, there has been much propaganda and misinformation circulated, much of it heralding the death of homeopathy, yet the evidence shows that interest in complementary and alternative medicine is growing.

In February, the "sceptics" campaign had a breakthrough—a report from the House of Commons Science and Technology Committee recommended no further NHS funding for homeopathy, despite a deeply flawed hearing.

The Society of Homeopaths—the largest body representing professional homeopaths—was refused permission to give oral evidence. Also notable by their absence from the panel were primary care trusts who currently commission homeopathy and representatives of patients who use homeopathy. Yet oral evidence was heard from a journalist previously investigated by the Press Complaints Commission for unsubstantiated criticism of homeopaths, and a spokesperson for a charity that has long publicly opposed homeopathy. It is significant that one of the four MPs asked to vote on the report abstained due to concerns about the lack of balance in the evidence heard.

Homeopathy is well-established in the UK, having been available through the NHS since its inception in 1948. More than 400 GPs use homeopathy in their everyday practice and the Society of Homeopaths has 1,500 registered members, from a variety of previous professions including pharmacists, journalists, solicitors and nurses.

And yet the portrayal of homeopathy as charlatanism and witchcraft continues. There is growing evidence that homeopathy works, that it is cost-effective and that patients want it. As drugs bills spiral, and evidence emerges that certain drugs routinely prescribed on the NHS are no better than placebos, maybe it's time for "sceptics" to stop the witch hunt and look at putting their own house in order.

It's all a far cry from the schoolgirl biologist who envisioned spending her life in a laboratory playing with bacteria.

Rachel Roberts is a homeopathic practitioner.

Harriet Hall

→ **NO**

An Introduction to Homeopathy: A Brief Guide to a Popular Alternative System of Remedies Based on a Nineteenth-Century Concept That Has No Scientific Validity

Homeopathy is an alternative system of medicine that was invented by a German doctor at the beginning of the nineteenth century. Scientific knowledge about chemistry, physics, and biology tells us it *should not work*; careful testing has shown that it *does not work*.

In 1800, conventional medicine was a disaster. Doctors weakened patients with bloodletting and purging, they poisoned them with mercury and other harmful substances, and they often killed more patients than they cured. Dr. Samuel Hahnemann was looking for safer, more effective ways to help his patients. He had an epiphany after he took a dose of cinchona bark and developed symptoms similar to those of malaria, the disease cinchona was supposed to treat. He extrapolated from this one observation to conclude that if any substance *causes* a symptom in healthy people it can be used to *treat* the same symptom in sick people. He formulated this as the first law of homeopathy, *similia similibus curentur*, usually translated as "like cures like." He diluted his remedies so that they would no longer cause symptoms; this led to his second law of homeopathy, the law of infinitesimals, which states that dilution increases the potency of a remedy. When he observed that his remedies worked better during house calls than in his office, he attributed it to jostling in his saddle bags, so he added the requirement of "succussion," specifying that remedies must be vigorously shaken (not stirred) by striking them against a leather surface at every step of dilution.

Homeopathic remedies are usually labeled with the notation X or C, corresponding to ten and one hundred. 15C would mean that one part of remedy was diluted in 100 parts of water, one part of the resulting solution was again diluted in 100 parts of water, and the process was repeated fifteen times. Hahnemann died before Avogadro's number was available to calculate how many molecules are present in a volume of a chemical substance. Today we can calculate that by the thirteenth 1:100 dilution (13C), no molecules of the original substance remain. Hahnemann typically used 30C remedies. At 30C, it would take a container thirty million times the size of the Earth to hold enough of the remedy to make it likely that it would contain a single molecule of the original substance. The most popular homeopathic cold and flu remedy is sold as a 200C dilution, and there are even higher dilutions. Above the 1,000C level there are remedies designated as multiples of M, where 1M=1,000C.

An example will clarify the mind-boggling implausibility of homeopathy. If coffee keeps you awake, according to homeopathy dilute coffee will put you to sleep. The more dilute, the stronger the effect. If you keep diluting it until there isn't a single molecule of coffee left, it will be even stronger. The water will somehow remember the coffee. If you drip that water onto a sugar pill and let the water evaporate, the water's memory will somehow be transferred to the sugar pill, and that memory of coffee will somehow enable it to function as a sleeping pill.

Later in his career, in order to explain the failures of homeopathy, Hahnemann came up with the idea that all disease is due to three miasms: syphilis, sycosis (gonorrhea) and psora (scabies, or itch). These could be inherited or the result of an infection; they had to be cleared before the homeopathic remedy could work.

Anything could be a homeopathic remedy. Soluble materials could be diluted in water or alcohol. Nonsoluble materials could be ground into powder (triturated) and diluted with sugar (lactose powder). Among remedies listed in the homeopathic *Materia Medica* are powder ground from pieces of the Berlin Wall, eclipsed moonlight, the south pole of a magnet, dog's earwax, tears from a weeping young girl, rattlesnake venom, and poison ivy.

To find out which remedy does what, they are tested—not by controlled scientific studies but instead by "provings." Healthy people ingest the substance and report *everything* that happens to them (for example, "my big toe itched at midnight, I got heartburn after eating a big meal, I felt angry"). There is no attempt to separate the ordinary vicissitudes of everyday life from symptoms caused by the substance. These reports are then compiled into a *Repertory* where the homeopath can look up a patient symptom or characteristic to see what remedies had been associated with it in provings. For instance, there are twenty-nine listings for a patient's facial expression, including astonished, bewildered, anxious when child is lifted from cradle, besotted, cold, and so on. A single remedy is listed for "cold"; seventeen are listed for "besotted."

The homeopath then consults a second book, a *Materia Medica*, for a list of symptoms that are associated with each remedy. For natrum muriaticum, the book lists symptoms in all these areas: mind, head, eyes, ears, nose, face, stomach, abdomen, rectum, urine, male/female, respiratory, heart, extremities, sleep, skin, fever, and modalities. Examples of symptoms listed under those categories include eyelids heavy; anemic headache of schoolgirls; constipation; diarrhea; sensation of coldness of heart; palms hot and perspiring; hangnails; dreams of robbers; oily skin; warts on palms of hands; chill between 9 and 11 AM, and so on for many pages. What is natrum muriaticum? Common table salt.

The initial consultation with a homeopath typically lasts an hour. He inquires about every conceivable aspect of the patient's life; keep in mind that for an accurate homeopathic diagnosis he must know about matters such as whether your eyelids are heavy or whether you have dreamed about robbers.

They pick the remedy that they deem to be the best match for you. If you get worse, they may tell you aggravations are a good sign. They will reevaluate you at every visit and change remedies as needed until one finally seems to do the trick or your illness runs its course and your symptoms have had time to go away on their own. If the treatment fails, they are never at a loss for excuses; they may tell you it's your fault because you inactivated the remedy by drinking coffee, not getting enough sleep, using a cellphone, or eating spicy foods.

In his book *Homeopathy: How It Really Works*, Jay Shelton examines all the evidence and concludes that homeopathy often "works," but not because of the remedies. The response to treatment is due to non-remedy factors such as unassisted natural healing, attention, suggestion, placebo effects, regression to the mean, the cessation of harmful or unpleasant treatments, lifestyle-assisted

healing, or a difference in perception of internal versus external reality.

Homeopaths have made numerous attempts to justify their remedies in the light of science. They have compared the remedies to vaccines, but vaccines are very different from homeopathic remedies because they contain measurable numbers of antigen molecules, they act by well-understood scientific mechanisms, and their results can be quantified by measuring antibody titers. Homeopaths have appealed to hormesis, a phenomenon whereby a low dose of a chemical may trigger the opposite response to a high dose. But hormesis is questionable, and if it exists in some cases, it's not a universal phenomenon by any means; it also describes a response to a *low* dose, not to *no* dose. Defenders of homeopathy have also invoked "water clusters" as a way water might store information; clusters of water molecules do form, but they only last for trillionths of a second, and there's no way they could register or transmit information. They have tried to attribute homeopathy's effects to quantum entanglement, with ill-informed Chopra-like speculations that would leave a quantum physicist rolling on the floor with laughter. They have done fatally flawed experiments trying to prove that water can remember, as if that alone would somehow validate clinical treatments. The most famous was Jacques Benveniste's study, published in *Nature* (see: http://en.wikipedia.org/wiki/Jacques_Benveniste), demonstrating that he could detect a biological effect of antibodies after they had been diluted out of a solution. A subsequent *Nature* investigation showed that the positive results were all from one technician and were best explained by poor controls and inadequate blinding procedures; attempts to replicate his findings failed.

Homeopaths sometimes argue that because homeopathy is individualized, it can't be tested in randomized controlled trials or judged by the same standards as conventional medicines. They are wrong: it can. Homeopaths could individualize their prescriptions as usual, the remedies could be randomized and coded by a second party, and they could be dispensed by a blinded third party who didn't know whether what he was handing out was what the homeopath ordered or a substitute. Homeopaths involved in designing homeopathy studies have conspicuously chosen not to design them this way.

The implausibility of homeopathy wouldn't matter if it could be shown to work. When penicillin was first used, no one understood *how* it worked; however, it was immediately obvious that it *did* work, so doctors started using it right away, and only much later figured out that it kills bacteria by interfering with their ability to manufacture cell wall components. If the evidence for homeopathy's effectiveness were as strong as the evidence for penicillin, it would have readily been adopted into mainstream medicine.

There have been a number of positive clinical studies of homeopathy, but the effects have been inconsistent and small in magnitude. We know that there are many reasons an ineffective treatment may appear to work in a study. The better the design of a homeopathy study, the more likely it is to have negative results, and the best-designed studies have been consistently negative. Systematic reviews fail to support homeopathy. A 1997 meta-analysis published in the *Lancet* concluded that homeopathy worked better than placebo but was not effective for any single clinical condition (on-line at http://www.ncbi.nlm.nih.gov/pubmed/9310601). That's like saying that broccoli is good for everyone—but not men, women, or children! In 2002 Edzard Ernst did a systematic review of systematic reviews that showed homeopathy was no better than placebo.

Homeopaths love to cite statistics from nineteenth-century cholera and typhoid epidemics where patients treated with homeopathy were more likely to survive than patients treated with conventional medicine. Those historical successes are easily explained. Doctors of the time were using remedies that often actively caused harm, but homeopathic remedies did nothing, so of course the results were better. Homeopathy was just a way of avoiding iatrogenic harm. Conventional medicine has made a lot of progress since then. The "What's the Harm?" website offers numerous modern examples of patients who died because they chose homeopathy over conventional treatment that could have saved their lives.

One real danger of homeopathy is in the area of vaccines. Unlike real vaccines, homeopathic vaccines contain no antigen molecules, so they can't possibly produce immunity. People are deluded into believing they are protected from vaccine-preventable diseases when they are actually putting themselves at risk and putting others in their community at risk by decreasing the herd immunity. In a United Kingdom study, experimenters posed as patients planning a trip to Africa and asked homeopaths what they should do to prevent malaria. Ten out of ten homeopaths advised homeopathic "protection" instead of conventional malaria prophylaxis. One said, "They make it so your energy—your living energy—doesn't have a kind of malaria-shaped hole in it. The malarial mosquitoes won't come along and fill that in. The remedies sort it out." (See http://www.badscience.net/2006/09/newsnight-sense-about-science-malaria-homeopathy-sting-the-transcripts/.)

There are other risks. Sometimes a homeopathic remedy is not dilute enough and has actual harmful physiological effects. A homeopathic teething remedy was recalled in 2010 because it contained varying amounts of belladonna and children taking it had suffered seizures consistent with belladonna poisoning. In 2014 several homeopathic products were recalled because they contained actual drugs: measurable amounts of penicillin. (See http://www.fda.gov/safety/midwatch/safetyinformation/safetyalertsforhumanmedicalproducts/uem390002.htm.)

Homeopathy is big business. The homeopathic flu remedy Oscillococcinum is one of the ten top-selling drugs in France, and it brings in $15 million a year in the United States. That one is particularly illogical, since the original substance never actually existed. A French doctor looked through a microscope at blood samples from victims of the 1918 Spanish flu epidemic and observed the phenomenon known as Brownian motion, where visible particles are jostled by collisions with water molecules. He didn't recognize it as Brownian motion but imagined he had discovered a hitherto unknown oscillating bacterium. He christened it Oscillococcus; then he imagined he saw the same bacteria in a sample of duck liver. The Oscillococcinum sold today is a 200C dilution of a smidgen of a Muscovy duck's heart and liver. The liver is long gone but the quack is still evident.

Too many people assume that anything on the shelves of a store must have been approved as safe and effective by the government and that false or misleading advertising claims are strictly prohibited and promptly punished. Unfortunately, this is not true. In the United States, prescription drugs must be proved safe and effective before the FDA will approve them for marketing, but homeopathic remedies are not required to undergo any kind of testing. The whole homeopathic pharmacopoeia was grandfathered in without question. Homeopathic remedies were exempted from federal regulation governing other medications by legislation passed in 1938 at the instigation of senator and homeopath Royal Copeland.

As early as 1842, it was obvious to thinking people like Oliver Wendell Holmes that homeopathy was pseudoscientific nonsense. He exposed its silliness in his classic essay "Homeopathy and Its Kindred Delusions," which is available on the Internet and is still well worth reading. Homeopathy has also been referred to as "Delusions About Dilutions." James Randi has a standing offer of $1 million to anyone who can distinguish a highly dilute homeopathic remedy from plain water, and he's in little danger of losing his money.

So, why is it still being used? There are several reasons. Many consumers have no understanding of what homeopathy actually is and even many medical professionals have only a vague impression that a homeopathic remedy is some kind of mild natural herbal remedy. The remedies are harmless, whereas real medicines have real side effects. The remedies are much less expensive than prescription drugs. Patients love the long appointments, individual attention that they don't get from their medical doctors. Or they enjoy the independence of choosing their own homeopathic remedy and treating themselves. Or they trust the testimonials of friends who believe it cured them. Or they have tried it and have become convinced that it works. Unfortunately, when people rely on personal experience, they are just not very good at determining whether a remedy works: that's why we need science.

HARRIET HALL is a retired Air Force physician.

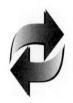

EXPLORING THE ISSUE

Are Homeopathic Remedies Effective?

Critical Thinking and Reflection

1. Why are homeopathic remedies popular despite the lack of scientific evidence they're effective?
2. Describe the basic principles of homeopathic treatments.
3. Why do so many people feel better after a visit to a homeopathic practitioner?

Is There Common Ground?

Most rigorous clinical trials and valid analyses of the research on homeopathy have determined that there is little or no evidence to support homeopathy as an effective treatment for any specific medical condition.

Homeopathy is a controversial topic in alternative or complementary medicine research. A number of the key concepts of homeopathy are not consistent with fundamental concepts of chemistry and physics. For instance, it's not possible to explain in scientific terms how a treatment which contains little or no active ingredient can have any effect. This creates major challenges to legitimate and rigorous clinical investigation of homeopathic remedies. It can't be confirmed that an extremely diluted medicine contains what is listed on the label, nor can one develop objective measures that show effects of extremely dilute remedies in the human body.

An additional research challenge is that homeopathic treatments are highly individualized, and there is no uniform prescribing standard for homeopathic practitioners. There are hundreds of different homeopathic remedies, which can be prescribed in a variety of different dilutions for thousands of symptoms. Each is tailored to an individual patient and his or her symptoms.

Despite the controversy, an estimated 3.9 million adults and nearly a million children use homeopathy in the United States each year. These estimates include use of over-the-counter products labeled as "homeopathic," as well as visits with a homeopathic practitioner. Out-of-pocket costs for adults were close to $3 billion for homeopathic medicines and $170 million for visits to homeopathic practitioners. Clearly, many patients appear to seek out this therapy despite its lack of scientific evidence.

Additional Resources

Medhurst, R. (2014). An update on recent research in homoeopathy. *Journal of the Australian Traditional-Medicine Society*, *20*(1), 46–49.

Pakpoor, J. (2015). Homeopathy is not an effective treatment for any health condition, report concludes. *British Medical Journal*, *350*(8000), 2.

Schmacke, N., Müller, V., & Stamer, M. (2014). What is it about homeopathy that patients value? And what can family medicine learn from this? *Quality in Primary Care*, *22*(1), 17–24.

Smith, K. (2011). Against homeopathy—A utilitarian perspective. *Bioethics*, *26*, 398–409.

Internet References . . .

National Center for Homeopathy (NCH)

www.nationalcenterforhomeopathy.org/

National Institutes of Health—Homeopathy

https://nccih.nih.gov/health/homeopathy

National Library of Medicine—Alternative Medicine

www.nlm.nih.gov/medlineplus /complementaryandalternativemedicine.html

Selected, Edited, and with Issue Framing Material by:
Eileen L. Daniel, *SUNY College at Brockport*

ISSUE

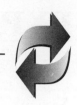

Do the Benefits of Statin Drugs Outweigh the Risks?

YES: Jo Willey, from "The Benefits of Statins 'Greatly Outweigh' Small Risks Say Experts," *express.co.uk* (2014)

NO: Martha Rosenberg, from "Do You Really Need That Statin?" *huffingtonpost.com* (2012)

Learning Outcomes

After reading this issue, you will be able to:

- Assess the overall benefits of statin drugs for patients without symptoms of heart disease.
- Understand the risk factors associated with heart disease.
- Understand the side effects of statin drugs.

ISSUE SUMMARY

YES: Journalist Jo Willey reports that statins' ability to prevent heart attacks and stroke outweighed any risks and that tens of thousands of deaths from cardiovascular disease could be prevented if all eligible adults took the drugs.

NO: Investigative reporter Martha Rosenberg interviewed physician Barbara Roberts, who claims that statins treat high cholesterol, which is a weak risk factor for heart disease, and that the side effects of the drugs negate any benefits, especially when taken by otherwise healthy adults with high cholesterol.

About 610,000 people die of cardiovascular disease (CVD) in the United States every year, which represents one in every four deaths. CVD is the leading cause of death for both men and women though more than half of the deaths due to heart disease in 2009 were in men. Coronary heart disease is the most common type of heart disease, killing over 370,000 people annually. There are a number of risk factors linked to heart disease including age, smoking, diet, and elevated serum cholesterol. Statins are a category of drugs prescribed to reduce serum cholesterol levels by blocking a liver enzyme that plays a central role in the production of cholesterol. The majority of cholesterol in the blood stream is manufactured by the body, primarily in the liver. Elevated cholesterol levels have been linked to cardiovascular disease (CVD) including heart disease and stroke. Statins have been found to reduce the risk of cardiovascular disease and mortality especially among individuals at high risk. The evidence

is strong that statins are effective for treating CVD in the early stages of the disease and potentially in those at elevated risk but without CVD. As a result, statin drugs are among the most widely prescribed drugs on the market, with one in four Americans over 45 taking them. While the drug has some important benefits, it also has side effects, which include muscle pain, increased risk of diabetes mellitus, and abnormalities in liver enzyme tests. In addition, the drugs have rare but severe adverse effects, particularly muscle damage. Some research suggests statins help with asthma symptoms, but a 2011 study found that some individuals with asthma who took statins had more symptoms and worse lung function than asthma patients who didn't take them.

While there are side effects associated with statins, the drugs are also considered by many to be one of the greatest public health triumphs of the past quarter century. During that time period, the death rate from heart disease in the United States fell by half, resulting in close to 350,000 fewer Americans dying from heart disease each year. Though the data are fairly spectacular, there is a debate over whether statins actually reduce death from heart disease among asymptomatic patients with no known heart disease. Statins have been proven effective for individuals who have already suffered a heart attack or stroke. The data on healthy adults is not as clear, though the drug is prescribed for both patients who have had a heart attack and those who are healthy but have high cholesterol, particularly high levels of low-density lipo-proteins. Interestingly, serum cholesterol levels are as not strongly predictive of heart disease as once thought and most current research indicates that these levels are actu-ally a fairly weak predictor of who will have a heart attack.

There is another possibility that statins might pro-vide benefits unrelated to cholesterol reduction. There is some evidence that they also decrease inflammation which, when it occurs in the arteries, is thought to increase the risk of heart disease. A 2008 study called the JUPITER trial tested statins in about 18,000 people with normal high-density lipoproteins but with an elevated marker for inflammation. Statins reduced the risks of heart attack and stroke among this group, leading proponents to con-clude that by working through an additional mechanism, lowering inflammation, not just low-density lipoproteins, statins were beneficial to people with normal cholesterol levels.

New American Heart Association guidelines released in 2014 expanded the criteria for statin use. Under these new guidelines, nearly 13 million more Americans, mostly over 60, will be eligible to take statin drugs. The American Heart Association guidelines expanded the criteria for statin use to include people with an increased risk of developing heart disease over a 10-year period.

In this study, researchers used data from more than 3,700 Americans, aged 40 to 75, to determine how the new guidelines would affect the number of people who use the drugs. A large increase in usage would occur among people older than 60, with 77 percent eligible for statins under the new guidelines compared to 48 percent under the previous standards. The use of statins among people aged 40 to 60 would increase only from 27 percent to 30 percent, the researchers said. Men aged 60 to 75 who are not taking statins and do not have heart disease would be most affected by the new recommendations, with the number who are eligible increasing from about 30 percent to 87 percent, according to the study, which was published in 2014 in the *New England Journal of Medicine*. The use of statins among healthy women in this age group would rise from 21 percent to 53 percent. On the other hand, the researchers also found that about 1.6 million adults who were previously eligible for statins would no longer be candidates for the drugs. Most of these people are young adults who have elevated cholesterol but a low 10-year risk of heart disease.

It has been standard practice among doctors for the last 50 years at least to treat serum cholesterol levels as a risk factor for heart disease, and to assume that there is a causal connection. Half of Americans over 65 are taking prescription statin drugs (and one-sixth of people between 45 and 65). It's clear that statins lower serum cholesterol, but whether the drugs lower risk of heart disease is less clear, and there may be no benefit at all for overall mortal-ity rate.

The above questions are difficult to answer because there is such a deep division of opinion in the medical community. The mainstream view, which has the best data and the best studies behind it, has been funded by the pharmaceutical industry, and statin drugs are a $35 billion dollar industry in America, growing rapidly. It may ulti-mately be determined that the drugs are not effective for healthy people despite their ability to lower cholesterol.

YES ↵

Jo Willey

The Benefits of Statins "Greatly Outweigh" Small Risks Say Experts

The pills taken by 8 million people in the UK have been given a clean bill of health by British researchers despite raising the risk of diabetes.

They found the pills may cause small increases in weight gain and blood sugar which in turn raises a person's chances of Type 2 diabetes.

But they said that statins' ability to prevent heart attack and stroke negated this danger—and that simple lifestyle changes could be used to balance out any problems.

Professor Colin Baigent, from the University of Oxford, said: "The magnitude of the benefits of statins arising from the prevention of heart attacks and strokes greatly outweighs any small risks of diabetes, so the current recommendations for statin use remain appropriate."

The backing came after researchers from University College London and the University of Glasgow discovered how statins increase the risk of diabetes and stroke.

They found that taking statins was associated with an around 240 g—or half a pound—weight gain and a 12 per cent increased risk of developing type 2 diabetes over four years.

In a separate comment on the research, Professor Baigent added: "Statins have previously been shown to cause a small increase in the risk of developing diabetes, and this study provides some clues about the biological mechanism by which this occurs.

"But although it is helpful to understand mechanisms, this research does not change our assessment of the safety of statins."

Statins work by reducing the efficiency of a liver enzyme involved in cholesterol production, which causes liver cells to trap more "bad" low-density lipoprotein (LDL) cholesterol from the blood and lower levels.

This is why the drugs are credited with dramatically lowering the risk of suffering a heart attack or stroke.

The research published in *The Lancet* looked at data on nearly 130,000 people from clinical trials that previously tested the effect of statins on heart disease and stroke.

It found those given statins vs placebo, or higher vs lower doses of statins, had a small increase in risk of developing Type 2 diabetes of about 12 per cent over a four-year period, and also to gain 240 g in weight.

Co-lead author Dr David Preiss of the University of Glasgow Institute of Cardiovascular and Medical Sciences, said: "Weight gain is a risk factor for diabetes which might help explain the small increased risk of diabetes observed in people taking statins."

The researchers found that commonly occurring genetic variants were also associated with a higher weight and marginally higher type 2 diabetes risk.

The effects were much smaller than from statin treatment, but enabled the researchers to conclude that the weight gain and diabetes risk found in the analysis from trials were related to the known mechanism of action of statins rather than some other unintended effect.

Co-senior author Professor Naveed Sattar of the University of Glasgow, added: "Previous analyses have indicated that the cardiovascular benefits of statin treatment greatly outweigh the risk of new-onset type 2 diabetes.

"Nevertheless, many patients eligible for statin treatment would also benefit from lifestyle changes including increased physical activity, eating more healthily and stopping smoking. The modest increases in weight and diabetes risk seen in this study could easily be mitigated by adopting healthier diets and lifestyles.

"Reinforcing the importance of lifestyle changes when discussing these issues with patients would further enhance the benefit of statin treatment in preventing heart attacks and strokes."

Professor Jeremy Pearson, associate medical director at the British Heart Foundation, which helped fund the study, said: "Statins offer substantial protection from coronary heart disease. This rigorous and extensive study looked at why people taking them have a small increased risk of diabetes.

"The researchers found a direct relationship between how statins reduce cholesterol production and small increases in weight gain and blood sugar. This could explain the slightly increased risk of diabetes—a risk that could be reduced through lifestyle changes.

"This study should reassure people that the benefits of taking statins far outweigh the small effect on diabetes risk. But the results also reinforce that, alongside prescribed medication, taking steps to maintain a healthy weight is essential to stay heart healthy."

Professor Tom Sanders, honorary nutritional director of HEART UK, said: "Statin treatment seems to result in a small weight gain and increase blood glucose resulting in an increased diagnosis of type 2 diabetes.

"Advice to maintain a healthy weight and physical activity, which are key to preventing type 2 diabetes, should accompany the prescription of statins."

The new research comes after Britain's leading heart doctors joined forces to state "the jury is no longer out" on whether the benefits of statins outweigh the risks, confirming that quarter of a century of research has provided clear and definitive evidence to back the use of the cholesterol-lowering drugs.

The heart pills have been mired in controversy after scare stories about their dangers which were later retracted.

In May, researchers were forced to withdraw "misleading" claims about statins published in the respected *British Medical Journal* which overestimated side effects 20-fold.

They later accepted the research, which claimed the drugs caused higher rates of diabetes, tiredness and muscle pain than had previously been scientifically proven, was incorrect.

At the time, medics warned that thousands of people could be needlessly putting their lives at risk if they stopped taking the life-saving pills because of the false claim that statins had severe side effects in a fifth of patients.

Although six leading scientists joined forces to declare the evidence is "substantial" that the pills are safe, they said people should not rely on the medication as a "quick fix" but be encouraged to adopt healthier lifestyles to lower heart attack and stroke risk and make an informed choice with a doctor about statins.

Statins are already used by eight million people in the UK.

In July, updated guidance from the National Institute for Health and Care Excellence said statins could soon be taken by as many as 17 million adults in a bid to prevent heart problems.

The pills are currently offered to people who have a 20 per cent risk of developing cardiovascular disease within 10 years.

But the NHS will now lower this threshold to include people with just a 10 per cent risk.

This could see an additional 4.5 million patients offered the drugs, bringing the total of all eligible people to 17 million—around 40 per cent of the adult population of England.

If everyone eligible took the drugs, Nice estimates that between 20,000 and 50,000 deaths could be prevented every year.

Jo Willey is a journalist specializing in health and medical issues.

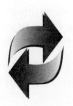

Martha Rosenberg   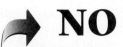 **NO**

Do You Really Need That Statin? This Expert Says No

This is an interview with Barbara H. Roberts, M.D., author of The Truth About Statins: Risks and Alternatives to Cholesterol-Lowering Drugs.

Statins are medications that lower cholesterol by inhibiting an enzyme involved in its production by the liver and other organs. First approved by the FDA in 1987, statins are arguably the most widely-prescribed medicine in the industrialized world today—and the most profitable, representing billions a year in profits to the drug industry. In fact, Lipitor was the world's best-selling drug until its patent expired recently. Yet most trials that prove statins' effectiveness in preventing cardiac events and death have been funded by companies and principle investigators who stand to benefit from their wide use. In February, the FDA warned that statins can increase users' risk of Type 2 diabetes and memory loss, confusion and other cognition problems.

Barbara H. Roberts, M.D., is director of the Women's Cardiac Center at the Miriam Hospital in Providence, R.I. and associate clinical professor of medicine at the Alpert Medical School of Brown University. She spent two years at the National Heart, Lung and Blood Institute of the National Institutes of Health (NIH), where she was involved in the first clinical trial that demonstrated a beneficial effect of lowering cholesterol on the incidence of heart disease. In addition to *The Truth About Statins: Risks and Alternatives to Cholesterol-Lowering Drugs*, she is also author of *How to Keep from Breaking Your Heart: What Every Woman Needs to Know About Cardiovascular Disease*.

Martha Rosenberg: Statins have become so popular with adults middle-aged and older in industrialized countries, they are almost a pharmaceutical rite of passage. Yet you write in your new book there is little evidence they are effective in many groups and no evidence they are effective in one group: women without heart disease. Worse, you provide evidence, including stories from your own patients, that they are doing serious harm.

Barbara Roberts: Yes. Every week in my practice I see patients with serious side effects to statins, and many did not need to be treated with statins in the first place. These side effects range from debilitating muscle and joint pain to transient global amnesia, neuropathy, cognitive dysfunction, fatigue and muscle weakness. Most of these symptoms subside or improve when they are taken off statins. There is even growing evidence of a statin link to Lou Gehrig's disease.

Martha Rosenberg: One patient you write about caused a fire in her home by forgetting that the stove was on. Another was a professor who experienced such memory loss on a statin he could no longer teach; others ended up in wheelchairs. The only thing more shocking than the side effects you write about is the apparent blindness of the medical establishment to them. Until half a year ago, there were practically no warnings at all.

Barbara Roberts: There is no question that many doctors have swallowed the Kool-Aid. Big Pharma has consistently exaggerated the benefits of statins and some physicians used scare tactics so that patients are afraid that if they go off the statins, they will have a heart attack immediately. Yet high cholesterol, which the statins address, is a relatively weak risk factor for developing atherosclerosis. For example, diabetes and smoking are far more potent when it comes to increasing risk.

Martha Rosenberg: One group you say should not be given statins at all because there is no benefit and significant risk is women who have no heart disease.

Barbara Roberts: In three major studies [1–3] of women without diagnosed heart disease, but who were at high risk (in one of these studies, each participant had to have high blood pressure and three other risk factors), 40 women out of 4,904 on statins had either a heart attack or cardiac death, compared to 44 women out of 4,836 on placebo.

That is not a statistically significant difference. Since the likelihood of experiencing a statin side effect is about 20 to 25 percent, the risk of putting a healthy woman on a statin far outweighs the benefit. Still, statins are routinely given to this group because the guidelines are shaped by Big Pharma. The guidelines are not supported by the evidence, and in the case of healthy women I don't follow them.

Martha Rosenberg: You give a story in your book about your 92-year-old patient who had a total cholesterol of 266, triglycerides of 169, HDL cholesterol of 66, and LDL cholesterol of 165. Her primary care doctor wanted her to take a statin, but you did not feel she needed to because she had no evidence of heart disease, had never smoked, did not have high blood pressure and was not diabetic.

Barbara Roberts: Yes and today she is 103.5—and doing fine, never having taken a statin.

Martha Rosenberg: In *The Truth About Statins* you explain pretty clearly how studies have made statins look more effective and safer than they are. How has this been done?

Barbara Roberts: First of all, the studies are of short duration, and some of them even have a "run in" phase during which people are given the drug to see if they tolerate it. If not, they are not enrolled in the study. Secondly, study subjects are cherry-picked to exclude the very elderly, people with liver or kidney disease or those with any chronic illness that might "muddy" the results.

Martha Rosenberg: In other words, the very people who will be taking them?

Barbara Roberts: Yes, and of course patients will also be staying on the drugs for life unlike trial subjects. Then, the data from the studies are usually given in terms of relative rather than absolute risk. The absolute risk of a cardiac event is only reduced by a few percentage points by statins and in some patients, like the women without heart disease we just talked about, the reduction is not even statistically significant. In some studies surrogate end points like inflammation or artery thickness are used but a favorable change in surrogate markers does not always translate into clinical benefit. In addition, many studies use composite end points, which include not only "hard" end points like heart attack or death (which are pretty hard to misdiagnose) but also "softer" end points like the "need" for revascularization or the occurrence of

acute coronary syndromes. For example, studies may be performed in many countries with very different rates of revascularization procedures, making use of this as an end point very problematic.

Martha Rosenberg: This brings to mind the JUPITER trial, which enrolled people without heart disease, with normal levels (less than 130) of LDL or bad cholesterol, but evidence of increased inflammation as measured by the hsCRP test and treated them with placebo or rosuvastatin. JUPITER stood for "Justification for the Use of Statins in Prevention," and both the study and its principle investigator were funded by AstraZeneca, who makes the statin Crestor. The principal investigator also holds the patent for the hsCRP blood test. Why was JUPITER regarded as medical science and not marketing?

Barbara Roberts: Actually, the JUPITER study was criticized to some extent. But you have to remember that medical journals depend upon Big Pharma for their ads and reprint orders just as medical centers and medical professionals rely on Big Pharma for funding. It is a round robin situation that probably won't change until the patients, doctors and the public demand change. As for CRP, it can also rise if a patient has a cold, bronchitis or is taking post-menopausal hormones.

Martha Rosenberg: You are very outspoken about the problem of industry shaping and influencing medical practice, yet you also admit that you accepted Big Pharma money yourself.

Barbara Roberts: In 2004, Pfizer asked me to become a speaker, specifically on Lipitor. I told the drug rep who invited me to be a speaker that I would be interested in giving talks on gender-specific aspects of cardiac disease, but not in just talking about their statin, and I gave lectures in restaurants and hospitals. Despite the fact that Pfizer was sponsoring my talks, I never failed to point out that there was no evidence that Lipitor—or any statin—prevented cardiac events in women who did not have established cardiovascular disease. They tolerated this until one day a regional manager came to one of my talks, and then I was disinvited. I was on the speaker's bureau for another company, Abbott, but when they began to insist that I use their slides rather than my own, I gave up being on any Big Pharma speaker's bureaus. I write in my book that even though my interactions with drug and device companies complied with ethical guidelines it does not mean I was not influenced.

Martha Rosenberg: In journalism, when a reporter takes money from someone she is writing about, she is regarded as no longer a reporter but a publicist. Yet doctors who consult to Pharma are not judged as harshly and most contend they are not influenced by industry money . . .

Barbara Roberts: They are wrong. An article in the *American Journal of Bioethics* in 2003 found that gifts bestow a sense of indebtedness and influence behavior whether or not the recipient is directly conscious of it. More recently, research presented at a symposium at Houston's Baylor College of Medicine called the Scientific Basis of Influence and Reciprocity mapped actual changes in the brain when gifts are received.

Martha Rosenberg: I was surprised to find recipes in your book and even more surprised by some of your dietary recommendations, such as avoiding a low-fat diet and eating a lot of olive oil. A lot of experts have recommended a low-fat diet.

Barbara Roberts: The first thing I prescribe to my patients who have low levels of the "good" or HDL cholesterol is two to three tablespoons of olive oil a day, and in every case the HDL increases. Olive oil is rich in polyphenols, which have anti-inflammatory and antioxidant effects. Several studies [4, 5] have shown that the Mediterranean diet reduces total mortality and especially death from cardiovascular disease, yet it gets little media attention. The Mediterranean diet is a plant-based diet that includes colorful vegetables, fruits, whole grains, beans, cheese, nuts, olive oil, seafood, red wine with meals, and very little meat.

Martha Rosenberg: You indict professional medical associations like the American Heat Association (AHA) for profiteering at the public's expense by calling harmful foods healthful in exchange for corporate money.

Barbara Roberts: For years, the AHA preached the gospel of the low-fat diet, calling it the "cornerstone" of its dietary recommendations though there was, and is, no evidence of its benefit. The AHA rakes in millions from food corporations for the use of its "heart-check mark." Some of the so-called heart-healthy foods it has endorsed include Boar's Head All Natural Ham, which contains 340 milligrams of sodium in a two-ounce serving, and Boar's Head EverRoast Oven Roasted Chicken Breast, which contains 440 milligrams of sodium in a two-ounce serving. High sodium intake raises blood pressure, which increases the risk of cardiovascular disease. In addition, studies have shown that eating processed meat increases the risk of diabetes and atherosclerosis.

Martha Rosenberg: You are not afraid to express strong opinions. You say that the AHA has "sold its soul," that medical centers conducting drug trials for Big Pharma have become "hired hands" and that one university medical center is Big Pharma's "lapdog." Are you afraid of retaliation from Big Pharma, medical centers or the colleagues you work with?

Barbara Roberts: I haven't received any communiqués from Big Pharma. A few colleagues have expressed dismay, but I am thick-skinned and hard-headed and don't care what they say. My main concern is the health and safety of my patients.

References

1. http://circ.ahajournals.org/content/121/9/1069.short
2. http://www.thelancet.com/journals/lancet/article/PIIS0140-6736(03)12948-0/abstract
3. http://fundacionconfiar.com.ar/capacitacion/Clase_5/Levels%20Results%20of%20AFCAPSTexCAPS.pdf
4. http://www.ncbi.nlm.nih.gov/pubmed/9989963
5. http://www.ncbi.nlm.nih.gov/pubmed/18071168

Martha Rosenberg is an investigative health reporter.

EXPLORING THE ISSUE

Do the Benefits of Statin Drugs Outweigh the Risks?

Critical Thinking and Reflection

1. Do the benefits of statins outweigh the risks?
2. What are the alternatives to statin drugs?
3. Who would most benefit from statins and why?

Is There Common Ground?

Cholesterol-lowering statin drugs are ubiquitous these days, with more and more being prescribed each year. But questions remain about their safety and effectiveness. While the medical literature does show that statins may help people with a history of a heart attack, stroke, or current signs and symptoms of existing cardiovascular disease (CVD), studies have found that people without a history of heart attack or stroke who take statin drugs do not live any longer than the people who take a placebo. This is particularly true for women, who have not been well represented in clinical research studies.

In a review of statin data published in the *British Medical Journal*, lead author John Abramson of Harvard Medical School says that people who take statins to prevent a first heart event don't lower their risk of dying from any cause, or from heart disease over 10 years. Not only do statins *not* lower the risk of dying early, but they also don't lower the chances of being hospitalized for a heart problem or other serious heart-related illness. The medication can lower—very slightly—the risk of having a heart attack or stroke. But that benefit is offset by the drugs' side effects. "For people with a less than 20% risk of having a heart event in 10 years, which is the vast majority for whom the statins would be prescribed under the new 2014 guidelines, we are not seeing a net benefit," Abramson says.

And while they're generally considered safe, statins have a variety of side effects, including decreased liver function, interference with the manufacture of coenzyme Q10 (CoQ10), rhabdomyolysis (the breaking down of muscle tissue), nerve damage, impaired mental function with prolonged use, possible increased risk of cancer and heart failure with long-term use, fatigue, diabetes, and weight gain. Fortunately, there are safe and effective lifestyle changes which can help lower cholesterol and reduce the risk of cardiovascular disease. These include weight loss, exercise, smoking cessation, blood pressure control, and eating a diet high in fruits and vegetables, especially the Mediterranean diet.

Additional Resources

Benefits strongly outweigh risks associated with statins. (2014). *Reactions Weekly, 1503*(1), 2.

Four myths about statins. (2015). *Harvard Heart Letter, 25*(6), 1–7.

Mlodinow, S. G., Onysko, M. K., Vandiver, J. W., Hunter, M. L., & Mahvan, T. D. (2014). Statin adverse effects. *Clinician Reviews, 24*(11), 41–50.

Murray, M. T. (2014). Saying "no" to statins. *Better Nutrition, 76*(12), 28–29.

Park, A. (2014). Who really needs to take a statin? *Time.Com,* 1.

Internet References . . .

American Heart Association

www.heart.org

Food and Drug Administration

www.fda.gov/Drugs

National Institutes of Health

www.nlm.nih.gov/medlineplus/heartdiseases.html

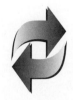